BREATHE FREE

To Louise,

Enjoy the read & I hope this helps you coach all those Sayue ladies

Best Wishes

BREATHE FREE

Breath Training for a Healthy Body,
a Strong Mind and a Great Life

LEO DANIEL RYAN

Any use of information in this book is at the reader's discretion and risk. The information given in this book should not be treated as a substitute for the advice of a qualified medical professional. You should consult a medical professional in matters relating to health, especially if you have an existing medical condition, and before starting, stopping, or changing the dose of any medication you are taking. Individual readers are solely responsible for their own healthcare decisions. The author and the publisher expressly disclaim responsibility for any adverse effects arising from the use or application of the information contained herein.

All efforts have been made to ensure the accuracy of the information contained in this book as of the date published.

© BREATHE FREE. Copyright © Leo Daniel Ryan. All rights reserved.

www.innate-strength.com

No part of this book may be used or reproduced in any manner whatsoever without written permission except in the case of brief quotations embodied in critical articles and reviews.

Email: leo@innate-strength.com

FIRST EDITION PUBLISHED 2023

Publisher: Innate Strength Publishing

ISBN: 978-1-7393516-0-1

Designed by: Karl Hunt
Cover Design by: Svitlana Stefaniuk
Illustrations: Marcus Quinn & Leo D. Ryan

For my wife, Joy, I love you always.

And to our children: Beatrice, Genevieve and Juliette,
you bring life to our lives.

We hope we support and guide you plentifully to enable
your growth through the stresses of life.

Remember always: breathe, smile and know who you are.

We love you.

CONTENTS

Foreword ix
Introduction – Why I Wrote This Book xi

PART 1 – THE INTERCONNECTION OF LIFE, STRESS AND THE BREATH 1

1. Breathing Free is the Goal 3
2. Unravelling the Language of the Breathing World 11
3. Understanding Balance 20
4. Modern-Day Causes of Imbalance 27
5. Stress and Breathing 36
6. The Human Performance Pyramid 58

PART 2 – BREATHE-ABILITY 93

7. The Way the Breath Works 95
8. Connecting the Breath with Specific Dis-eases 133
9. Breathe-Ability 201
10. Understanding Breathing Techniques 218

PART 3 – THE INNATE-STRENGTH BREATH TRAINING PROGRAMME — 229

11	Roadmapping Your Success	231
12	Breath Training Programme Considerations	253
13	Personalised Breathing Assessment	271
14	Phase 1 Training Design – Breath Mechanics	290
15	Phase 2 Training Design – Breath Resilience	331
16	Phase 3 Training Design – Breath Rhythms	344
17	The Magic of Breathwork	360
18	Complimentary Breathing and Lifestyle Habits	366
19	Breathing for Life Performance	389

Epilogue — 407

Appendix – 21 Life-Changing Learnings from Breath Training Clients — 411

Glossary of Terms — 415
Bibliography — 420
Acknowledgements — 434
About the Author — 439

FOREWORD

When Leo asked me to write the foreword for his book, I was hesitant. There are a lot of books on breathing out there (I have read most of them) and they are all basically the same. I changed my mind when I read Leo's book. *Breathe Free* contains a lot of information – and deep knowledge – that does not appear in any other breathing books.

His insights into the human experience, and his vast repertoire of techniques, methods and, most importantly, principles, make this book unique. Leo Ryan has written a primer for breath work and breath training that I believe will be considered the authoritative text book on the subject.

Breathe Free takes you step by step through the process of mastering your breath. It doesn't matter if you are a doctor or a new reader interested in breathing; this book presents the information in a way that not only helps you to understand the difficult topic of breathing physiology, but also teaches you how to apply that information in your everyday life. Leo guides the reader, step by step, from beginner to advanced client, with techniques and practices that are easy to apply in any situation.

This book is written for the lay-person, physiologist, therapist, medical doctor and counsellor. I include counsellor because this book also teaches you how to release mental, emotional and physical stress through the framework of breath work. *Breathe Free* can also be used as a textbook for teachers in any profession involving therapy.

It should be the gold standard for the application of breathing programmes and it is a must-read for any coach, trainer or therapist involved in health care.

Breathe Free takes breath training to a new level. I sincerely hope it finds the audience it deserves.

Eric Serrano, MD.

WHY I WROTE THIS BOOK

> *It is our light, not our darkness, that most frightens us...*
> *we were all meant to shine... we were born to make manifest*
> *the glory of God that is within us... and as we let our own*
> *light shine, we unconsciously give other people the*
> *permission to do the same*
>
> MARIANNE WILLIAMSON

Inspire – breathe it all in; deep and full, belly, chest and head. Breathe in the air in and fill your ribs 360°. Fill your lungs with air and with the wisdom of these pages. This is a story about modern life, a quest to breathe free, regain your health and enhance performance. The suffering of pain, the joys of health, the discipline of training and the pursuit of a great life are the common themes of this book.

By getting to know your breath, training and developing it, you too can make your way from your comfortable, modern, sedated and sick life to becoming energised, vivacious, healthy, and living your great life. It is my hope that you will use this book to find the inspiration and the tools to develop your breath, then use it for the betterment of your life, whether that is as a tool for achieving glory in sport or simply to live your life better.

The origins of *Breathe Free* date to a personal training client I worked with back in 2013 and 2014. Unbeknownst to me at the time, she altered the course of my coaching career and became the catalyst for this book. When she began with me, she weighed over 220 lbs and wanted to lose a significant amount of weight. In our first consultation she told me she led a good life but a very stressful one. Her husband owned a contract business and she ran much of it. He made the sales; she ran the projects and worried about the finances. Wining and dining the clients was part and parcel of the business. To alleviate the stressors of her life, she often ate and drank heartily. Those choices of course led to longer-term problems for her that she couldn't foresee. She didn't exercise much, had few pastimes, and didn't sleep too well either.

For nine months, she trained hard with me and improved her nutrition steadily. She trained with me three times per week, played curling, and added extra cardio sessions regularly. She reduced alcohol, calories, processed foods and carbohydrates in her diet. Throughout that time, she gained a tremendous amount of energy, her blood markers improved, her cardiovascular health improved, and her strength and fitness improved. However, she lost a grand total of five pounds. She was distraught at the results. She was frustrated with her physical appearance and her lack of visible progress. I could have continued down the path of improving nutrition and exercise but I knew something deeper was at play. I needed more data and I needed support. I started by wanting to find out two things:

1. Why was her body holding onto excess fat?
2. What did she need to do to realise her goal faster?

My plan was to get some numbers on her physical health and then bring additional support into our training. I made three suggestions to her: I wanted her to get a doctor to run some bloodwork tests, I suggested she attend a counsellor and I wanted her to get a sleep test done. I told her she could not expect to achieve her goals with me without this information and support.

She duly fired me.

It was a shock to me that she fired me, but I was content too. I was ok knowing that I didn't string her along, take her money, train her more, and pretend she might get results with me. I knew she needed to get to the root cause of her health, and I knew I needed additional support too.

Three months passed, and one day I received a call from her. She told me she had done the sleep study during the intervening time. It turns out she had chronic obstructive sleep apnoea. Sleep apnoea is a condition where you stop breathing in your sleep until your oxygen levels drop so low that your brain wakes you up. It has correlations with all major lifestyle diseases, such as cardiovascular disease, diabetes and cancer. The onset of sleep apnoea is not unlike most diseases of our modern life. First, you are overwhelmed by life. This is the stage where your body or mind is stressed and unable to cope. You feel like you don't have much energy compared to your youth. Some people are prone to picking up niggles, injuries, colds and flus during this phase. Next, the body adapts to your new way of life, and dysfunction sets in. You move differently, think differently and your immune system weakens further. Finally, you develop a disease. It could be sleep apnoea, like my client, asthma, like me, or any other diseases we commonly suffer from today. Essentially, it's a state of being that's so far from healthy that you require medical intervention to live a half-decent life.

To help my client breathe at night, she was placed on a CPAP machine. This medical intervention worked. She was doing much better, she told me. She'd lost twenty-eight pounds and was continuing to progress with her health. She thanked me for sending her on the right path and I thanked her too. You would think I'd be happy in the weeks after I took the call, but something nagged at my mind. I knew there was a limit to how much the CPAP could help her. I knew that if she wanted to really thrive once more, as she had in her youth, she needed to address more of her lifestyle. She needed to breathe better, think better, continue to exercise, continue to nourish her body and mind and live better as a whole. I knew she had to dive deeper again to fulfil her goals but I also knew I didn't have the skills to help her at the time.

Drawing on past education, I knew that sleep apnoea is directly related to sleep-disordered breathing, and sleep-disordered breathing is an adapted breathing pattern – it is the result of poor breathing habits. I knew all of this because I was a severe asthmatic as a child and young man. This was my start in the health and fitness industry, long before I was a personal trainer. Back then I used the Buteyko Breathing Method to cure my asthma, optimise my immune system, improve sports performance, and live my great life.

LEO'S ORIGIN STORY

As a child and teenager, I loved sport. For most of my life, I weighed no more than 9.5 stone (that's old money for 61 kg or 134 lbs if you're from North America). I was small and skinny but incredibly fit – when my lungs were healthy. Often, I was sick with asthma attacks and chest infections. Since the age of three, I'd been on medication for asthma. Like the weather here in Ireland, some years were better than others, but there was always a gloomy grey cloud over my life. I can still remember, when I was a little boy, maybe seven or eight, my GP administering medication to me in the middle of the night, after my mam had rung him, panicking that I'd taken another attack. There were also times when I was hospitalised, maybe three or four of them. One in particular stands out in my memory.

My parents went on a weekend holiday, and I was staying over at my cousin's house. We played chasing and football and kids' games all day long outdoors. I was having great fun, as any other child would. That fun carried into the evening with a pillow fight. By the time it was bed-time I had turned from a very active and playful boy to a sack of stones, heaving, panting, and wheezing for my breath.

Asthma is a funny old disease like that. One minute you can be full of life; the next, you're fighting for every breath. Your lungs are caving in, your body is groaning and your mind panics. With every breath you take, the grasp of the attack becomes tighter and tighter, like a snake choking its prey. Before long, there's a rattle in your chest that sounds like you're an old man taking his last, heaving breath before he passes over to the next life. Then comes the relief.

My parents were called, and I was rushed into Children's University Hospital, Temple Street, one of Ireland's primary children's hospital. After a quick assessment, I was put on a nebuliser. It's the equivalent dose of 25 puffs of a blue Ventolin inhaler. On that occasion, I remember staying in hospital for several days. Once I was well enough, I was sent home and life returned to normal, with the exception of having an even bigger bag of medication to take every day. The culmination of my childhood asthma came in my nineteenth year.

By this stage, the asthma was mostly 'under control', and by this, I mean I was taking several puffs of two inhalers three times per day. I still had attacks a couple of times per year and chest infection always followed these. The chest infection was probably the worst of it because that would knock me out for two weeks at a minimum. By the time I was nineteen I had been on that much medication and such a variety of meds I could have been my own doctor. I knew the potency of all the inhalers, steroid medications and anti-biotics I used. I knew which ones would work well with a given dose and which would not. Sometimes, a stand-in GP in the surgery would try to prescribe me a lighter medication for another attack/infection. I often argued with them, knowing it wouldn't work but they insisted, and with the doctor being the authority, he won over. Until I came back the following week, still sick and needing even more meds.

From 2003-2004, I spent an aggregated six months in bed sick with asthma. I was well for a few weeks, and then I would have an attack and become bed-ridden for two weeks. No matter what medication I took and the dosage I was given, this cycle repeated itself again and again. That year I took 14 courses of anti-biotics, 400+ prednisolone steroid tablets, and a daily dose of three inhalers to try to quench the ravages of chronic asthma. But it was no good. By this stage, I was extremely unhappy with how my life was unfolding. I was studying a career I hated, my life's dream of becoming a Dublin footballer was flowing down the drain with every asthma attack, and I was losing my sparkle for life. During one of my now bi-monthly visits to the GP, I asked him what he thought of a career change for me. I hated computers; I loved sport. I realised I may never become a footballer, but I thought I could have a career in the fitness world and so I asked him what he thought about my chances of becoming a fitness trainer. My GP told me that nothing more could be done for me. He said he'd get me an appointment with Mr. Richard Costello, one of Ireland's leading respiratory consultants, but knowing the medical system in Ireland, that could take a while. To this day, I still remember his words ringing vividly in my ears:

> *Leo, there is no hope for you. If we lock you away in a room and wrap you in bubble-wrap until you're twenty-five, I cannot say that you will get better. We are doing everything we can for you, there is nothing more to be done.*

That was his response.

At this point, I was broken. I could feel it in my heart. 'Fuck you!' was all I wanted to shout to him. I pictured myself standing up and flooring him with one punch, 'fuck you, doctor,' and walking away from it all. But that was a fantasy. That's not how real life works. Life went on as normal for another month or so. More meds, more attacks, more doctor's visits, more time in bed, less time playing ball and even less time studying. My life was all about to change, however, as towards the end of 2003 my mam found a breathing course that would change my life.

> *When the student is ready,*
> *the teacher shall appear*
>
> DR. WAYNE DYER

Patrick McKeown had recently returned from Russia to teach the Buteyko method. The method was based on the life's work of Dr. Konstantin Buteyko. Dr. Buteyko originated his method to cure his own fatal diagnosis of high blood pressure, developing the method and theory to help thousands of people perform similar miraculous feats. The Buteyko method is different to most other breathing methods. It was developed by a medical doctor, it had a plausible theory to support it and by 2003, it had three clinical trials with asthma patients to support its effectiveness. All the trials showed positive results; it could be used to help treat people with asthma. It showed that, with the method, you could reduce and possibly eliminate the need for asthma medication.

Like me, Patrick heard about the method and in 1999 he left Ireland for Russia to become one of the first Western practitioners of the method. Patrick used the method to alleviate life-long dysfunctional breathing patterns, mouth breathing, symptoms of chronic fatigue, sleep-disordered breathing, anxiety and poor mental function, amongst other symptoms. In 2002 he began teaching workshops on the method and started to promote the idea of breathing as an adjunct therapy to traditional medical methods for the alleviation of asthma symptoms. Since then, he's worked tirelessly to promote the method to the medical establishment in Ireland and beyond with the Buteyko method and his own *Oxygen Advantage*.

The Buteyko method claimed it could reverse asthma symptoms by addressing the underlying breathing dysfunctions. This was something I had to try. I attended Patrick's workshops one morning a week for three weeks. Here I learned all about the method and its breathing techniques. I loved that it had a measurement of progress scale and that the scale was related to your breath quality and symptoms of disease. With goals firmly set, a desperate motivation to improve my life, and the actions steps required to make a difference, I was good to go.

I performed the breathing exercises three times per day for twenty minutes, combined with lifestyle alterations to breathing patterns, food, exercise and sleep. I recorded my scores diligently and watched in awe as my symptoms gradually disappeared over the course of weeks and months. During the first session, I felt some relief from the chronic wheeze that was now plaguing my life. It was not a lot but it was enough to inspire me to continue the program. Within six months of taking the first workshop, I was completely symptom-free. It was unbelievable. I was still on my inhalers, but hadn't had an attack in over six months; that meant no extra steroids or anti-biotics.

By the time my appointment came around for Mr. Richard Costello, my life had turned on its head. I had been symptom-free for almost six months, and I had completely changed my breathing and way of life. What's more, I had a journal documenting my training and gradual progress. As Floyd Mayweather says, 'Men lie, women lie, numbers don't lie'. It was hard for anyone to refute the impact that breath training had had on my life. Mr. Costello was a gentleman when I met him. He sat down and listened to what I had to say. He had heard of Patrick and the method, and he wanted to know what was next for me.

'I want your permission to come off all medications, please', I said.

After listening to me and reviewing my journal, he granted my request on condition that I did so slowly and kept my medication on hand just in case I needed it. And so, I did. Within eighteen months of beginning my breath training I was asthma symptom-free and medication-free. That is essentially the definition of a cure. I had cured my asthma. It was astonishing to me.

> *You will face many defeats in life but*
> *never let yourself be defeated*
>
> MAYA ANGELOU

As a side note here, that doesn't mean I took a magical pill, and all was well with me again forever more. I knew that if I returned to breathing and living in the same vein as I had before, then my symptoms would return, just the same way that a person with heart disease can reverse the symptoms through lifestyle or a person can lose and gain weight. Asthma, therefore, is an epigenetic disease, in my opinion, much like most other diseases. It develops as a consequence of your genetics combined with your lifestyle. With this perspective, I have learned that you can do nothing about your genes, but there is a hell of a lot you can do about your lifestyle. In this vein, I also acknowledge that it took me the guts of ten years to build resilience into my immune system and raise my confidence enough to remove the crutch of having medication on hand altogether. Health is not a twelve-week transformation, especially after having a small life-time of disease and medication. I still had much work to do.

After I cured my asthma, I set off on a path to become a fitness trainer and I returned to playing football. One of my sweetest memories of this time in my life was the winter of 2005. Playing traditional Gaelic Games in Ireland, we have a culture of training outdoors in the mud and cold all winter. This one night I remember vividly. We were running repeat 80 m sprints in the heavy mud. The floodlights were on and the rain jackets were zipped up tight as it was lashing rain. But none of that mattered. I ran those sprints as if it was high noon on a summer's day. Sprint after sprint, I finished five metres in front of my teammates. Nobody could keep up with me. It was like walking on water, gliding over the mud instead of being stuck in it. By the time I finished each sprint, I would turn around and canter back to the start line, refreshed and ready for the next one. I could have lived that whole night for a year.

It was a strange and beautiful feeling, working so hard but feeling like I had a never-ending gas tank. It wasn't until 2017 that I fully realised what was happening in my body that night. How I was able to be so fresh yet work so hard. Even though I had cured my asthma and I was back playing good football, I was scarred from the whole experience. Psychologically I was wounded from spending so many years sick and, once I tasted good health, I didn't want to lose it. I lived in fear that I might ruin my health again if I pushed my body to its limits, as I often would in GAA, and so I backed off. I suppose this fear was the seed for my lack of belief in myself and the resulting de-motivation to train hard and hone my craft. I see that now, I understand it and I accept it. It's all a part of my path in life that's led me to who I am today. This is why I am so passionate when I speak about breathing and health to people. On the one hand, it destroyed my confidence in becoming an elite athlete, whilst on the other it gifted me the ability to be the man and coach I am today. I went from depending on medication to survive and being bed-bound with asthma for a total of six months to returning to sport, increasing lean body weight by over twenty kilograms, climbing mountains bare-chested in below-freezing temperatures, running marathons without training and achieving a black belt in Judo. I also became a coach who understood my client's position. Thanks to breath training, I had experience, sorrow, empathy, skills, insights and success. I had learned from first-hand experience the importance of breathing for overall health and performance, but it was not something I shared openly with my clients so much up to 2014.

After working with this lady, being fired by her, hearing how the CPAP improved her health and her performance in life, and knowing what I knew about breathing, it was time for me to become educated in methods of breathing and help more people.

Since that time, I've qualified in many methods. I've read tens of books and hundreds of journal articles. I've learned from some of the pioneers in the modern breathing world, and coached hundreds of people to breath free, become healthy, and live their great lives. With all this education and experience, I've come to learn something which very few other people seem to know – breathing is the fundamental tool to knowing and managing your health. It is a skill which can be trained, learned, and experienced by everybody. It is at the heart of every activity you practice with your body; it's linked to every process in your brain, and is innately connected to your spirit. In fact, I think it is the fundamental skill every human being in this age needs to acquire if they want to improve their health and optimise performance. Why? Because when your stress-load overwhelms you to the point that your breathing adapts, then nothing else in your body and mind functions well. To illustrate this point, I adapted a 13th Century proverb to suit the case of breathing and health. It highlights the impact of the little details of the breath on the grand scale of a great life. It highlights the importance of breathing for health, life, and longevity.

For want of a breath, his natural centre was lost.

For want of his natural centre, his health was lost.

For want of his health, his mindset was lost.

For want of his mindset, his behaviours were lost.

For want of his behaviours, his goals in life were lost.

For want of his goals, his desire for a better future was lost.

For want of his desire for a better future, meaning in his life was lost.

For want of meaning in his life, he became lost.

All for the want of his breath.

THERE'S MORE TO BREATHING THAN MEETS THE EYE

Even today, most people think breathing is either just something you do or a technique you perform to get a specific result. But there's much more to it than that. Breathing is a mirror for stress in your body. It shows you two things:

1. how you respond to stress
2. how well your body is coping with the stress load of your life

If your breath is adapted or changed because of life's stressors, it is a sign that every single cell in your body is failing to cope with the way you lead your life. Breathing is the most fundamental part of being a human being, and if that adapts, then everything else changes with it.

All is not lost, though. The breath can be trained, restored and renewed. You too can breathe free once more. By training yourself to breathe free, you gift yourself the opportunity to become healthy, pursue your goals, find meaning in life and live your great life. This is another gem most breathing experts don't realise. Yes, it takes persistence and patience, but it can be done. I am living proof of it and so are many of my clients. This is the crux of what I've come to learn.

UNDERSTANDING BREATH TRAINING

Essentially, if you want to restore your breathing system, you need to understand that all breathing techniques fit into a framework of training governed by principles. These principles are rooted in biology, human behaviour and in the art of breathing. As we stand today, science is not yet evolved enough to understand exactly how breathing can be restored. However, the experience of many people indicates that it is only a matter of time before science discovers the mechanisms for what is known by many people today. Scientific research is catching up fast. It is now beginning to understand the mechanisms of breathing for physical and mental health. It connects breathing with fear states, anxiety traits and your ability to focus, concentrate, and relax. It is now obvious to people in the know that breathing affects more than just the respiratory system. It is hugely important for your overall physical and mental health.

This book is a distillation of all that I have learned about breathing and health. It fills in the gaps in the science to connect breathing with your lifestyle and disease. It shows you how breathing works in practice and it lays out the framework for you to breathe free. Sometimes, however, knowing what to do is not enough. Often we need to be coached and supported in our journey to self-improvement. That is why I have included many stories from my coaching life to help you along the way.

WHO WILL BENEFIT FROM THIS BOOK?

I want to see you live a better, healthier, and greater life. Breathing free is the foundation of that process and this book will guide you on your journey. In this vein, the type of people who will find the most value in this book are people who want something more for themselves in life. They want to breathe better and become healthy; they want to understand the process of breath training and they want to use those skills of breathing and health to achieve a great feat of physical fitness for themselves. Some examples of people who want more for themselves are found in the clients I've worked with over the years.

I've coached people with cardiovascular disease, lung diseases like asthma, sinusitis and hay fever, type 2 diabetes, obesity, rheumatoid arthritis, fibromyalgia, sleep apnoea, panic, anxiety and mental health disease, to name a few. I've worked with people with chronic pain in their back, hips, knees, shoulders and neck. Some clients were massively successful in their training, while others were not so successful. The successful clients found a way to breathe easier, feel better, become healthier, and enjoy life more. Some of them completely cured their disease, while others reduced the severity of their pains significantly and returned to living a joyous life. This is the natural world of health coaching. If there is anything I have learned along the way it is this:

> *If you want to improve your health badly enough, manage pain and even cure it, then you can do it. You just have to really, really, really want it, be prepared to put the daily work in for a long time and find out what your body needs to return to health, for health is a natural state of the human body.*

The second type of client I work with wants to achieve some physical feat. I've worked with people at all levels of sport. Olympians, ultra-endurance competitors, an NHL hockey strength and conditioning coach, professional tennis players, local GAA teams, recreational athletes and people who want to take on cool challenges like the

Channel swim or climbing Mount Everest. The same principles apply to these people as to those looking to improve their health:

> *The goal is to place the body in a position of health so the body will work for you. It will be at ease, free of pain, and willing to perform well regardless of your pursuit.*

Essentially, I wrote this book for the boy who was told his illness was all in his genes, was told nothing could be done for him, and was given no hope. I wrote it for the boy who found better ways to live life.

I also wrote the book for people like that boy. People who find themselves in a tough spot mentally and physically. People who have 'tried everything' and are willing to try one more thing to help themselves feel better and become healthy.

I wrote it for the sportspeople and high performers of this world looking to get the edge on their game.

I wrote it for the health coaches and trainers out there seeking ways to improve the lives of their clients.

Most importantly, I wrote this book for you, the person who picked it up and has read this far. There is a reason you were inspired to read this book. Follow that instinct, act on it and breathe into it.

Breathe Free.

Leo Ryan, 13/11/2021

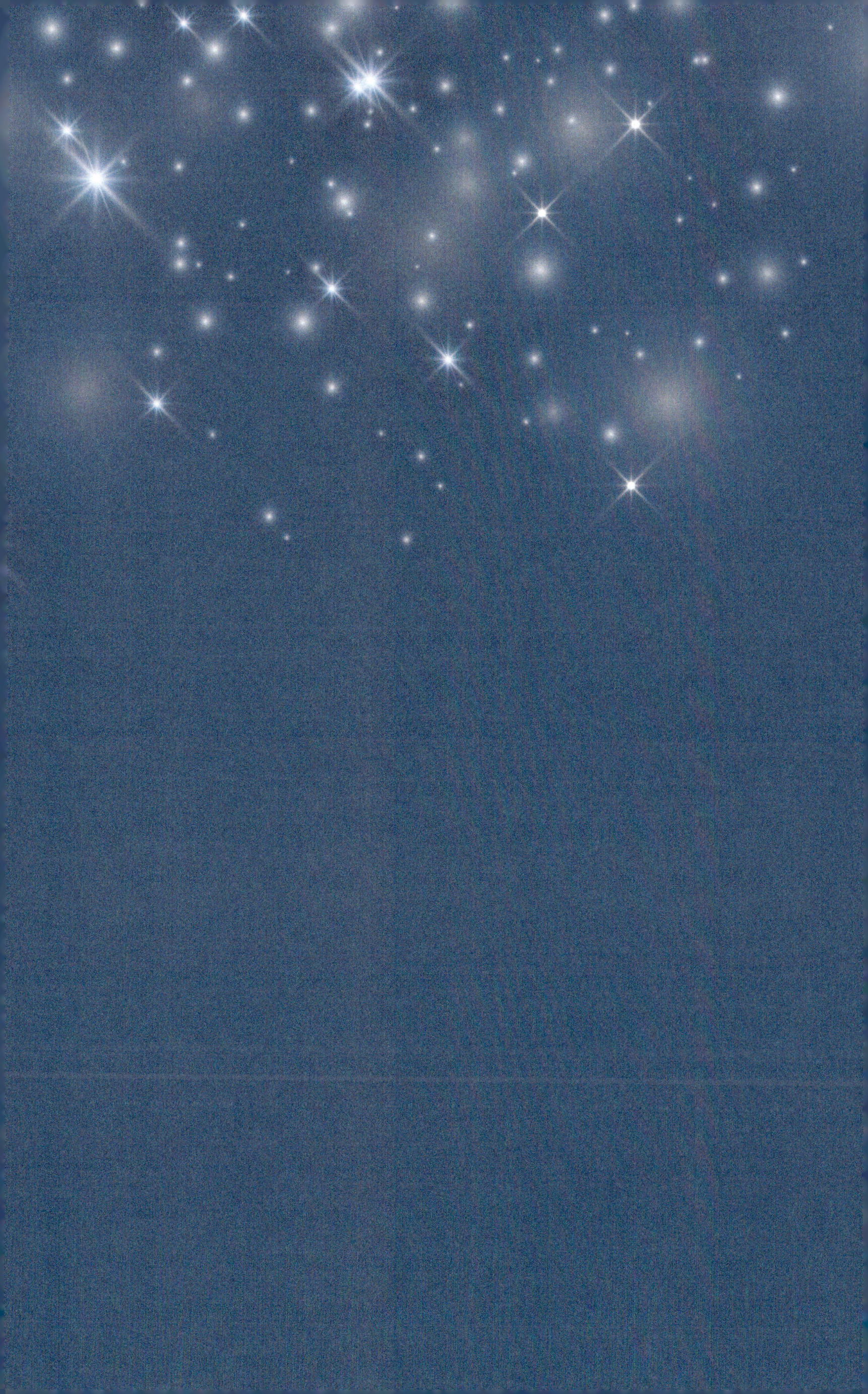

PART 1

THE INTERCONNECTION OF LIFE, STRESS AND THE BREATH

BREATHING FREE IS THE GOAL

Most of the important things in the world have been accomplished by people who have kept on trying when there seemed to be no hope at all.

DALE CARNEGIE

Breathing free is like any other significant accomplishment. It takes faith, hope, courage, focused training and most important of all: consistency of effort. Having a vision for what you want to achieve, many reasons for pursuing it and a plan to get there are all vital components to breathing free. Breathing has a unique place in our world, for it is the subtlest and most overlooked practice you could ever undertake to enrich your life. If breathing had a role in a Hollywood movie, it would star as the Ring of Power in Lord of the Rings – the one ring that binds them all. It is as simple as this: without your breath, you die; all diseases are made worse by adapted breathing patterns; health follows breathing freely; breathing together solidifies bonds and performance in life and sport flows easier when you train your breath. As I say to many of my clients:

> *Without your breath, you have but one dream and with it, you have thousands of dreams*

EXERCISE IN BREATH AWARENESS

Breath awareness is the first step in breath training. Familiarise yourself with your breath by checking in with it regularly. Journal what you notice and check back in with your journal every now and again to see if anything has changed.

Take a moment right now to become aware of your breath. Find a quiet room if possible. Lie down on the floor with knees bent and relax.

- How does the breath move through your body?
- Is it stuck, tight and constricted or is it relaxed and effortless?
- Big or small?
- Fast or slow?
- Do you breathe with your nose or your mouth?
- Is it enjoyable?
- How do you feel emotionally/physically/mentally as you breathe right now?
- Remember to journal your answers to these questions.

YOUR GOAL: BREATHE FREE

Ultimately, your goal to building the quality of your breath is two-fold. The first is to breathe subtly in and out of your nose at rest, during sleep and during low to moderate-level activity; I call this breath a *naturally centred breath*. Secondly, your breath can be used purposely in trauma therapy, vocal performance, physical training and/or to enhance performance in life and sport. This is breathing intentionally, or deliberately. In this sense, breathing free is the foundation goal of all breathing techniques, methods, and practices. Using your breath deliberately, for a specific purpose, is a secondary goal. When you want to:

- Improve any lifestyle disease (physiological or psychological) – breathe free
- Understand your life more and find meaning in it – breathe free and deliberately
- Deepen your connection with loved ones, friends, community, and nature – breathe free and deliberately
- Enhance creativity – breathe free and deliberately
- Improve sports performance – breathe free and deliberately

To breathe free with a naturally centred breath is to nasal breathe subtly at rest, during sleep, and in low to moderate activity. By breathing free you naturally cultivate awareness and sensitivity in your responsiveness to life. You sense more (touch, taste, smell, hear, see and intuit), react less and respond with clarity to the stressors of life. Breathing free requires the use of proper breathing mechanics, a base level of carbon dioxide tolerance, and a gentle, subconscious breathing rhythm. Add this to specific breathing protocols for releasing emotional blockages, aligning your body and mind, and learning to use your breath for specific purposes and you breathe deliberately. In the pursuit of breathing free you will meet several unexpected successes on the road.

THE SEVEN GREAT OPPORTUNITIES BREATHING FREE OFFER YOU ARE:

1. Knowing a subtle breath
2. Reducing fear, panic, anxiety and the need to breathe
3. Realising that it's possible to cure chronic diseases and become healthy
4. Becoming resilient and sustaining a highly energetic lifestyle
5. Being fit, strong, clear-minded and calm under the great pressures of life
6. Improving sports performance and maintaining it for longer
7. Showing you that you have the potential to live your greatest life

To embody breathing free – that is, to know it for yourself – you need to train the foundations of breathing for health and meet the following objectives:

BREATHING FOUNDATIONS

Breathing Free I – Unravel your Breathing Mechanics

To breathe a full breath with ease and free of restriction: lying on your back in a quiet, comfortable place, you inhale through your nose; the belly rises, followed by the chest. The chest rises upwards and expands laterally. You can breathe a full breath without restriction in the lower ribs, mid or upper chest. Finally, the exhale is 'let go'. It springs forth from the top of the inhale and is completely relaxed. In the exhale, there is no muscular tension in the jaw, tongue, throat, shoulders or upper chest. In this analysis the breath can be exhaled through the mouth. Breathing mechanics requires the following training:

- Restore full diaphragmatic breathing
- Restore costal breathing
- Train the exhale to 'let go' and relax
- Perform some stretching techniques to add length and the feeling of freedom to the breath

Breathing Free II – Ingraining a Subtle Breath at Rest

All breathing at rest, in low to moderate activity and during sleep, is performed innately through the nose. The subconscious breathing rhythm is quiet, calm and gentle. You cannot hear the breath and you can hardly feel it move. The breath waves through the body at ease. The lower ribs and belly area move naturally and subtly as you breathe; there is no conscious control of either inhaling or exhaling. This objective requires the following training:

- Nose breathing habits during the day and night
- An introduction to breath work to align the body, spirit and mind
- Breath-holding techniques to develop higher levels of carbon dioxide tolerance
- Calm breathing rhythms to teach the brain to breathe subtly automatically
- Complimentary lifestyle habits to improve breathing

BREATHING FOR PERFORMANCE

All these objectives are built on top of developing your breath foundations. Skipping the basics and jumping straight to this aspect of training may benefit you somewhat, but you'll never realise the full potential of your breath. If anything, learn the foundations and you'll gain more than 90% of the benefits of breath training.

Breathing Deliberately I – Response to Life

Your body naturally opens the breath in response to life's challenges and in sport. As your metabolic demands increase, your breath responds accordingly. You have built on your breathing foundations to develop a range of techniques that help to regulate your body as needed in life. You have developed the skill of breathing to downregulate your system or upregulate it required by life.

- Develop the foundations of *Breathing +*
- Specific 'in the moment' techniques to upregulate and downregulate your system

Breathe Deliberately II – Expressing Emotions

You can consciously use your breath and voice to express emotions without inhibition, build confidence, and communicate with others.

- Develop the foundations of *Breathing +*
- An introduction to breathwork to balance emotions and express them freely

Breathe Deliberately III – Life Performance

You have used your breath to discover more about yourself, unearth creativity, and find the greatness which lies inside you. With the breath you are more creative and you are discovering how to share your gifts with the world. You have learned to connect more deeply with loved ones, friends, and your wider community.

- Develop the foundations of *Breathing +*
- An introduction to breath work for visualisation
- An introduction to breath work to connect with others

HOW TO WORK THROUGH THIS BOOK

The book is divided into three major parts: the why, the what and the how of breath training. The major parts are subdivided again into further sections to enable bite-sized reading times and allow plenty of time to digest the wisdom in the pages.

The Why

What you are reading now forms Part 1 – the Why. The first section of the book aims to show you the connections between life, stress and the breath. It connects the three through neuroanatomy, neurophysiology, somatic education and life as we know it. It offers fresh insights on the interactions between the breath, body, mind and spirit. Structured diagrams illustrate the systematic effects of breathing to help you see life, stress, breathing, health and performance a little differently.

The What

Part 2 shows you what happens to the breath when life becomes too much. It shows the effects of adapted breathing on the body and mind and explains the associations between common disease states and adapted breathing. After the adapted breath, it shows you what a quality breath looks like.

The How

Part 3 is the *Innate Strength Breath Training Program*. It contains coaching perspectives and a step-by-step guide to training your breath from rehabilitation to performance. It is structured in a manner that delivers the most efficient and effective results for you. It includes supplementary techniques, explains the practice of breath work, and layers in lifestyle practices complimentary to breath training. In this part, I show you the baseline fundamentals you require for a quality breath and then guide you to the techniques that will work best for you.

When reading this book, I suggest you read it as it is laid out and then review certain aspects as needs be. I also acknowledge that not everybody learns like me. Some like to dive straight into the practice and pick up the knowledge as they go along. If this is you, then start with Part 3; this is the essential training component of this book, and it contains your goals and your training program for health. As you train, you may want to gain deeper insights into your actions. If this happens to you, then read and review Part 2 of the book, where I explain the connections between your breathing and the health of your body and mind. If you lose motivation along the way, return to Part 1 – remembering the powerful impact breathing can have on your life. Remember that what it has done for others, it can do for you too, if you continually apply yourself to the programme.

Throughout the book, you will find highlights in each chapter. These are boxes containing key points of interest relevant to the chapter.

PART 1 THE INTERCONNECTION OF LIFE, STRESS AND THE BREATH

Coaching insights for you to contemplate, exercises to perform, stories to bring the breath to life, and points of interest to keep you engaged. I encourage you to take your time with the highlights. Think on them, play with them, and journal about them.

The book also contains QR codes for some of the most essential exercises. Scan these codes with the camera on your phone and you'll be directed to a demonstration of the technique online.

Remember, this is an active learning book and only through experience with reflection will you grow as a person and learn to breathe free.

UNRAVELLING THE LANGUAGE OF THE BREATHING WORLD

2

> *A language we do not know is a fortress sealed*
>
> **MARCEL PROUST**

As a brand-new field of interest on the international stage, there is no unified language in the world of breathing. Different breathing practices, cultures, professionals and the various strands of the scientific community all have their own stamp on the language; it can be very confusing for people new to the breathing field. A quality breath is undefined, the meaning of the term 'dysfunctional breathing' is disputed and not even a 'deep breath' is well defined. For example, I remember when I began my breath training in the Buteyko method and I visited the GP one day. In the assessment, the GP put the stethoscope on me and asked me to take a deep breath. I did what I was trained to do; I took a deep breath by inhaling gently into my stomach using my diaphragm. The GP didn't notice anything and asked me again to breathe deeply. By this point, I copped on and decided to play a game, so I did the same thing again. Irritated, he turned to me and told me to take a deep breath again. Innocently I replied, 'I have been taking deep breaths. I think you mean a big breath, like this.' and I proceeded to take a big breath and fill my lungs. 'Yes,' he said, 'that's the one!' I'm not even sure he noticed I was fooling around. The GP was not the only one confused by breathing terminology. Even today, I listen to many experts talk about big and deep breathing and there is no unified definition for it. Personally, I think of filling a container when I think of deep versus big. A deep breath is one that moves low into the body; typically the belly will expand with a deep breath but it is possible to manipulate this movement, keep the belly still and expand the ribs laterally. On the one hand, a big breath is one the fills the whole respiratory cavity with air. The belly protrudes, the ribs expand 360° and the top of the rib cage fills with air. Beyond deep and big breathing terminology, I think it is important to define the goals of a breathing practice, the roles of the people involved in breathing, and to clean up any remaining doubt for you. To start with, let's find out what breathwork is and the difference between it and breath training.

Breathwork is the term traditionally used to describe any breathing practice for the last sixty years. It is thought the word has its origins in Qi Qong. Breathwork involves the use of any breathing technique to change your state. However, the more recent use of the term refers to longer sessions such as Holotropic Breathwork, Wim Hof breathing, Rebirthing or Soma breathing sessions. Longer sessions are emotionally, psychologically and spiritually deeper experiences, and they are usually facilitated by an experienced guide. During the longer and deeper sessions, the participant uses their breath to go deep into their mind with the aim of 'becoming whole', as Dr. Stan Grof would say. Breath training, on the other hand, is very different.

Using the term breath training was a natural progression for me given my training background. I differentiated breathwork and breath training because I felt breathwork and its intentions were somewhat different from my formalised approach to breathing. For me, breathwork is an adjunct aspect of breath training. It is part of the system, but it isn't the be-all and end-all of breathing. Short breathwork sessions are often used as a 'hack' for stressed people to help them relax or think clearly. Meanwhile, long breathwork sessions can become trauma therapy sessions for people who've ignored their body signals for a long time. In both cases, breathwork can become a crutch for you if you don't take the time to restore your breathing fully. A handful of people are able to restore their breathing with breathwork alone but almost all people need to train their breathing system as a whole to restore their breath. *Breath Training* is a structured approach to optimising your breathing. Typically, it cultivates an awareness of your breath, both at rest and in response to life. It involves many daily practice sessions until certain goals are reached and the body returns to its natural centre. The training adheres to the principles and laws of any other physical training modality, such as the FITT, Individualisation, Recovery, Adaption, and SAID principles. Breath training aims to optimise the breathing system in a structured manner until your breath is restored. Only then do you truly have the ability to use your breath effectively for a specific purpose, such as in a highly stressful scenario, in life or in sports performance. I want to diverge for a moment to explain the principles of fitness which underpin breath training.

PRINCIPLES OF FITNESS UNDERPINNING BREATH TRAINING

Frequency Intensity Time Type (FITT). The FITT principles refer to the variables of training which can be manipulated to change the effects of your training session. Every type of physical training has an ideal combination of these factors to create a specific training effect.

The amount of training you perform in a week is termed the Frequency, and it is probably the most crucial factor when it comes to training your breathing foundations.

Next, intensity is defined as how hard you push your session relative to your maximal ability. Note that Intensity is probably the most commonly misunderstood variable in this training principle. There is a world of difference between something you feel as intense and something that is actually intense relative to your maximal ability. For example, if your personal best for a 100 m sprint is 10.5 seconds and you run it in 10.5 seconds then you have run at maximal intensity. However, if you're doing a training session with five repeat 100 m sprints then it may seem difficult or 'intense' but you will generate nowhere near the same speed you did for your personal best. All weight training is managed similarly relative to your single rep max. In the same vein, holding your breath for a maximal time is different from holding multiple rounds of a lesser breath hold. They both may feel intense, but intensity is truly managed relative to your maximum.

The third variable is Time. It refers to the amount of time you spend in a training session. For example, performing 60 minutes of breath training differs from performing three blocks of 20 minutes. Training time would be 60 mins in the former and only 20 mins in the latter but you would have increased your frequency from one session to three that day. Time and Frequency are different. Later on, you will see a minimum threshold of 10 minutes time in each breath training session, but ideally, you train two to three times per day. This is vastly different from training one session for forty to sixty minutes.

Type is the final variable of training. Every exercise produces a different effect on the body (sometimes it's a slight difference, sometimes a large one). The exercise you choose usually fits into a block of similar activities. Running, cycling and swimming are typically categorised as 'cardio' training (although I'd debate that one!) whilst weight training and calisthenics are forms of strength training. More specifically, a barbell squat and a deadlift are resistance training exercises. Both produce very similar whole-body results in the sense that they both target improvements in the neuromuscular system. However, their effects on the postural system are very different. The squat strengthens the knees more, whereas the deadlift focuses on the hips and back. Breath training is no different to any other physical training. It can be classified grossly as respiratory training but every technique also fits into sub-categories, such as breathing mechanics, resilience, and rhythms.

Individualisation. If all people had the same life experience and thought about life the same way, then a technique would have the same effect across the board; but because our lives are all unique techniques work on us differently. This is the principle of Individualisation.

Having said that, techniques work on a continuum. If you are a well-balanced person, then the technique has a similar impact across all people, mostly relaxing or energising in the case of breathing. If, for any reason, you are a stressed person with an adapted centre (I'll explain this term), then techniques work differently on you. Almost all the untrained people I've come across in my work operate from an 'adapted centre'.

It is because of the principle of Individualisation that the Wim Hof breathing technique, or any technique for that matter, produces very different experiences. Some like it, some hate it. Understanding why it's working on you the way it does is paramount to choosing the right techniques for you.

Adaption is the process of change the body undergoes in response to a stimulus. There is a specific and a general adaption that takes place. The specific response is relative to the tissues directly involved in the technique and the general response is also commonly known as the stress response; it is how the overall system reacts to a stimulus – that is body, mind, and spirit. You can grow or shrink as a result of a stimulus depending on its potency, how you perceive the stimulus and your ability to recover. As the famous Swiss physician Paracelsus once said, 'Everything is a poison; the dose makes it so'.

Recovery is what happens between training sessions. How you sleep, eat, think, and live outside of your training all modulate, or impact, the effects of a training session. If you want to gain maximal benefit from your training, then the session is only half the battle; recovery is the other half. The world-renowned Olympic strength and conditioning coach, Ian King, taught me a simple formula to produce great training results: Training + Recovery = Training Effect. If you only focus on one half of the puzzle, then you're missing out on many of the benefits and wasting your time. This is especially true for breathing. The more adjunct practices you can bring in to complement your training and reset your body, the more effective your training becomes. Sleeping well and adding heat training are two such practices which aid breath training.

Specific Adaptation to Imposed Demand (SAID). You can only ask the body one question at a time. The body answers that question by adapting or responding to it. The response is directly related to the characteristics of the questions – its size, shape, length of time etc. The way you ask questions of the body is with movement and techniques. For example, developing maximal leg strength in the gym requires the right mix of all variables. An appropriate exercise like a barbell back squat is chosen. The tempo of the movement matters; the intensity (weight), repetitions, sets and rest periods are all structured to elicit the benefits sought from session's, the goal that is, the development of maximal leg strength. If performed with the correct technique and adequate recovery the body responds to the training accordingly by developing maximal strength in the legs. It does this by improving neuromuscular control and possibly growing additional muscle tissue. Similarly, if you perform a walking breath-hold programme with appropriate guidelines and recovery strategies, then the body answers by improving the physical response to a rise in carbon

GEM #1 PRINCIPLES OF PHYSICAL TRAINING APPLY EQUALLY TO BREATH TRAINING

Sports coaches and therapists tend to forget that breathing adheres to the same principles and rules of training, the same as muscles and the energy systems. FITT, SAID, Adaption, Specificity and Individuality principles, for example, all apply to breath training. The way you breathe in and around training also directly affects the results you gain from any given physical training session.

dioxide and the psychological response. Alternatively, if you were to choose a seated breath-hold programme, the body responds by mostly improving the psychological reaction with little improvement to the physical response.

THE BREATHING SYSTEM

The Breathing System is a term I use to describe every aspect of the body and mind which enhances the breath. It encompasses so much more than the respiratory system alone, and it involves every system in the body: respiratory, neuro-myofascial gut, skin and skeletal systems. When we use a breathing technique, a stretch or even a nutrition protocol, the idea is to improve that one sub-part as well as enhance the overall system. Speaking of which, that is how I also think of the body and mind in totality.

ONE BODY, ONE MIND, ONE SPIRIT

The body, mind and spirit are connected as one. There is no such thing as mind training without involving the body and spirit. The reverse is also true; the same can be said for health. Mental health and physical health are one. Since the advent of scientific materialism, we tend to slice up the body and mind into parts and talk about them as if they are separate, but they are not. Take a look at your right hand. Now look to your left foot and tell me where they are separated. They are not, right? They are connected. You are connected. You are one human being from head to toe and everything in between. From now on, when I speak about health, I'll refer to your whole body-mind-spirit simply as your 'biological system' (in other words, everything contained inside your skin). If I want to emphasise a particular aspect of that system, then I will speak directly about that part. Once the breath is restored, the focus of breath training shifts to conditioning the breath for a specific purpose, such as life or sports performance.

The final terms I'd like to unpack for you are those of breathing *Guide, Instructor, Teacher* and *Coach*. Each of these terms is used intermittently throughout the world of breathing. Some people apply different terms to their practice depending on the person they are talking to. Traditionally, breathwork practices use the term *Guide* or *Facilitator* to describe what they do. A *Breathing Guide* is a person who leads a breathwork session. They create the environment for the breathing participants, nurture the atmosphere, create a safe space for participants and help integrate the breathers experience. Breathing guides are responsible for the safety and wellbeing of their participants for the duration of the breathwork session, and they should provide support afterwards.

A *Breathing Teacher* (or *Practitioner*) is more oriented to the education side of breathing. They typically know a lot about the science of breathing, and are usually immersed in a method such as the Buteyko method or a physiotherapy-based method, like the Bradcliff method. Usually they impart the knowledge of the breathing programme to participants and ask them to go away and practice the method independently. A good breathing teacher will provide long-term support to their students.

A *Breathing Coach* is more hands-on than a teacher. They manage the programme a lot closer, communicate a lot with their clients and light the path for the client until the client is ready to train on their own. Like a sports coach, a breathing coach is there to inspire and empower you to achieve your goals with your breathing programme. As Michael Jordan once said, 'A coach is someone that sees beyond your limits and guides you to greatness'.

I fall into all these categories! I am a Breather, a Guide, a Teacher and a Coach, depending on the demands of the individual. I believe, a guide, teacher or coach is the only short-cut you will find in helping you achieve your goals faster. There is no other magic pill. Only experience teaches us to be better. In all my years coaching clients, as a personal trainer first and then as a breathing coach, I have gained many insights into the worlds of health, performance, progress and breathing. Throughout this book I'll share some of those insights with you to speed up your progress along your path.

UNDERSTANDING BALANCE 3

THE GAME OF HEALTH AND HOW TO PLAY IT

One of the most important concepts I have learned over the years is that long-term health and performance is the game of balancing the opposites in life. The Chinese philosophy of Taoism describes it in a symbol as Yin and Yang. It is a concept of dualism which explains that everything has the seed of its opposite contained within it. The Star Wars movie franchise depicts this concept of Yin and Yang wonderfully, as the lives of the movie heroes and villains unfold from the experiences they are exposed to and they make choices at each significant moment.

In the franchise, Darth Vader is one of the main villains and his son, Luke Skywalker, is the hero. In the beginning, Darth Vader has the seed of goodness in him and Luke has the potential to follow his father to the dark side of the Force (aka evil). As the plot develops, Darth Vader succumbs to fear, anger, hatred and suffering, becoming an apprentice to the Dark Lord himself. Meanwhile, Luke chooses hope, faith and love to remain on the light side of the Force. Like Luke and his father, Yin and Yang are not total opposites, they are relative to each other. The philosophy behind Star Wars and the Yin Yang symbol contains kernels of truth for how life works in practice. Darth Vader was not entirely evil and Luke absolutely good. Both had the potential to shift to either side of the Force at several major turning points in the plot if they wished to do so. I believe this philosophy holds as a principle across all domains of life. I have seen this concept not only in Hollywood movies and Chinese philosophy but also in the sporting, physical, financial, wellbeing and relationship domains of human life. It is evident in practical aspects of life like in the sport of judo, current explanations for the neurobiology of stress, somatic education, movement practice, raising my children and in breathing itself. As I reflect on each of these domains in light of this philosophy, I can more clearly see how the human body works as a whole and how all interventions can be used to improve one's health and performance. I want to share those insights with you now to reveal to you how your biological system and breathing works.

JUDO REFLECTS STRESS IN LIFE

For every action in judo, there is an opposite reaction from your opponent. In its simplest form the goal of judo is to create a reaction in response from your opponent so that you can break their balance and throw them. The success of any throw is found in the preceding counter-movement. With the flick of a wrist, a high-level judoka is able to sense a range of potential reactions three or four moves ahead of time, the same way a master chess player will plan a check-mate several moves ahead. In judo, you achieve this result by pushing or pulling your opponent out of their centre. As you initiate an attack your opponent either moves with your attempt or resists it. Your goal, then, is to use their movement against them. You apply a force in a different direction to break their balance and throw them. For example, you may resist my attempt when I pull you forward. You stay rooted in the same place, but your body's centre of gravity has shifted backwards in your effort to resist my pull. This is a 'perceived centre'. I can sense this resistance. I counter your resistance by swiftly pushing you backwards and throwing you to the mat (*Judo and Life*, Jigoro Kano). You are smart, though. You learn from this experience and adapt to my moves by developing your own set of counter-movements. With eight major movement patterns and more than fifty throws in the core syllabus, the game of pushing and pulling to break balance becomes infinitely complex, thought-provoking and enjoyable. Judo is a way of life. Its philosophy is based on the same premise as the Force in Star Wars and in the Yin Yang symbol. Judo philosophies, its value system and standards are as much a part of the process of becoming a worthy judoka as learning the skills of the game itself. It takes many years to become proficient at the game, let alone achieve a high level of expertise, and it can take a lifetime to understand its nuances. The wisdom gained from judo transfers directly to the rest of life. In life, we have a centre of balance, and an innately intelligent whole-body mechanism known as allostasis, which maintains balance through life's challenges. How allostasis works is the game of health we all play. The changes in life, and our lifestyle, are the forces that push and pull us to break our balance and move us out of our natural centre. If it is a continuous small force, we are transferred to a perceived centre, less in balance with ourselves but continuing on with life. We know this as being stressed. If it is a significant force, we fall down, sometimes with pain, disease, illness or a mixture of all of them.

FINDING THE CENTRE IN HUMAN HEALTH

In 1864, Louis Pasteur succeeded in convincing the scientific community that germs were the cause of all illnesses. Claude Bernard was a contemporary of Pasteur. Although he shared many of Pasteur's beliefs, he didn't believe in Pasteur's germ theory. Instead, he thought that the body's state was the most important factor in disease. On his deathbed, Pasteur acknowledged Bernard's idea and reneged on his own theory when he said, 'The germ is nothing, the terrain is everything,' which I think is funny given the fact that the germ theory has been the dominant position of conventional allopathic medicine for almost 150 years. Meanwhile, Bernard's beliefs were largely ignored. In 1865, Walter Canon proposed the idea of homeostasis. He claimed that everything in the body worked to maintain a static position.

Homeostasis was the ideal health goal of the day. Even today, many pharmaceutical interventions work toward this goal of maintaining a static norm by suppressing extreme responses. However, this model cannot explain many complaints of modern life, such as hypertension and metabolic syndrome, and so a new model was proposed – allostasis. Allostasis can be defined as 'remaining stable by changing'. It describes the workload the body must perform to re-establish homeostasis. When the body has to work too hard, it becomes over-loaded and the results can be detrimental to the body. The allostasis model can better explain chronic conditions such as asthma, obesity and diabetes.

Allostasis is a predictive model of efficiency for the body. In allostasis, the body is continuously reading your experiences in life. It senses your thoughts about the past, present and future as happening now. It combines those thoughts with the inputs from your lifestyle and your genetics to produce an efficient way of dealing with your life. The allostatic response is a systems-wide change in the body. If you thought fifty throws built from eight movement patterns in judo was complex, can you imagine how many allostatic processes the body must manage to keep your body in balance? The body has a relatively high level of flexibility in response to life's challenges. Still, after a while, the maintenance of allostatic changes, where the body fails to revert to its natural centre, leads to overload and begins to have consequences. The consequences result in dysfunction as we experience it: pain, illness and disease.

Breathing is a good example: during the day, our breathing rate is typically 12-15 breaths per minute (bpm) at rest. It can surpass 60 bpm in times of extreme physical activity and drop to 3.5 bpm or less during deep rest. None of this is pathological. However, if the demand for breathing is constantly set at a higher level, due to long-term stress, for example, then the natural centre will be reset to a higher 'perceived centre'. This new normal is the adaptation response and although it may lead to disease or pain, it is not necessarily inappropriate, nor is it due to dysregulation. External lifestyle factors have been responded

PART 1   THE INTERCONNECTION OF LIFE, STRESS AND THE BREATH

to in a normal, efficient manner by the body. It is the external lifestyle factors (or even your perception of them) that are dysregulated and inappropriate, not the response. If the physiological and psychological response is normal, where should therapeutics intervene? Current interventions aim at the body's reactions, rather than the insults of the reactions. But this can cause several more problems:

1. Every signal has a domino effect of reactions
2. The brain drives the body's response – altering the response causes the brain to compensate by driving other mechanisms harder
3. Blocking responses to a set level reduces the ability of the body to respond to changing needs, thus blocking physiological responses

Drugs, surgery, supplements, even massage and other forms of therapy, may force the response back to normal, but the body will once more over-compensate and find its 'new norm' in relation to all the information it receives. A straightforward example is when the chronic pain in your back disappears after a physical therapy session but returns a day later and persists twice as strongly. The problem is not the body but the things we do in our lifestyle that cause our body to respond with pain, illness and disease. The solution is not physical therapy, drug intervention or surgery, but moving more often through our day in a variety of ways.

To further illustrate this point, chronic disease is widely regarded to be on the rise exponentially in the USA and across the Western world, despite the annual investment of billions of dollars in healthcare. What fascinates me is that all people with chronic physiological diseases (like hypertension, diabetes, anxiety and asthma) present with elevated resting breathing rates. Simultaneously, it is interesting to observe that the 'normal' breathing rate for US citizens has risen from 12-15 breaths-per-minute to 17-20 breaths-per-minute in the last year. This is allostasis in action and it doesn't just end with an increase in breathing rate. Everything in the body is affected by the increased breathing rate.

In the beginning, big and fast breathing dramatically change blood pH – in as little as two minutes. If you continued to over-breathe throughout the course of the day, the brain upregulates other organs, like the kidneys, to keep your blood pH in balance. If you continue to over-breathe for days, the brain gets your message that it had the wrong set-point in the first place, so instead of simply recruiting the kidneys to help, it re-sets the set-point for breathing. The brain accepts that you want to breathe more and it redefines the amount of air you need to breathe subconsciously to survive. Now that your set point has changed, you have less pressure on the kidneys. However, the lungs aren't exactly working as normal. You subconsciously breathe more than you require. At first, on a conscious level, you don't notice this. It may take years to develop that awareness, but you find that you are more sensitive to breathing-related issues. You are more sensitive to allergens in the air and food. You develop itchy skin and a dry scalp. You become more prone to viral and bacterial infections. Over time anxiety and panic attacks occur more often. Chest infections become recurring. Fatigue and mental fog become a norm for you.

When we live a stressed life, our bodies adapt to that lifestyle. The body tries to bring us back to our natural centre but, if you continue to live a stressed life, the body resets its systems to a new normal. The consequences of this newly perceived centre usually result in chronic pain, physical and psychological disease. Maintaining a natural centre in the body is similar, then, to maintaining balance in judo. The body and the judoka alike are moved away from their natural centre by a combination of previous choices and external force. Both the body and the judoka try to maintain that centre by adapting to the choices/force. Eventually the will of the choices/force creates a perceived centre in both the judoka and health – they look stable but they are off-balance. If the choices/force is too powerful or comes from too many directions, then both the health of the body and the judoka's balance will be broken. The result is that the judoka gets thrown and the health of the body deteriorates.

GEM #2 UNDERSTANDING BALANCE

Your body and brain have a natural centre – a place of balance to which they return following a stressful event and a recovery period. Acting from a natural centre gives you the potential to stress the body more (act more) and recover fully.

When we continuously push our body in one direction, it shifts our natural centre to a perceived one. Now we are more likely to develop pain, a host of chronic diseases and injury.

MODERN DAY CAUSES OF IMBALANCE

4

Imagine living in the Palaeolithic era. Your primary goals in life are to survive, mate, relax and have fun with your tribe. When the sun goes down, you either rest your head and go to sleep or you light a fire, dance, play music, sing, party, have sex and go to sleep. By day you hunt, forage, eat, and set up protection for your people. If you are unsuccessful in these simple daily tasks, you and your tribe will pass out of existence. You will die.

Daytime hunting involves many hours of walking and following animal tracks. Food may be scarce or abundant depending on where you live and the time of year. Often, you go hours and even days without food when times are tough. When food is in rich supply, you eat your fill and share the leftovers; but you can't save your leftovers as you have no way to store the food. To be a successful hunter or gatherer, you need to develop skills that put you in touch with nature. You need heightened senses – vision and hearing – to locate animals in the distance. Your sense of smell is developed with your sense of taste to choose non-poisonous foods and track animals a little closer to you. Your sense of touch is deftly defined, enabling you to step quietly, run swiftly and move over the physical landscape at speed. You are an optimised hunter-gatherer. You passed trials of pain and endurance as a young tribesperson and you have become one of the strongest and fastest in your tribe.

One day, during your hunt for life-sustaining food, you come across a bear wandering around outside her den; her newly-born cubs are playing nearby. The bear senses you are near. She sticks her snout in the air, takes a whiff and then turns her head to you. As she eyeballs you she stands up tall on her hind legs and lets out a roar. She drops onto all fours again and charges for you. What do you do? How does your body react?

If you value your life, then let's begin with what you don't want to do. You don't want to stay and analyse the situation. You don't want to know if the bear is 7 ft tall or 8 ft tall, the bear's shade of colouring or her weight. Instead you run or you play dead – the famous 'flight or freeze' response. The analysis of the situation occurs in the thalamus region of the emotional mammalian brain. In a split second it sees the danger for what it is – life or death. The thalamus sends two signals out. One signal is sent upwards to reduce the blood flow to your slower, thinking, rational brain. The thinking forebrain is shut down to save energy and allows you to act on instinct. The other signal is sent down to the fast-acting reptilian brain. Within milliseconds of seeing the bear coming for you, your reptilian brain secretes a huge dose of adrenaline and nor-adrenaline hormones. As these hormones course through your blood, they prepare your whole system to run. Your breathing quickens and deepens; your heart rate shoots through the roof; muscles are lit up to get you out of there. Every organ and bodily function that is unnecessary in that moment of need is also reduced. Blood flow to essential organs of long-term health, like the sexual organs, stomach and gut are turned down to funnel all energy and blood back to the systems you need working now. Your mouth dries, eyes narrow and digestion slows. You are prepared to run as fast as you can or die. What this means is that the fear of the bear hurtling towards you up-regulates your whole body and mind to get you out of that situation. This is Human Stress Response and it still works the same for you today as it did for your ancestors. It is a generic response to all major perceived stressors (real and imaginary) as discovered by Hans Selye in the 1930s. Stress is viewed as 'anything that disrupts the body's homeostasis'. It is not simply the feeling of pressure or anxiety. Rather it is a much broader definition which encompasses everything physical, mental, emotional and spiritual that disrupts the autonomic processes of the body at rest. The stressors acting on people in modern society are different, and more prevalent, than those acting on our ancestors.

MODERN STRESSORS

The variety and intensity of our modern-day insults are vast. Yet no single insult is so potent that our bodies can't handle it. For example, the organ which produces most of our stress hormones, the adrenals, is said to be able to deal with stress for a lifetime of more than 200 years. Our bodies can handle any one stress, and even many multiples, quite easily; but when we accumulate stressors one after another over many years, they can eventually overwhelm our system. The result is pain and chronic disease.

You fall asleep after midnight while watching TV, only to be woken up by a social media alert on your phone. Eventually morning comes around and you crawl out of bed after hitting the snooze button for a third time. A quick shower, throw on some clothes and make yourself half-presentable. Down a quick cup of coffee and shove a bowl of cereal down in three gulps: breakfast of champions, you think. Then you're out the door and into an hour of rush-hour traffic, if you're lucky. Sitting there you have time to decompress. Then you feel that all too familiar feeling of a headache building in your forehead. You hate traffic. Road rage, polluted air from the fumes of the vehicles; nothing but negative news and garbage celebrity stories feature on the radio again. All the sights, sounds and smells of a normal morning in the life of a modern person. Then the workday begins. It opens with thirty emails and a to-do list the length of your arm. Your boss is already screaming at you because you're late with yet another deadline. As much as you'd like to tell him to shove the job up his ass, you don't, because you know the rent is due on Friday and you can't afford to be out of work for more than a few days. Instead you bite your tongue, swallow your pride, nod and smile. The rage inside you is suppressed for now as he's moved onto his next victim. The moment has passed and you breathe a huge sigh of relief that today was not the day you told him to go jump off a cliff!

Exercise, too, is another form of modern stress. The term given to this process in science is hormesis. The training process in the gym is hormesis at work, so is taking an ice-bath; going for a run or doing a yoga session. In each case, we stress our body by doing something with it. After the session we hope to recover, adapt and get better. The idea is that our bodies learn from the experience and it changes everything in the body – a hormetic effect. Take weight training, for example. When we perform a session and receive an adequate recovery it is long-established that nerve-signal speed alters, the quality and quantity of muscle fibres can change, the length-tension ratio of a muscle adapts and the flexibility of our cardiovascular system is adjusted. The hormone system adapts and all biological systems make changes thanks to that one session. When we expose ourselves to a weight session again, our body remembers what happened, and it now requires a greater degree of stress to adapt again. Problems arise when we do not give adequate recovery to the system in terms of time and support, or when we search for large gains from the session and we over-cook the session itself. Pushing our system a little too hard for too long is called over-reaching and pushing it way too hard without adequate recovery ends up with your biological system becoming over-trained. The result is a whole series of negative symptoms such as chronic fatigue, pain, moodiness, exacerbation of any underlying health conditions, chronic inflammation throughout the body, loss of appetite, sleep inhibition, immune suppression and more. Sounds familiar, right? These symptoms are not reserved for elite athletes pushing their bodies to the limits. They are common to almost everybody. The reason we suffer from symptoms of over-training throughout our lives is because we expose ourselves to many insults and our body constantly adapts to them.

City life, fast living, poor relationships, no purpose or meaning in life, disrupted biological rhythms: these are all by-products of our imagination. We created this world and there is a cost to the recent evolutionary path we've chosen. We were not built to thrive or even survive in this landscape. Our biology has remained the same as our ancestors'; our stress response is the same. It's our environment that's changed. Our modern-day insults can be likened to the Chinese torture of death by a thousand cuts. Up to the start of the 1900s a person found guilty in Chinese courts could be drugged, beaten and tied to a post in public. Over the course of several days, the transgressor would be sliced and nicked thousands of times. In the beginning, the torturer would cut body parts with low blood supply like the kneecaps and elbows. As the torture continued it would move to more painful areas

LIST OF COMMON MODERN-DAY INSULTS

Difficult birthing process	Disconnection from humans, nature and animals	Social media
Lack of safe and loving upbringing	Micro-organisms (pathogens, viruses, bacteria, parasites etc.)	Exposure to artificial light and lack of sunlight
Parental attachment issues		Overheating – living indoors and clothing
Physical, sexual or emotional abuse	Mundane psychological work practices	Lack of movement or excess training
No meaning or purpose in life	Technological stressors (Wi-Fi, microwaves etc.)	Alcohol, cigarettes and drugs
Lack of meaningful social connections	Financial hardship	Over exposure to pharmaceutical drugs
Physical weakness and an inability to fend for oneself in society	Air pollution	Adapted postures due to sitting, driving & commuting
	Water pollution	
	Poor nutrition quality	
	Excess calories	

such as the nipples and stomach muscles. After days of this torture, the convict eventually bleeds out and dies, or dies from the amount of pain endured. A horrific process no doubt, but are we inflicting a less painful but equally dangerous torture on our own bodies with modern living? I think so. We are inflicting the same type of torture on ourselves each day of our lives without even realising it (at least in some cases). You may think I'm being a bit extreme but look at the list of stressors on the previous page. They are common to almost every one of us nowadays. They were not common to anybody all those millennia ago.

As shown in the table on page 31, this list of possible insults is comprehensive. Every one of us in the modern day is exposed to many of these stressors, multiple times, every day of our lives. The list covers all aspects of human lifestyle – growth, development, meaning, work, remuneration, rest and play. Traumatic events, global events and daily habits all have a role to play in how healthy and strong you become. Most of all your perception of how these things impact you has a huge role to play in their effects on your body. You may not even think of some things on this list as a stressor. You may think of it as 'just life'. To an extent you are right. Shit happens in life. It's how you think about it, your body's reaction to it and your response that counts the most. In creating this list, I am not trying to get you to eliminate these stressors entirely. Instead, I want you to acknowledge that they may be causing your body, mind and performance issues. You know if they are harming you by the reaction of your body and mind to them. Identifying which stressor you should keep or eliminate may be easier said than done, as they all produce the same stress response in the body. Instead, you may want to start by looking at the sum effect of all these stressors on your body.

Our biological reaction to each of these insults and to the sum of all stressors is the same response as our ancestors. Adrenaline and noradrenaline are secreted and cortisol is upregulated. All processes unnecessary to survival are turned down and the energy is redirected to support the stress response, including sex hormones, digestion and complex logical thinking. All of this happens in the blink of an eye. Without the need for a conscious thought, your whole biological system is on red alert and prepared to run as hard as it can to survive. To make matters worse, we don't use that energy to run and survive. Instead, we sit in the stew of stress and our response to it. We compound matters by then exposing ourselves to even more stresses. We feel sorry for ourselves and so we numb our pain with food, sex, alcohol, drugs and medications in a bid to suffer less. We train to extremes and live to extremes. And, although these substances/practices work for a time, they are only a band-aid on the real issues we are not addressing. Eventually this chronic lifestyle of stress becomes too much to handle and our biological body breaks down. Our breathing adapts, our posture changes, our mind stops working well and our internal organs deteriorate drastically. Pain, disease and mental illness can all ensue. It doesn't happen over the course of a day, a week or even a year. This allostatic process can take twenty or thirty years to manifest.

> *'I am a trainer with over 20 years' experience in the fitness industry. I am a mother, I am 44 years of age and I took up athletics at age 40. I also suffered with auto immune diseases since the age of 15...*
>
> *As I trained my breathing with Leo, I started to realise the main issue for me was that my body and mind was always in a stressed state. When you look at me you would never think I am stressed. I come across as the most calm and relaxed person you could meet. But I found when I took time to really connect with my breath it told me so much more about myself even on a daily basis.*
>
> *Through Leo, I found the power of the breath on improving stress and that power is huge!'*
>
> **MARTHA MOUSSALLY. INNATE-STRENGTH CLIENT**

NESTING OUR STRESS

The diagram below beautifully illustrates the nesting of insults, traumatic or otherwise, in our body. Whenever we have unresolved stress in our biological system, it is built upon and embedded into the next event. Our body adapts around that stressor, integrates it into the shape of our breath, our movement and the internal workings of our organs. Though we may forget that we even had that original insult and adaptation from it, it is still present in our system; it has still changed us. Where our natural centre was position one, it now becomes position six in the diagram. We have a new 'perceived centre' instead of our natural centre. This is a concept I adapted from Taoist philosophy, playing judo, my understanding of the somatic nervous system and observations in coaching and life. The concept was reaffirmed for me when I read Gary Ward's view on posture and movement. Gary views human movement from the foot up (Ward 2013). As foot mechanics change due to modern living, Gary sees a shift in our centre of mass and an adaptation to a new perceived centre. I view the body both from a movement and a whole biological system perspective. In this

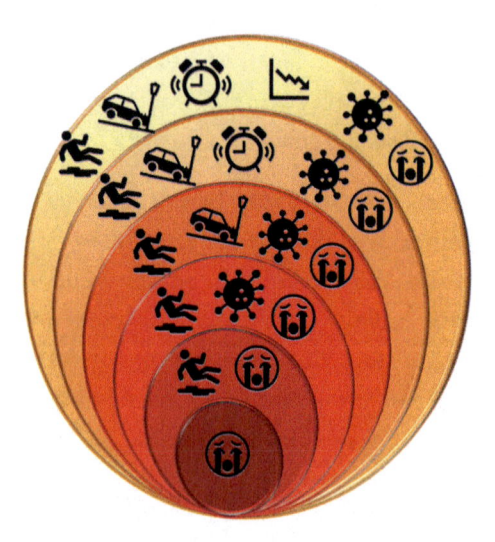

Nested Stress in humans. The idea that unresolved traumas are embedded into us, one on top of the next, and carried with us over time

sense, the body can adapt to its environment because of foot mechanics but it can also adjust its perceived centre to general stress and life via the autonomic nervous system. This shift is best observed from a breathing perspective because of breathing's connection to the regulation of general stress in the body. Through this lens, we become that Jenga tower – still standing tall, but liable to collapse with the next play in the game.

We breathe more into one area, lengthen certain areas of our postural muscular chain and increase blood flow to produce particular hormones. As we move further away from the original centre, these same parts of our body become loaded with added work and pressure, whilst the other parts atrophy due to lack of use. As one stressor builds on top of another, our body becomes overwhelmed, distorted beyond its natural shape and eventually shows signs of pain and disease. This perceived centre affects all domains of the human body and brain: the nervous system, brain waves, heart rhythm, breath, posture and hormone levels. An endocrinologist observes changes in blood work numbers. A psychologist witnesses a shift in one's mindset. A neurobiologist may see altered blood flow patterns in brain scans to different brain regions. A movement specialist identifies adapted posture and walking gait and a breathing coach observes these adaptations in the flow of breath.

Talk to anybody in their mid to late thirties nowadays and you'll find out almost everyone is in pain. They often have one or more diseases and take some form of medication. We are a world of sick people who are sedating our way to an early grave. Perhaps the most challenging aspect to swallow about this whole process – and yet the most beautiful – is that we have the power to reverse this entire process. With our combined knowledge and experience, we can turn the tide on stress in this modern world. And it all starts with understanding how our body works, the foundations of which is learning to breathe better.

STRESS AND BREATHING

5

Breathing is essential to every moment of our life. We all know that without our breath, we die. Doesn't it make sense, then, that life and its stressors can affect the quality of our breath and our breath can also impact the vitality of our life? In our caveman biology, breathing played a very important role in helping secrete adrenaline, give you a boost of energy and get you out of a stressful situation. We still have that same biological system in place today. What's different is our life, our stressors and how they impact the breath over the long term. Let's get more specific in this section and detail just how stress can impact your breathing. Remember that bear story from the last section? Put yourself back in that scenario. The bear spots you. What happens in your body in that instant?

> *Your breathing increases, your pupils constrict and your heart starts pounding. You are energised to run and get out of the situation. These responses are the first signs of an immediately upregulated sympathetic nervous system.*

Now, let's say you escape from the bear. You run five kilometres at top speed and lose it somewhere in the forest. You are safe. What happens now?

Your breathing slows (to below normal), your eyes dilate to take in the new surroundings, your heart rate calms, and your muscles relax. The more you sit there recovering, the deeper you drop into relaxation. You may yawn, stretch, and even take the liberty of a little nap after all the excitement. After your body has relaxed and recuperated, it returns itself to its natural centre once more. Often, we learn from our experiences physiologically and mentally. When we return to centre, we return with a stronger sense of self and become more robust in our ability to handle stressors. To use the bear analogy once more: after we've evaded the bear, rested and recovered, we reflect, and learn from the experience. We may develop better strategies for tracking bears or learn how to evade them better. Our bodies may also have adapted by becoming physically fitter from our run. These are the signs of a functioning biological system.

The repeated experience of perceived life-endangering events, combined with rest, recovery and reflection, helps us to build a strong natural centre and a broad comfort zone. A strong natural centre is the foundation of our ability to explore the edges of our comfort zone and be ok with it. The ability to explore the edges of our comfort zone and beyond is critical to our growth as human beings, and it leads to a healthier, more robust, more fulfilled and greater life.

From my experience in life and as a coach, I recommend we visit the inside edges of our comfort zone in both training and life. We could, of course, just use everyday life as a training ground; but the potential chaos of life, combined with the relative comforts of our modern lives, can leave many of us broken. Training is an ideal way to build a strong natural centre, and it enables you to explore the edges of your comfort zone in a controlled environment. This training then prepares you better for life. The sense of self you've developed in your training, along with your skills, knowledge and attitudes, are tested in the crucible of life, sport, and adventures. The caveat to training is that we perform it in the spirit of pushing ourselves as far as we are physically, mentally and spiritually ok to do. I call this place the inside edge of our growth zone. This exploration requires three things:

PART 1 THE INTERCONNECTION OF LIFE, STRESS AND THE BREATH

Natural Centre

4. Stronger Centre Built & Return to Natural Centre

1. Stressful Experience

Comfort/growth Zone

Outside your Zone

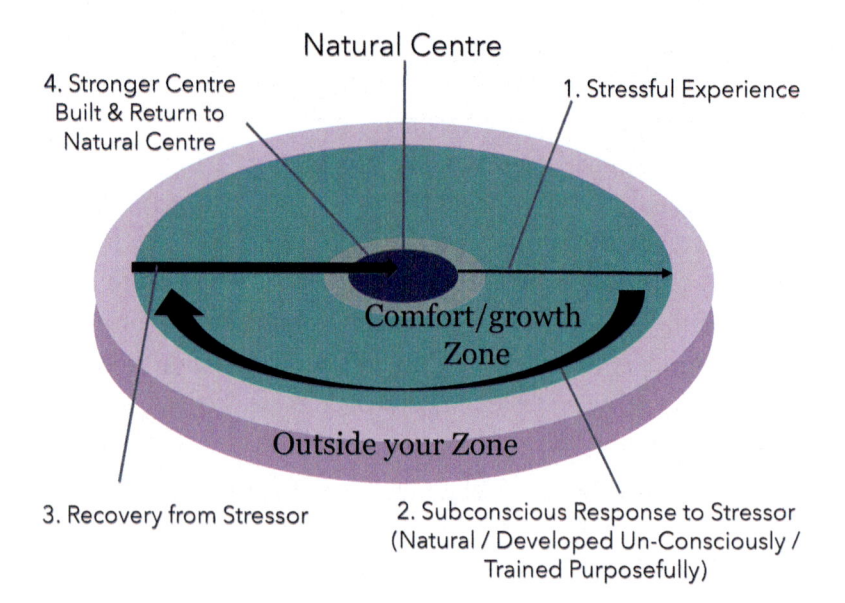

3. Recovery from Stressor

2. Subconscious Response to Stressor (Natural / Developed Un-Consciously / Trained Purposefully)

Depiction of Human Growth: As we live through stressful experiences, we move from our centre to the edge of our growth zone. Afterwards, we rest and recover. The combination of experience and recovery builds a strong centre and expands our growth zone.

1. Courage to step up to the edge of your growth zone
2. A high degree of interoception to feel the moment for what it is
3. A high degree of agency so you can make rational judgements in the moment of fear. Are you afraid because what you are doing is stupid or are you fearful because it is a brand-new experience for you and your brain is trying to keep you safe? Are you willing to explore even further or is it time for rest, recovery, and reflection?

After every visit to the edge of your growth zone, the idea is to rest, recover and reflect on the experience. Our system automatically bounces us into a parasympathetic or lowered state after an event. With both the stimulus and recovery combined, we gain confidence in expanding and exploring those edges more liberally. This process builds our strong natural centre, giving us even more power to explore our edges. Over time, as we become competent with knowing our body, mind and spirit, we begin to step more outside our comfort zone. This, for me, is the secret to developing your life and your breath.

The popular alternative for growth is to go outside your comfort zone. However, I have found that when my clients and I take this approach, people often wander too far without developing the skills to survive out there. The result is often an experience of heightened fear. When we experience fear that we cannot relax into, our body subconsciously retracts from this experience reducing our ability to explore our edges in the long run. We begin to shy away from new and challenging life experiences. We retract into ourselves. Our body and mind hear this message and keep you in this state of retraction for safety. The less we do, the more afraid we are to try anything new. At the same time your body and mind will signal you to do less and fear more. Our posture adapts, our thinking becomes erratic and our breathing patterns are altered; it becomes a perpetual vicious cycle. We enter an adapted state of being, acting from a perceived centre, full of fear and an inability to access the edge of one or other states of arousal. Some are 'switched on' consistently and unable to downregulate themselves. Others are severely depressed or 'switched off' and unable to motivate themselves.

This is how that whole process of life, stress and your adaptation to it appears from a breathing perspective. When you see the bear, you breathe bigger and faster. This big and fast breathing is registered by the brain almost immediately. The brain then sends a signal to the autonomic nervous system – it secretes adrenaline in milliseconds. The adrenaline sets off a cascading effect to down-regulate the functions of the parasympathetic nervous system and shift energy to the functions of the sympathetic nervous system. All parts of the stress response are then kicked into action from a nervous system perspective. This response happens in milliseconds. It enables you to react to the bear and save your life. This whole response begins with bigger and faster breathing. In research, the effects of bigger and faster breathing are shown to also dampen pain and cold sensitivity and improve immune function. This is the exact same biological response that a sports person experiences in competition, a boxer experiences in a fight, a mother has when she can't cope and an executive experiences in a board-room argument.

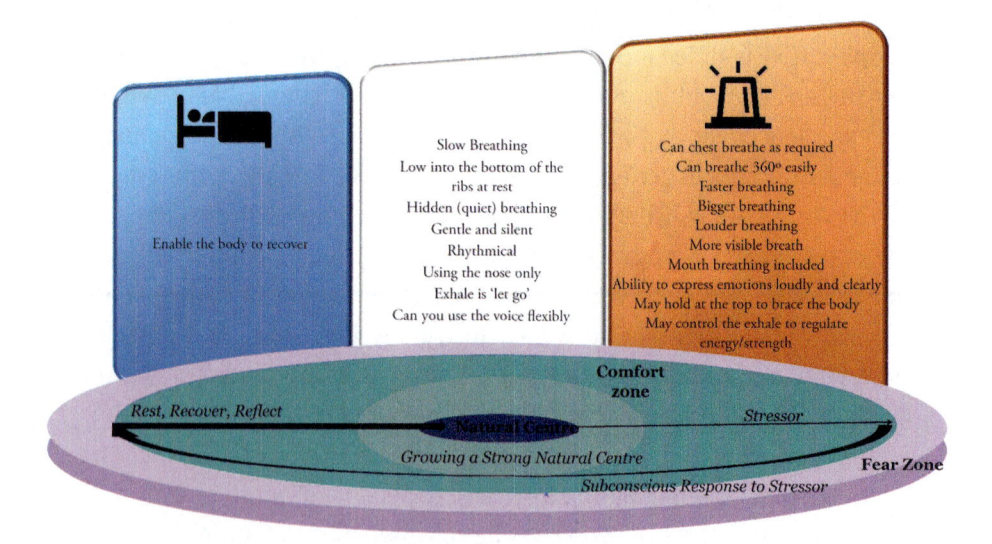

| Enable the body to recover | Slow Breathing
Low into the bottom of the ribs at rest
Hidden (quiet) breathing
Gentle and silent
Rhythmical
Using the nose only
Exhale is 'let go'
Can you use the voice flexibly | Can chest breathe as required
Can breathe 360° easily
Faster breathing
Bigger breathing
Louder breathing
More visible breath
Mouth breathing included
Ability to express emotions loudly and clearly
May hold at the top to brace the body
May control the exhale to regulate energy/strength |

Comfort zone

Rest, Recover, Reflect — Natural Centre — Stressor
Growing a Strong Natural Centre
Subconscious Response to Stressor
Fear Zone

The Human Growth Model layered with the Breathe Ability Model

The only difference in our modern life is that our biological systems aren't regulated as efficiently as our ancestors; our baselines have been lowered due to the potency, quantity and frequency of multiple stressors. We tend to hold onto that original stress response, keep it active all day long then, over time, we can't react as well. We act from a perceived centre. Remember, we generally don't have bears roaming the streets in the modern day. Instead, we have lots and lots of little triggers which elicit a chronic stress response. This chronic stress response can lead to a long-term over-breathing pattern.

THE TOP 6 CAUSES OF CHRONIC OVER-BREATHING

1. Poor nutrition and excess calories
2. Excessive talking
3. Psycho-emotional stress, including trauma
4. Sedentary lifestyle
5. Big breathing as a sub-conscious pattern
6. Increased temperatures

The way we live today is akin to a child playing with a light switch. On, off, on, off, on, off, the light switch goes. The child continues to play with the switch. Eventually, the light switch gets stuck in the on or off position and the light bulb remains in that position too. The child notices this – and feels it's ruining his game. So he starts flicking the switch twice as fast until, BOOM, the light bulb blows. The same happens to our biological system with modern stress. A little bit of poor-quality food, poor air quality, sedentary living. Throw some viruses in. Add in some alcohol and coffee. Mix in some unresolved conflicts, add the pressure of social media, technology, and a career you don't love and – voila – your system gets stuck in an on (hyperactive) or an off (depressed) position. On-off-on-off-on-off until, POP, the light bulb blows.

Before it blows, though, you experience a range of signs which inform you your body is breaking down. This is the 'stuck' phase. In this phase, your body can't regulate itself normally. You will either feel low and experience symptoms of suppression or feel heightened and over-aroused, depending on who you are and the lifestyle you have led. In fact, you may begin to lose your sense of 'normal' as you lose interoceptive abilities in these states. Just like big and fast breathing is one of the first responses of the body to ellicit the stress response, so it is the first sign that the body has that it is holding that response and burning itself out rapidly. The difference is that, now, an altered breathing pattern is your normal subconscious breathing rhythm. The other shapes of an altered breathing pattern become important too. Holding your breath at the top, controlling your exhale and breathing into your chest only or your belly only are all signs that your breathing is stuck in a perceived centre state. You can be stuck in a lowered or heightened state. These patterns are commonly referred to as 'dysfunctional breathing patterns' in research, but there is nothing dysfunctional about the pattern itself. The pattern is doing exactly what it is supposed to do – keeping you safe the best way your biological system knows how. What is dysfunctional is the life experience which promoted the pattern in the first place. For this reason, I call these patterns *Adapted Breathing Patterns*. The adapted breath is a long-term subconscious pattern that has changed its shape in response to the stressors of your life. It has adapted to your life.

ADAPTED BREATHING PATTERNS

Our natural breathing pattern shifts in one of two directions in response to life. These routes reflect the two reflexes of the somatic nervous system, affecting our posture and strength, and they also reflect states of autonomic arousal in the nervous system (flee or freeze). The heightened breathing pattern reflects the fixed end-state of the Green-Light-Reflex and Fight-or-Flight. It is like leaving your nervous system switched on the whole time. In reality, it is never on the whole time, but it certainly has a high sympathetic tone and a low parasympathetic tone. Initial symptoms of adaptation, which reflect a heightened breathing pattern, are high levels of arousal, inability to get to sleep, waking up during the night, dominant personality, and voice, go-go-go all the time.

ADAPTED HEIGHTENED BREATHING PATTERNS
↑ Mouth breathing
↑ Big breathing
↑ Loud breathing
↑ Chest breathing/ reverse breathing
↑ Sighing
↑ Breath holding after the inhale
↑ Emotional outbursts
Controlled exhale by constricting the mouth, jaw and/or neck muscles
↓ Ability to breathe into belly
↓ Ability to breathe full breaths

Adapted High Breathing Pattern

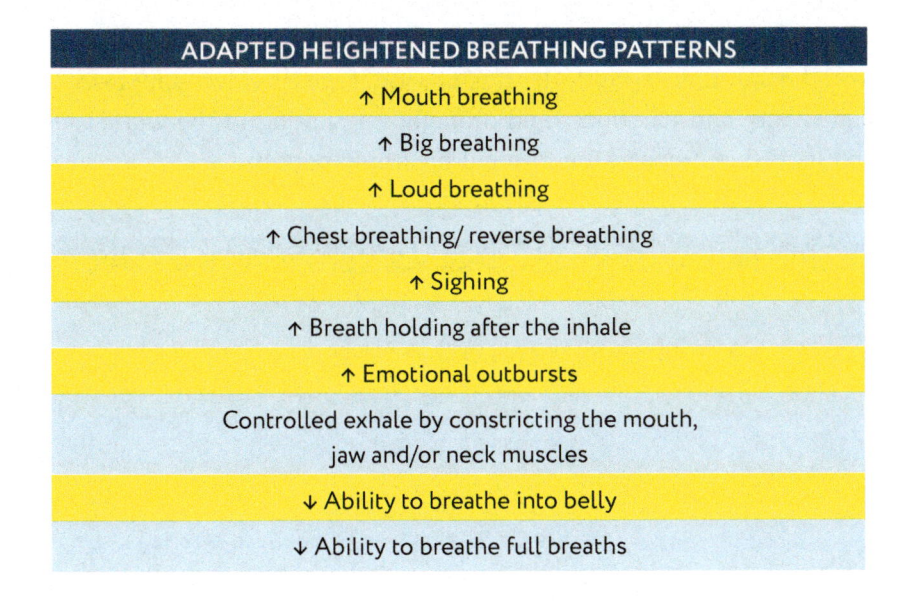

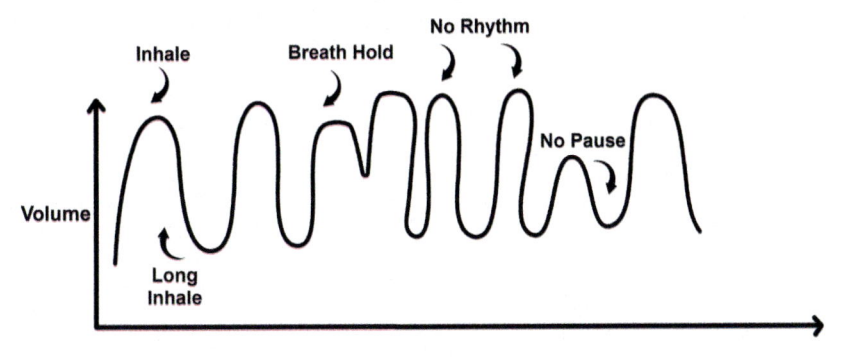

[Diagram showing an irregular breathing waveform labeled with: Inhale, Breath Hold, No Rhythm, No Pause, Long Inhale, Volume]

The Adapted Heightened Breathing Pattern is agitated. There is no rhythm to the breath. Some breaths are short, some big, some long, some short and there can be intermittent breath holds without any conscious awareness. Usually this breathing pattern is accompanied by mouth breathing/big/chest breathing at rest, and some possible tissues restrictions.

On the opposite side of the coin is the 'lowered breathing pattern'. The lowered breathing pattern reflects the states of the Red-Light-Reflex in the SNS or the stooped, old-man posture, and withdrawal states in the ANS. This is still a stressed breathing pattern; however, the symptoms manifest completely differently from the heightened breathing pattern. Withdrawal, low arousal, depression, low tone of voice, suppressed personality and emotions, and difficulty in relating to the world are common symptoms of the lowered breathing pattern.

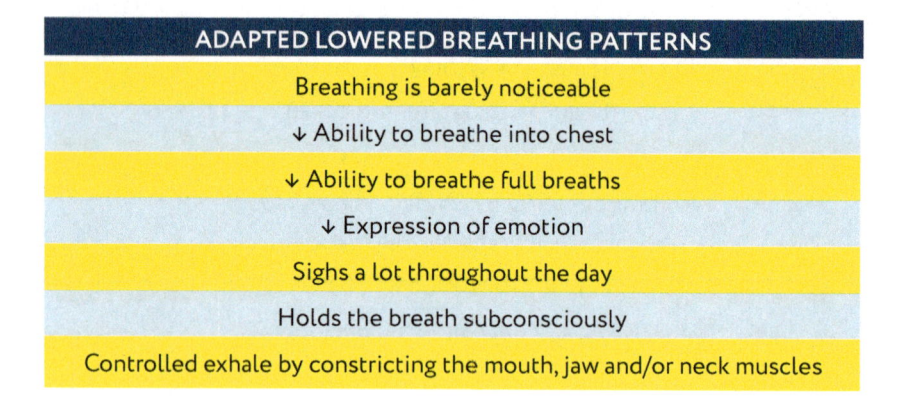

ADAPTED LOWERED BREATHING PATTERNS
Breathing is barely noticeable
↓ Ability to breathe into chest
↓ Ability to breathe full breaths
↓ Expression of emotion
Sighs a lot throughout the day
Holds the breath subconsciously
Controlled exhale by constricting the mouth, jaw and/or neck muscles

Adapted Low Breathing Pattern

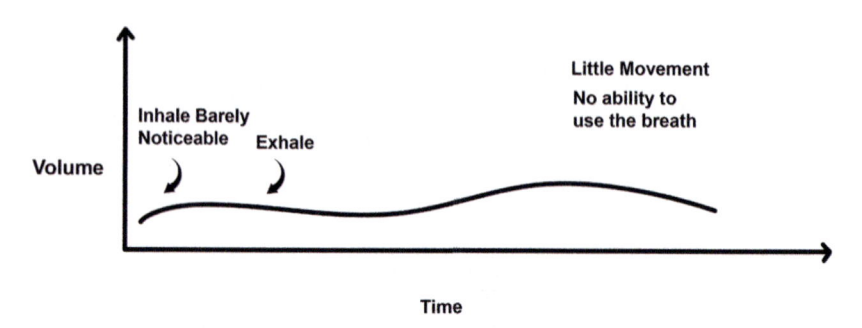

The Adapted Lowered Breathing Pattern is suppressed, and it is hardly noticeable. Usually it is accompanied by restrictions in muscle tissue and the inability to express the breath freely.

The third response is where the system balances between the two opposites. This is the natural centre of the human biological system. It is a finely trained biological state. One where you have the ability to upregulate or downregulate your system consciously.

STRESS AND BREATHING

BREATHE-ABILITY	
Naturally Centred Breathing Pattern at Rest	**With the ability to…**
Slow breathing Low into the bottom ribs at rest Hidden (quiet) breathing Gentle and silent Rhythmical Using the nose only Exhale is 'let go' Can use the voice flexibly	Use the full breath when required Chest breathe as required Breathe 360° easily Faster breathing Bigger breathing Louder breathing More visible breath Mouth breathing included Ability to express emotions clearly and loudly May hold at the top to brace the body May control the exhale to regulate energy / strength

Breathe Ability

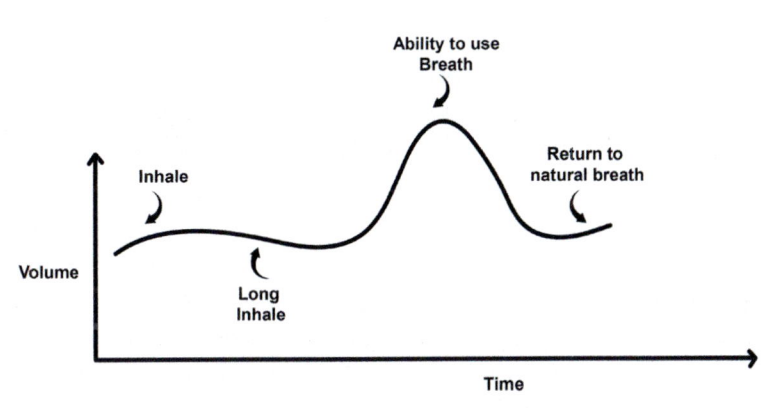

A representation of Breathe Ability. Calm, gentle and quiet breathing using your nose at rest, <u>combined</u> with the ability to use your breath when required. Then a return to a naturally-centred breathing pattern at rest.

45

PART 1   THE INTERCONNECTION OF LIFE, STRESS AND THE BREATH

THE WAY THE BREATHING CONTINUUM WORKS

The person with a naturally-centred breath can tip into either one of the two opposites sides of breathing at any point in time. However, if you present with an adapted breathing pattern, you shift your natural centre to a perceived centre. This means that you experience more of one side of the continuum, and you are unable to access either deep rest or the opposite side of breathing. You can have a perceived heightened or a perceived lowered centre.

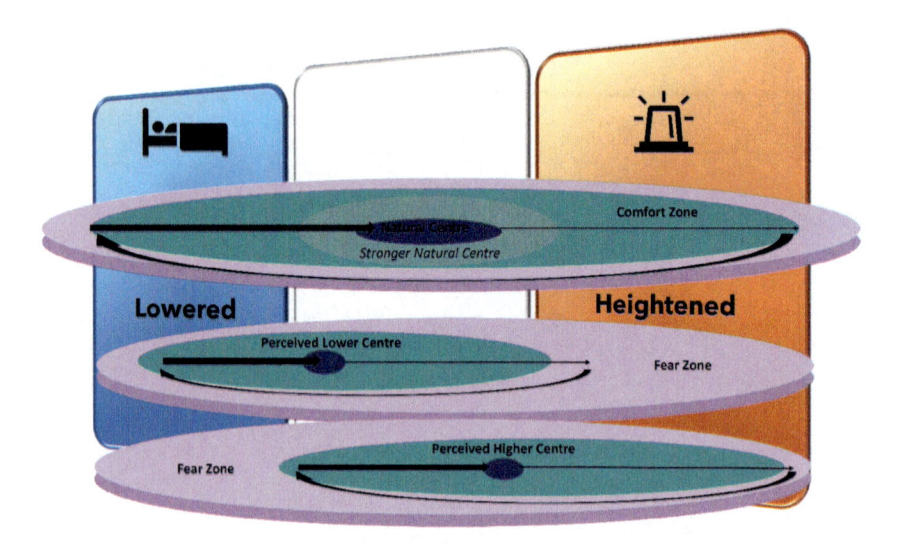

Comfort Zone
Stronger Natural Centre

Lowered   **Heightened**

Perceived Lower Centre
Fear Zone

Perceived Higher Centre
Fear Zone

'Centred' and two 'Adapted' states of living relative to the nervous system. In the Centred state, you have access to both sides of the nervous system and stress has a positive effect on you – building a stronger centre, once you've recovered. In the two 'Adapted' states stress negatively impacts growth resulting in smaller centres and growth zones. People in a 'Perceived Lower' state find it difficult to get motivated and do things in life. People in a 'Perceived Higher' state are always on the go and find it difficult to rest and recover. Both perceived states are adaptions to a state of mind and body. They lead to a more narrow life experience, filled with fear, anxiety, disease and/or pain in the body, mind, and/or soul.

Centred and Adapted Breathing Patterns

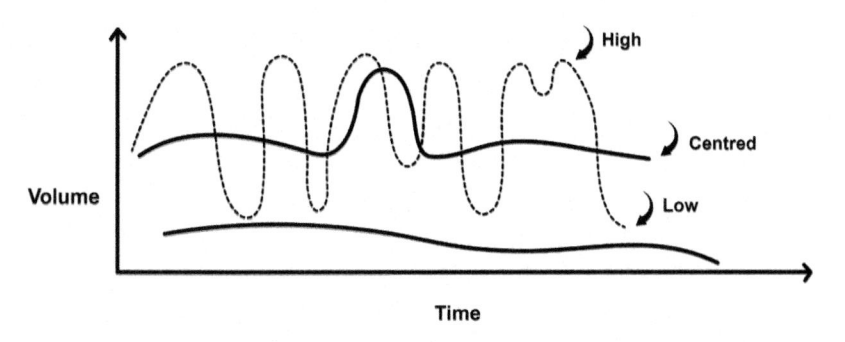

Representation of breathing patterns seen in people living in each of the three states of being – centred, lowered, and heightened

THE BREATH IS A MIRROR FOR OUR PERCEPTIONS OF STRESS

In this way, I think human beings are like a growing tree. In an ideal world, a tree grows tall and full, given the right conditions and nutrients. However, the sun's position, the wind direction, storms, animals and nutrients usually affect the tree's growth. So instead of the tree growing tall and full, it adapts to the situation and grows as best it can. If a branch is broken off, the tree will heal and scar the damaged area. The tree always remembers the broken branch but it never grows the same way again. Regardless, the tree continues to produce new branches in a different area. Similarly, if the wind howls from the east for several years, the tree leans westward and continues to grow in that direction until the wind changes again. Each of these events in the life of a tree influences how tall the tree grows, how strong it becomes and the overall lifetime of the tree. In this sense, humans are no different from trees.

There is no such thing as a perfect environment for a tree or a human to grow. Stress is the rite of passage we must pass through to become all we want. If we want more for our life, we need to grow. We need a stimulus to initiate that growth. Stress, in any of its forms, is that stimulus. My greatest blessing and teacher in life has always been stress: asthma, cold exposure, financial crisis, arguments with loved ones, being underweight, and not being good enough. Without these stressors I would not be the man I am today. Without the death of his beloved wife, the world-famous breathing expert, Wim Hof, may not have influenced the world so positively and powerfully. We may not like it, but the sooner we accept stress as something we can learn from and grow from, the quicker we can pass through this phase and grow from it to the next one. Observing our breathing patterns is similar to observing the shape of a tree as it grows in response to its life. Your breathing pattern is a mirror for the sum of all your stressors in life. If your breathing is adapted, high or low, it signifies that you are finding it difficult to cope with the demands of your life. However, a naturally centred breath signifies that you are strong, healthy and resilient to life's stressors.

REFLECTIONS OF ADAPTED LOWERED BREATHING PATTERNS

Usually, people present with a range of these adaptations, depending on the length of time their breathing has been adapted, and the reasons for subconsciously changing their breath. Today, lowered breathing patterns are less common than heightened breathing patterns or, perhaps, they are just better hidden from society. They are not as noticeable because the people with those patterns make less of a fuss. After almost twenty years of experience, I am someone who instinctively analyses people's breathing everywhere I go, and even I find it more difficult to notice a lowered breathing pattern than a heightened one. It is often easier to see this breath pattern when it is exaggerated in people's posture. Shoulders are rounded, spine is curved over and eyes look down. This posture is also referred to as the Red-Light-Reflex in Somatic therapies, and it is synonymous with a lowered breathing pattern. Mostly, though, this pattern becomes obvious when the person needs to express their breath. As subtle as they are, lowered breathing patterns are still just as destructive to your health as heightened ones are, particularly for the health of your mind. My experience would suggest that lowered breathing patterns are reflective of people having complex mental health issues. Typically these people are struggling to cope in life; they are withdrawn from the world, they have a negative attitude, the world appears to be against them and they are afraid to express their feelings about their world. Disquiet, anger, hatred, and fear are all internalised. They become less able to express love, joy, and excitement and become more reclusive in the confines of their own mind. Eventually a lowered breathing pattern reflects anxiety, panic, major depressive symptoms and mental illness. In my own practice, by the time they see me, many clients with lowered breathing patterns have done a lot of work on their psyche with psychologists. They feel a lot better but still find it difficult to cope in the world. A part of the reason for this mindset is because they have changed the 'thought level' on the human performance pyramid (discussed in Chapter 6), but the emotions and feelings are still in their body. By changing their breathing patterns and in helping them to express their emotions and breathe life more fully, these people unravel another very important part of the puzzle of coming to terms with their lives.

REFLECTIONS OF ADAPTED LOWERED BREATHING PATTERNS		
PATTERN	**EMOTIONAL REFLECTION**	**CONNECTED DISEASE STATE**
↓ Ability to breathe into chest ↓ Ability to breathe full breaths ↓ Expression of emotion Sighs a lot without satisfaction Controlled exhale by constricting the mouth, jaw and/or neck muscles	↓ Expression of emotion ↓ Both positive and negative thoughts and feelings get trapped inside ↓ Thoughts turn quite negative	Anxiety Panic Depression Pain in the body, particularly the jaw, neck and chest Headaches and migraines Mental disease

REFLECTIONS OF HEIGHTENED BREATHING PATTERNS

Breathing more than your body needs or chronic hyperventilation; mouth breathing; chest breathing and subconscious breath control, are all shapes of the heightened breathing pattern. Embodying this style of breathing leads to an up-regulated nervous system and the state of 'always being switched on'. People find themselves over-sensitive to the pressures of life – they are 'stressed'. Like a pot boiling with the lid on, when you raise the temperature one more degree, the water explodes out of the pot. One more trigger, one more thought and people, in this state, tend to emotionally, physically and mentally break down. The extreme end of the arousal pattern is the host of

REFLECTIONS OF ADAPTED HEIGHTENED BREATHING PATTERNS		
PATTERN	**EMOTIONAL**	**CONNECTED**
↑ Mouth breathing ↑ Big breathing ↑ Loud breathing ↑ Chest breathing/ reverse breathing ↑ Sighing without satisfaction Controlled exhale by constricting the mouth, jaw, and/or neck muscles ↑ Breath-holding after the inhale ↓ Ability to breathe into belly ↓ Ability to breathe full breaths	Overly sensitive to life's demands Boiling with frustration and anger	Asthma, rhinitis, sinusitis Anxiety, panic Sleep apnoea, type 2 diabetes, obesity Lower back pain Pain in and around the diaphragm Recurring hip and lower limb soft tissue injury in sports people

stress-based diseases that are all too prevalent today, such as sleep apnoea, type 2 diabetes, obesity, cardiovascular disease, anxiety, and panic disorders. Lower back pain, and respiratory diseases like asthma, bronchitis, sinusitis, and rhinitis are all more prevalent in people with a long-term heightened breathing pattern.

Of course, there are other factors that go into the mix with these diseases, like genetics and other lifestyle habits. However, arousal breathing appears to sit at the heart of the matter. When the arousal breathing habit is broken, symptoms of pain and disease lessen and in some cases stop altogether. People's emotions become more regulated, and they find themselves become more resilient to life's demands. They find themselves calmer in the midst of a raging storm.

TRAUMA IS A UNIQUE STRESSOR

Within the realm of stress, we have a more insidious insult called trauma. Trauma, by definition, is unbearable and intolerable stress. You don't have to be a soldier or experience an unimaginably tough childhood to suffer trauma. It happens regularly to ordinary human beings, our friends and families. When those who suffered trauma in the past even think about the event they try to push it out of their mind because it is too painful. It takes a considerable amount of energy to simply survive the memory of terror and the shame of weakness and vulnerability. While we may want to move beyond the trauma, there is a deep part of the brain, devoted to survival, which stores rather than denies the pain. Long after the experience is over, it can still re-activate those memories and feelings of terror, shame, and vulnerability. It upregulates your whole system at the slightest hint of danger to a state of extreme arousal. Feeling overwhelmed, fearful, panicked, anxious, and losing control are common feelings for someone who once suffered a trauma that hasn't been dealt with.

Bessel Van Der Kolk is a world-renowned psychiatrist, researcher and educator in the field of post-traumatic stress. He authored the

PART 1   THE INTERCONNECTION OF LIFE, STRESS AND THE BREATH

international best-selling book, *The Body Keeps the Score*. The book details how trauma impacts our life and how we can befriend it to live fully alive and present once more. In the book, he states, 'Nobody can "treat" a war, or abuse, rape, molestation, or any other horrendous event; what has happened cannot be undone;' instead, 'what can be dealt with are the imprints of the trauma on body, mind and soul'. According to Bessel, for most people this involves:

1. Finding a way to become calm and focused
2. Learning to maintain that calm in response to images, thoughts, sounds or physical sensations that remind you of the past
3. Finding a way to be fully alive in the present and engaged with people around you
4. Not having to keep secrets from yourself

The fundamental issue in resolving traumatic stress, then, is to restore the proper balance between the thinking and emotional brains, so that you can feel in charge of how you respond and conduct your life. Breathing is the simplest way to change how you feel and think, not only about trauma but about all insults to your body, mind, and soul.

> *Learning to breathe calmly and remaining in a state of relative physical relaxation, even while accessing painful and horrifying memories, is an essential tool for recovery*
>
> **B VAN DER KOLK**

To understand the impacts of trauma and stress on the body and the role breathing has in healing it, I interviewed some experts in the field to get their perspectives. Morgan Shepherd is a collegiate tennis coach in the USA with a masters in sport and exercise psychology. Through sport he became interested in the impact of human relations on the person and their performance. In Morgan's words, "a lot of work in sports psych is based on the mind and a lot of things I was seeing were the physiology of the body and this seemed to limit myself and others." His interest on the impacts of physiology and relationships on the psychology of his athletes took him back to study as a counselling psychologist, and licensed family and relationship therapist. Eventually, he wound up specialising in a blended approach called somatic psychology. Morgan's main field nowadays is coaching tennis and relationship counselling from the somatic psychology perspective. Somatic psychology offers a different perspective to traditional models by enabling people to look at holding patterns in the body. Dancing, shaking, music, breathwork and movement are all used in therapy, depending on the experience of the therapist and the person's needs and wants. At the heart of Morgan's work is following the person he's working with. "They know the answer within them," he told me.

Morgan sees himself as a guide to help people experience what is happening in their own body through the relationship. "Opening up, unwinding and finding the answers is the goal even if we don't know what the question is." The awareness of how and where people put our awareness is at the centre of Morgan's studies and experience. "The nuances, complexities of reflexes are infinite. Each person's embodied study is very individual and so is our experience." For Morgan, the solution for people with high stress and trauma is "feeling". "How much do you feel right down to the cellular level? Each part of the body, each cell, organ, muscle and joint has resources to offer us. You can do it through movement or visualisation, and each way we direct our awareness gives us a different experience, a different way of understanding our body and more options to move, do or be in relationship with whatever we want to do in life."

Similarly to Morgan, Wim Hof explained to me his thoughts on how the breath and cold therapy help people return to themselves after trauma. Wim is a person who has first-hand experience with trauma. He was a happily married man with a young family. Over several years his wife, Olaya, developed a disease of the mind and fell into a deep depression. The medications she was given only made matters worse. "Deeper and deeper into the darkness she fell," is how he describes her descent in his book, *The Wim Hof Method*. He goes on to recall the day he received the call from Olaya's brother to say she had kissed her children goodbye and jumped out the window of an eight-storey building. Wim was left broken-hearted and traumatised by the demise and death of his beloved. Yet he still had a young family to rear. The only thing that saved him was "the cold" and through the cold he learned to use his breath to control his mind.

> *I was in the ice first, Leo. The first thing you learn is to go deeper within yourself. When you go into the ice, then naturally you do 'fully inhale, exhale', that's what you do. That's what you learn. From there, the cold is your teacher and with the deeper breathing I became the alchemist over my blood pH levels, over my biochemistry. I could activate deeply in the adrenal axis, I learned to be stronger. Just through breathing and using the cold as a mirror.*

Wim used the breath and ice to heal himself. From there, he began a career setting 26 Guinness World Records, including a marathon in the Arctic wearing only a pair of shorts and sandals, climbing Mt. Kilamanjaro in record time, climbing to the death zone on Mt. Everest in just a pair of shorts and boots and setting several ice bath records. Towards the end of his adventure career, he turned his attention to using the method to create 'happy, healthy and strong people'. That's his motto now for life.

The Wim Hof Method has set the world alight in the last decade. Thousands of people now practice his breathwork and cold therapy. Joseph Fiennes is set to direct a movie based on his life. He has rapped with Jay-Z, taught Beyoncé to breathe and coached pro-athletes, TV personalities and actors alike. There are books written about him, physiology textbooks re-written because of him and his name is becoming synonymous with health empowerment. Through his method, Wim and his instructors teach you to become healthy, happy and strong. They achieve their goal through the breath, cold and mind to train your nervous system to deal with stress, reduce chronic inflammation and become resilient to life. "People who are coming to me, they are able to really de-traumatise. I teach them," he told me.

Wim believes that 'trauma is stored deeply within our brain'. He also considers the storage of trauma to simply be "a chemical storage facility in our brain". The idea behind his method is that you can access that chemical storage of the trauma by changing the brain's chemistry. As Wim told me, "There's sort of a storage facility in our brain of a moment or situation we could not cope with. It's quite difficult to get into it." The way to change brain chemistry, according to Wim, is through breathing. "Everybody has the capacity to deal with their own trauma and the breath is the bridge. The breath is able to get there (to the storage of the moment). Through the breath we change the chemistry and then we are able to influence deeply."

For some people, though, it can be very difficult to get to the trauma. The brain is extremely clever. The pain of the original insult is so hurtful to you that the brain somehow rewires itself and the blood flow to protect you from it. When your brain begins to feel that chemical storage of the trauma being accessed once more through breathing, it can re-awaken the feelings and thoughts associated with the original insult. Wim's solution is to "slow down. Slow down. It'll work out anyway, this breathing is very effective and strong. It needs tuning with those people. They need to be brought by feeling. Relax, Relax." Wim used the analogy of "standing in front of an oak door" for people who struggle to deal with a trauma. The door is too heavy to open alone because they don't want to deal with what's behind it. Instead of seeking the key and opening the door, people would rather live oblivious to the door and what lies within. However, it is the same door that will set them free from their inner demons. In this analogy, Wim says they have to "learn to find the key, to go back to find the courage, to find the tuning within, to open the door." According to Wim, the key to unlocking the door is the breath combined with a determined mind. In all of this talk of trauma and breathing to heal, Wim was keen to tell me that there is no fault or blame. Trauma is part of the mysteries of one's life. We all have some aspect of it and it is natural to us all as human beings. Finding your way through the trauma to live your best life needs nothing more than "breathing and using it well. Learning to tune to a way where you do not fall but determinedly go deep within yourself." In Wim's words to me:

> *Happiness is the control of the hormonal system. Health is the control of the immune system and strength is the control over the metabolic mechanisms – the cells creating energy, and we have proven the point through science so, if you love somebody, there is possible control over all these systems to guarantee happiness, strength and health. That's love. Everybody now is able to tap into it and I am doing the science and neurology to prove it. It shows that we can demystify what has been taught – how to bring love, how to radiate. Now we know conscious control over the autonomic nervous system is within everybody's reach. And what I did was to show everybody in brain scans, in blood samples, in fMRI's and all that.*

Admittedly, the mechanisms of how breathing techniques impact our long-term breathing patterns, stress, and trauma are not yet fully teased out in research. It is still a tiny, microscopic area of scientific research. And although breathing therapy has been around for 5,000 plus years and everybody seems to be doing it nowadays, I don't think breathing is understood very well at a practitioner level yet, either. There are only a few people I have come across who deeply understand how breathing works in rebalancing your body, mind and spirit to potentially return you to health. Therefore, all approaches to restoring your breathing are a mini-self experiment, an 'n = 1 experiment' as Brian MacKenzie refers to it. However, the science is a slow-burning machine and influencers are very influential. Many people start breathing practice and enter it at the wrong point because they've been influenced by somebody who doesn't really know what's happening with the breath. In the next chapter I want to offer some guidance on this by introducing you to the Human Performance

Pyramid (HPP). The HPP is a model for understanding the role of breath training for health and performance above all other practices. With this understanding, the HPP will help you to understand where to begin your practice.

THE HUMAN PERFORMANCE PYRAMID

6

I watched this human performance model in action during Wimbledon 2019. I walked in while my wife watched Souza from Portugal playing Evans from Great Britain on television. It was the first set and the stakes were high for both men. Each wanted to progress to the second week of the competition for the first time. Evans was up and looking dominant but I saw something different. There and then, I bet my wife that Souza would win and Evans would lose, in the final set, due to his own mistakes.

My wife, thinking me half-mad but knowing me better, wouldn't take the bet. We watched the match unfold anyway. Evans won the first set, Souza, the second. Evans won the third set and Souza the fourth. In each set Evans broke Souza and took the lead. He appeared to be the dominant player but he was losing his mojo. Souza was calm, cool and collected throughout the proceedings. Evans, on the other hand, was wild. He would ride the atmospheric wave of the crowd when things were going well for him and looked to his coach when things didn't go according to plan. He seemed to have no hold on his own physiology. His breathing was erratic. His movement was jerky. His decision-making was unpredictable, and his habits around his play were inconsistent. Still, he was in with a shout. In the fifth and final set, Evans again took the lead and Souza bounced back. Souza broke

Evans for a second time and led the match five games to three. In the final game, Souza played a blinder. Always calm and collected, he hit a crosscourt backhand to Evans. In what should have been an easy return, Evans scuppered his shot and missed. Souza won.

'How did you know that would happen?' my wife asked me afterwards.

'I could see it in the way he was breathing, in his movement, in his inability to control his body and mind.' Within thirty seconds of seeing both men play, I could make an educated guess about the outcome. What I did was not magic; it was knowledge of the effects of breathing, particularly on a person's energy and state of mind.

I have used breathing in my own sport, to know when to put pressure on an opponent as well as to know when to pull back, when I am fatiguing. All of this can be used by you too. Breathing is the highway through the entire human performance pyramid in life and sport.

I am unsure why God placed such power in the breath but it is there nonetheless. Breathing weaves its magic through each level of the human performance pyramid. It can be used as a barometer to measure your health. It can be used to assess one's state of readiness. It balances both sides of the autonomic nervous system (ANS) and it directly and powerfully influences the somatic nervous system (SNS). Breathing in a certain way can relax you or arouse you. We become more in tune with our body, emotions and feeling when we become more aware of our breath. We settle more into our body. Our mind comes to ease and we can think more clearly with breathing. New habits become easier to ingrain into your life. Performance levels increase in life and sport. Creativity flows as we breathe better and in certain ways; finally, we can become more aligned with the vision of our life when we begin to breathe better. All of this goodness is possible for me, you, and everyone. It simply requires some focused training, and time to make it happen.

The innate indicators of your stress are found in your body. They are built into your physical body as a self-management tool. The only place you will find your answers is inside. Working backwards, they are: performance, habits, thought patterns (mindset), feelings and emotions. These layers of self-regulation form what I call the human performance pyramid. The pyramid forms natural self-regulation heirarchies the same way as the brain arranges structures, language, and perceptual systems (Dilts 2015). The effect of each level is to organise and control information on the level below it (in the brain it works the opposite way around). Changing something on the upper level alters the experience on the lower levels; however, changing something on a lower level can, but does not necessarily, affect upper levels. A change in emotions impacts feelings, mindset, habits and performance. An altered mindset changes habits and performance but does not always affect feelings and emotions. Breathing, as it so happens, is one of the fundamental tools; it powerfully slices through all layers of the pyramid.

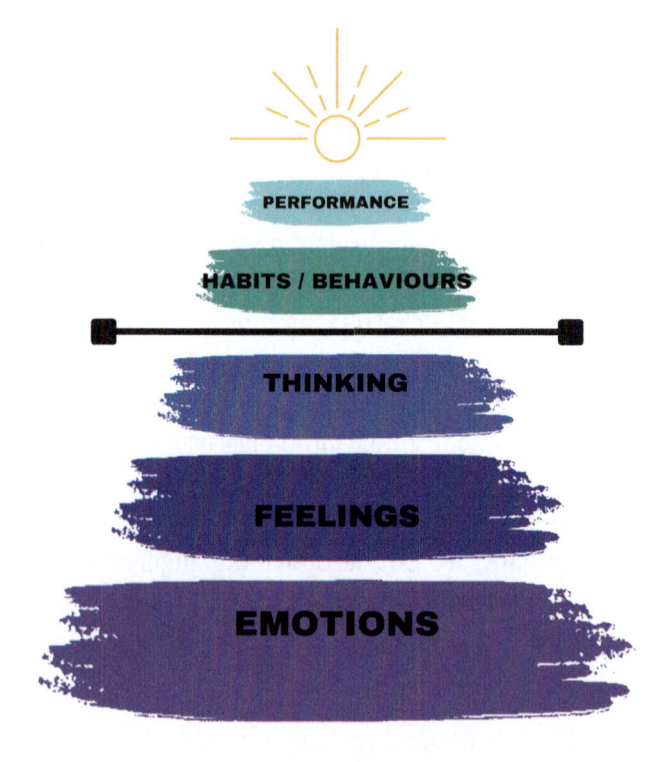

The Human Performance Pyramid

THERE'S A HIERARCHY OF PERFORMANCE IN YOUR BODY

Human functioning is arranged into a natural hierarchy in our brain structure. It is influenced by the sensory inputs into our brain and the levels of experience flow upward into all other systems in the body. The effect of each level is to organise and control the information on the level above it. Changing something on an lower-level changes thing on the upper levels; changing something on a upper level can, but will not necessarily, affect the lower levels.

Think of our organisation like that of a manufacturing plant. If something goes wrong at the worker level (like a muscle), it is fixed at that level, but it may not necessarily influence what happens up the chain in other areas of the plant. By contrast, the CEO's (the brain) decisions impacts everyone in the organisation, including upper, middle, and lower management levels, as well as the workers.

EMOTIONS

Emotions are the raw data coming into the body and being interpreted by the body. The great business guru Tony Robbins phrases it beautifully: Emotions are 'Energy in Motion – e-motion' (Robbins 2000). Air, water, food, exercise, sunlight, work environments, social circles, childhood conditioning, major life events – everything. These are your external inputs being internalised. The way this data is regulated works subconsciously for the most part. We have discussed these inputs and how they affect our biological system in the previous chapter. There are two important things to note here. The first is the emotions are external factors in your environment which come into your life. This means that health and performance are impacted by everything around you in your life. The second point to note here is that emotions sit at the bottom of the pyramid. Remember our biological system is built in a natural hierarchy of experiences. When we change our inputs (emotions) we affect everything upstream in our biological system. However, that is not necessarily true for other levels of the pyramid. This is primarily why changing your thought pattern, or habits alone, are such difficult practices to perform. First, we need to understand our emotions, change that level and then work upstream from there. Before we go into changing our emotions, let's look at the other four levels in the human performance pyramid.

FEELINGS

Feelings are our awareness of these emotions. Porges (2011) coined the termed that describes this awareness as 'interoception'. Feelings are subjective in that they are built on our own first-person experience. Feelings can relate to one specific input or they can give you a sense of your overall state of being. The overall state of being forms an emotional guidance system (Abraham, Hicks and Hicks 2004). Scientists initially thought there were only six distinct human emotions: happiness, sadness, anger, surprise, fear and disgust. This has now been extrapolated to 27 distinct feelings or at least words describing your state of being. In reality, all of these words describing our feelings uncover gradients of emotion, from positive to negative, on one continuous scale. Every feeling fits on either side of that fence to a varying degree. Feelings can merge into one another, so it becomes difficult to separate and define them. What is always true is that a feeling is either positive or negative inside you. Unless you are Irish, of course, then every feeling is neutral!

In response to how they feel about almost any event, most Irish people will say, 'I'm not so bad.' I used to do it myself but what does that sentence mean in reality? In its strictest form, 'I'm not so bad,' is a double negative. In English, it means 'I'm good'. You ask an Irish person to rephrase that sentence as 'I'm good', and it'll feel very irritating to them – they won't like it. Why? Because in reality, they do not feel good enough to tell you they feel good and they also don't feel bad enough to tell you they feel bad. They also don't say 'I'm ok' because they know that is a nothing answer and it will ellicit further questioning from their colleague, like, 'you sure you're ok?' In other words, they don't know what they feel because they haven't checked into themselves. If they do check in with themselves, and they still speak in this double-negative language, it is because they have over-ridden their feelings with thinking, and now they are thinking how they feel, not feeling how they are feel. The Irish way of communicating our feelings is true not only for our language but also for the way people feel their feelings. When we experience long-term stress or trauma, we often lose the sense of feeling in our body. This is true not only for the Irish; it is very common for many people, especially those who have suffered trauma and high levels of stress in their life. Both trauma researchers and somatic educators have noted this for years. Re-instilling our senses of interoception and proprioception (our sense of physical time and space through posture and movement) is critical for balancing this layer of the human performance pyramid and influencing every layer above it.

Any positive feeling leads to an upward spiral of feeling good and creating a positive life for yourself. Negative feelings will do just the opposite. One event of extreme joy may have the power to pull your whole system in the direction of health and performance instantaneously, whereas feeling the emotion of fear can do just the opposite. In energy medicine circles, it is said asthma is the fear of disease, cancer is the disease of unresolved conflict, a muscle tear represents an inability to move forward and depression is the lack of joy in one's life. These conditions are not viewed as diseases and an irreparable breakdown of the body. Instead, energy medicine sees them as dis-eases, where the body is no longer at ease. Therefore, the dis-eased state is an exaggerated biological state due to the inability to deal with a particular chronic stress. So, in the beginning you have negative feelings; next come feelings of fear. Once that fear has been ingrained into the body, the body will continue to feel that fear subconsciously. The body will adapt to this stressor, and any other stressor placed on top of it, by changing how it breathes, moves, feels, and works inside. With enough time, the body will exhibit pain related to that fear; finally comes the dis-ease. This process can happen almost in an instant if the stressor is large enough, or it can happen gradually over twenty, thirty, or forty years. Often, the events that kick off this response system occur in childhood and are compounded by events throughout the rest of life.

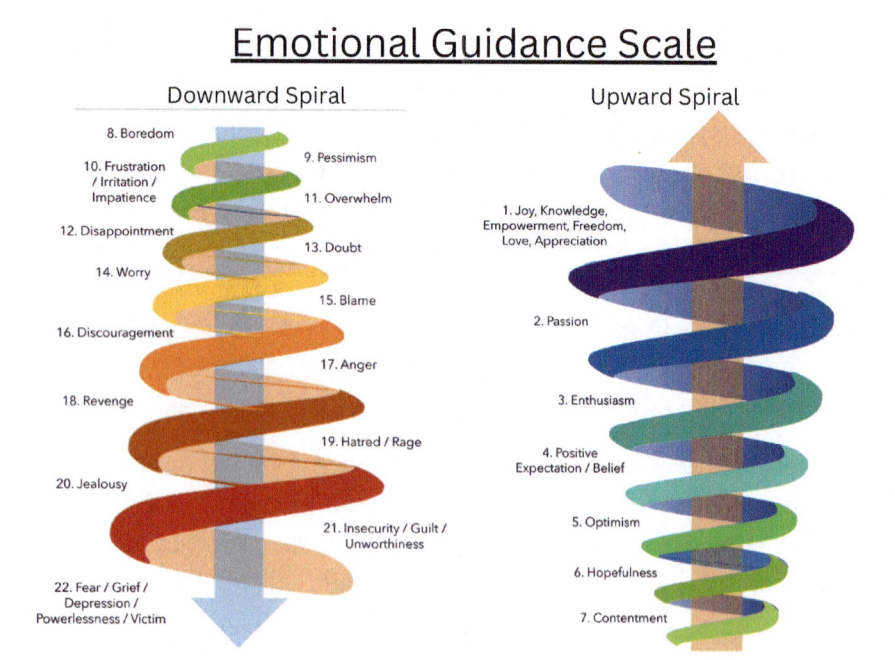

Emotional Guidance Scale

Downward Spiral
- 8. Boredom
- 9. Pessimism
- 10. Frustration / Irritation / Impatience
- 11. Overwhelm
- 12. Disappointment
- 13. Doubt
- 14. Worry
- 15. Blame
- 16. Discouragement
- 17. Anger
- 18. Revenge
- 19. Hatred / Rage
- 20. Jealousy
- 21. Insecurity / Guilt / Unworthiness
- 22. Fear / Grief / Depression / Powerlessness / Victim

Upward Spiral
- 1. Joy, Knowledge, Empowerment, Freedom, Love, Appreciation
- 2. Passion
- 3. Enthusiasm
- 4. Positive Expectation / Belief
- 5. Optimism
- 6. Hopefulness
- 7. Contentment

The spiralling of emotions up and down the scale expressed as feelings. Energy medicine practitioners believe that unresolved long-term emotions are ingrained into the body and mind leading to pain and disease.

THE ENERGY CONTINUUM INDICATES YOUR ALIGNMENT TO YOUR LIFE PATH

There are only two aspects of feelings that matter – positive and negative. Every other feeling falls onto a continuum of positive and negative (some are more extreme than others). The more negative feelings you experience, the worse your life appears. The more positive feelings you experience, the better your life becomes. Once you realise there are only two then you can begin to change how you feel. The power of emotion tells you how strongly you are in favour of one side over the other. It does not matter if something or someone else responds differently to you. The most important thing to remember is that you feel either positive or negative in response to an event. It is your perception that is key to a feeling.

If a tree falls in a forest and no-one is around to hear it, does it make a sound?

The centuries-old philosophical question could apply to feelings too.

Do feelings exist if you do not feel them? Do the feelings still exist if we have ignored or over-ridden them with thinking? To answer this question, let's extrapolate out that same line of conversation to more severe events and see what you feel about the response.

EVENT + RESPONSE	
EVENT	RESPONSE
You have disturbed sleep and low energy for years	It's normal for me, I just need a coffee to wake me up
You have chronic lower back pain and can't sit for periods	I'm ok, I'll keep going, I have the physio next week
There was a world economic crash and you can't pay your mortgage	I'm grand, sure everyone is in the same boat
You experienced sexual abuse as a child	It wasn't so bad, it was a long time ago

How do the responses feel to you?

They might be common responses but do they feel right in your body?

Can you see that our response is masking how we are really feeling? We are tricking ourselves into believing everything is ok when it is not. The power of thought can literally change how we feel about something, and it is not until we change those feelings that the thought can become reality. In this sense, I often see people mask their feelings with their chosen language. Here is a list of some ways people use language to trick themselves into believing all is ok:

I just/only had one bar of chocolate – making your choice seem insignificant and a one-off when in reality it is a much more important choice and occurs more frequently than you are telling yourself.

I need balance in my life – said with respect to making changes and wanting to keep old patterns. The word 'need' implies you can't do without, and 'balance' suggests you think you're working really hard and deserve some of the old things.

I deserve a break – mixing up priorities in life. Doing things you know you shouldn't be doing but covering it up because you feel pressured by all the changes you are making.

Everybody else . . . – makes it seem that what you are doing is ok because many others are doing it too, even though you know it doesn't feel good to you deep down.

Research says . . . – similar to the last statement but now you are using science to 'back up' your choice and hide the reality of its consequences. Admittedly, this can be a slippery statement because sometimes it may be true.

I had no choice . . . – there is always a choice. They mightn't be nice ones but there is a choice. If it really is a limited choice, ask yourself what decisions you made in the run-up to the final choice that could have broadened your options and made life easier for you.

Inasmuch as we can trick our conscious brain and change our perception of reality, our subconscious mind can still remember the stressful event and the original thought pattern, if it was strong enough. As adults we often continue to act out teenage behaviour patterns even when they no longer serve us. It is why you go for the cookie when you want to lose weight; it is why we return to our screens for a hit of social media when we checked it just minutes previously. We have convinced ourselves that our response is natural but in reality, it is far from natural.

YOUR BODY REFLECTS YOUR LIFE

Every trauma we suffer, every stress we endure, and every time we veer from our life path, our bodies keep the score. From birth and all through childhood right to the present day, our emotions are etched into our physical body, our movement pattern and especially our breathing pattern. Our breathing pattern is typically the first physical manifestation of the event's distress, and the last to be unwound.

THINKING/MINDSET

Our physiological state governs our thoughts and mindset. When we are shut down or aroused, the blood flow to our rational brain is altered. As we become more fatigued and stressed, our ability to think clearly, creatively and logically decreases. It's the old story that we wake up late for work and can't find our car keys. We spend a half hour searching frantically for them without luck. As the search time increases, we become more and more stressed about the keys. In the end, they are inevitably found in the last place you look, like the trouser pocket you searched three times or the kitchen table. The keys were there the whole time; you just couldn't see them because your rational brain was shut off from seeing them. You were in a state of high arousal. This state is good for you if you want to run from an angry bear. It is not so constructive if you need to think clearly, find your keys, and get to work! Your first job in this instance should have been to calm yourself by changing your feelings and emotions, then create a plan of possibilities to search.

Once the physiology is in balance, the development of your imagination and having a growth mindset becomes another critical layer in the human performance pyramid. Your mind does not know the difference between the past, the present and the future. It only knows what is happening now (real or imagined). This is the premise of how movies can change how we feel. The best movie directors are masters in taking a concept, creating an imaginary storyline and making it feel real to its specific audience. Through acting, CGI, picture, sound and experience they connect us with a story which evokes emotion in its audience; we laugh, cry, invoke anger, hatred, love or laughter at will. *Gladiator*, for example, is one of my favourite films of all time. I've watched it tens of times over and I still love it. Why? Because the story of a general, who became a slave, who turned into a gladiator, who overthrew an empire, is one that sings to my soul. I connect fully with the story in body, mind and soul. I see elements of me in Maximus and I see elements of Maximus in me. *The Last of the Mohicans*, *Braveheart* and *Star Wars* are movies I love too. But did you ever notice that some movies you love don't impact your friends the same way? Take my wife for example; she doesn't care much for *Gladiator*. The story doesn't connect with her the same way it does me.

She doesn't like the violence, bloodshed and hero story the same way I do. The reason she doesn't connect with *Gladiator* is that the picture of her life and her roles in life do not match those of the movie; she's not the right audience. Great movies know their audience and connect their story deeply with them. The movie needs to be written well, produced and directed with super quality too. When a movie feels more 'real' it connects deeply with its audience. When it comes to creating our own life, we can utilise the same tools as a Hollywood movie to project the life we want to live and shape the way we feel. First, we need to move beyond our past and our current set of circumstances.

THE POWER OF WORDS

To observe the power of our words on our reality, you should check out the movie on YouTube called: The Power of Words.

In the short movie, there is a blind man begging for money on the streets. He has a sign that reads "I'm blind, please help". Throughout the day he is receiving little to no loose change and is becoming despondent. Then a businesswoman appears to him. She takes the sign and rewrites the message for him. For the rest of the day, the man receives lots of money from passers-by.

At the end o the day she returns to see how he got on. He recognises her and asks, "What did you do to my sign?" Her response was:" I wrote the same ... but different words."

If you want to find out what exactly she wrote, check out the movie for yourself on YouTube by scanning the QR code below.

Your life right now is a product of your thinking and living in the past. You created the life you are living in the minutes, hours, days, months, and years leading up to now. If you are overweight now, it's because you ate too much, moved too little, slept too little, and experienced too high stress levels in the past. If your breathing is adapted now, it is because an accumulation of stress in the past created that adapted breathing pattern now. Usually our upbringing and history conditions us to think and live a certain way. We close ourselves off to the possibility of a better life; we think life happens to us instead of for us. Life becomes a struggle without a glimmer of hope for the future. All you see is more of the same. This way of thinking is what Stanford psychologist Dr. Carol Dweck termed a 'fixed mindset' (Dweck 2017).

A person with a fixed mindset is stuck in a rut. They are frustrated, critical, negative and limited. No longer can they see the possibility for better nor do they seek out change. They are afraid and consumed by fear – fear of what might happen if change is to come. People entrenched in a fixed mindset don't like to be challenged. They are content with life even if they are suffering great pain. Life is not fair for them; it's hard and will always be this way. The grass is always greener for everyone else. Life is easier for them because . . . If only I could . . . But then I am not willing to change to make it happen. These are common traits of the fixed mindset.

When we live in long-term states of withdrawal or arousal, the blood flow to rational and creative parts of the brain is reduced. These parts effectively become shut down. The brain does not operate in its natural, relaxed rhythm and the mindset becomes fixed. We can't imagine a better life for ourselves. Negative thoughts dominate our thinking and actions. We limit ourselves and close off opportunities for growth. Just like when we can't find our keys when we're in an acute state of stress, we can't find solutions to our problems so easily when we're in a chronic state of anxiety. This negative, compartmentalising and closed mindset is a response to our natural self-preservation reaction to stress. It keeps us alive in times of immediate major stress and pressure, like when a bear is chasing you; but it ultimately harms your quality of life if you maintain that state over time. When we hold onto that same closed mindset in the long term we further suppress our feelings to both the big stuff and the little stuff, to the point that we don't even listen to them anymore. We develop sensory-motor amnesia, as Thomas Hanna put it. We lose proprioceptive and interoceptive awareness. Our body adapts its posture and internal processes to the shape of the stressors and the mindset. States of arousal or withdrawal become fixed into our somatic and autonomic nervous systems, and the process of disease and decay takes hold in your life. Every new experience in life confirms the already closed mindset, and so the mindset becomes even more entrenched in your body and brain. It's like rolling a wheel down a hill. In the beginning it takes a lot of energy to get the wheel rolling. As momentum gathers, the wheel picks up speed. The longer and steeper the hill, the faster the wheel turns. The momentum of negativity works the same as the wheel rolling down the hill. In the beginning, negative thinking starts slowly. As you experience more stress in life you develop a fixed mindset. Life becomes hard for you. As the pattern builds momentum, it becomes more deeply ingrained in your system. The speed and momentum of the fixed mindset then dominates your life. The brain, nervous system, hormones, and postural systems are all affected. Breathing becomes adapted and the net results are negative consequences for our habits, health and performance in life.

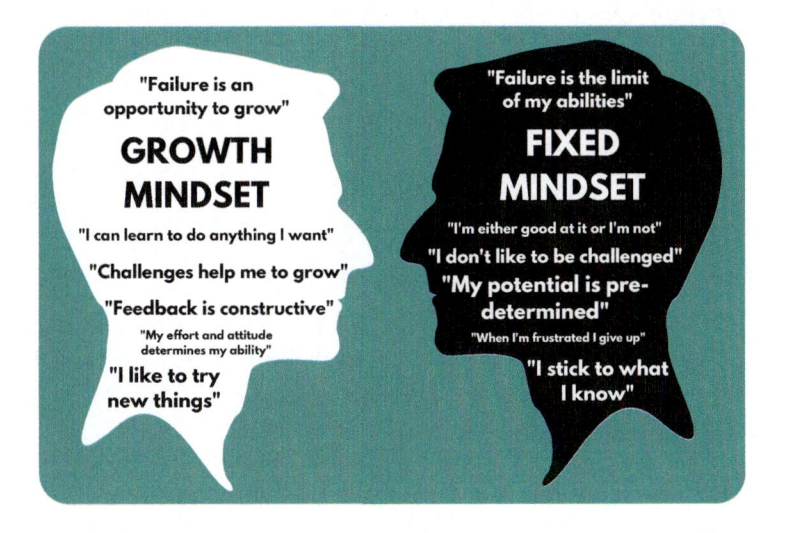

"Failure is an opportunity to grow"

GROWTH MINDSET

"I can learn to do anything I want"

"Challenges help me to grow"

"Feedback is constructive"

"My effort and attitude determines my ability"

"I like to try new things"

"Failure is the limit of my abilities"

FIXED MINDSET

"I'm either good at it or I'm not"

"I don't like to be challenged"

"My potential is pre-determined"

"When I'm frustrated I give up"

"I stick to what I know"

From a health perspective, a closed, negative and compartmentalising mindset leads to dysfunction, pain and a host of lifestyle diseases over time. This can include everything from anxiety, panic, depression, asthma, cardiovascular disease, and diabetes, to inflammatory diseases. It is not a matter of *if* you will get a disease; it is a question of *which disease* you will get if you continue to suppress your feelings with thought in the long run. All of these disease states have a huge influence on your breathing patterns. From a performance point of view, you will find yourself less able to execute the skills and habits of your craft. Habits and behaviours change because of a fixed mindset, and ultimately, you crumble under the pressure of more challenging environments.

A growth mindset is quite the opposite. It is an empowered mindset. The growth mindset is positive, self-affirming, creative, and imaginative. It views life as a challenge, sees opportunity in every situation, seeks out solutions, acknowledges limitations and strives for better. With a growth mindset we use our imagination and positive thinking to create the future we desire by thinking it and feeling it first. We influence the direction of our life with our thoughts the same way a Hollywood director shapes the story of a movie. This is not just about positive thinking; it's more about making the most of life, no matter what it throws at you.

Healthy and loved children tend to have more of an open mindset than adults. Most adults don't tend to have either a fixed or open mindset regarding to everything in life; rather they usually have fixed ways in relation to important areas in life and remain open in other areas. As people age, their patterns of life and thinking are ingrained into their system and they become more fixed in their thinking about any other approach. If you have suffered trauma, been filled with fear, or lived in a heightened stress environment for a period of time, you become more fixed in your mindset to help you survive.

Survivors of concentration camps, people with terminal illnesses, happy people content with their 'average' lives, high performers and ultra-successful people all have one thing in common – they've been known to cultivate a growth mindset. You too can do the same. Do as the saying says: 'When you're given lemons, make lemonade.' Taking time out to cultivate your growth mindset, to train it, is important when you want to ingrain that way of thinking into your life.

HABITS AND BEHAVIOURS

*We become what we repeatedly do.
Excellence then is not an act but a habit*

ARISTOTLE

It is true to say that habits and behaviours ultimately determine our health and performance. Habits entrain behaviours and behaviours are expressions of how we are feeling and thinking. This is the first level of our biological state that can be seen from the outside. Behaviours are a physical manifestation of our emotional inputs, feelings and mindset. Habits are the processes we repeatedly use to create our lives. Every behaviour starts out as a conscious act to get something we want. We know a baby is hungry for the first time because it cries. Pretty quickly, both parent and baby realise that crying is the means the baby uses to get their food. Crying becomes a habitual behaviour, a habit. Every time the baby wants food, they cry. As the baby grows to become a child, it wants for other things, like parent's attention or a toy. Crying worked for getting fed so the baby thinks it might work to get other things too. The more attention success the baby has with crying, the more it uses crying as the means to get what it wants. As a parent it can seem quite tricky to change the behaviours and habits of young children. Ingraining a new behavioural habit takes time, skill and patience. But young children are very adaptable, they depend on their parents for survival, they trust them and their brains are quite flexible to change. Usually children ingrain a new habit quite quickly (even if that may seem like an eternity to the parent). As the child grows to become an adult, though, their brains become less flexible and they are more self-reliant for change. I used to hear that it takes 21 days to build a new habit. When that concept was challenged by research, it became widespread knowledge that it actually takes 66 days to make a new behaviour automatic. However, that's still not the truth. The research said the median time it takes to ingrain a new habit is 66 days but the spread of time it could take a person to automate a habit lay between 18 and 254 days. That means if you happen to be one of the unlucky people, it may take you nearly a year of repeatedly doing the same daily act before it becomes subconscious.

Often times, a person isn't even aware of their self-sabotaging habits until they are written out in front of them. Similar to Porges' idea that we lose interoceptive abilities when stressed and Hanna's idea of proprioceptive loss, I see in my coaching practice that people become numb to the number of negative acts they repeatedly perform. Many people know that chocolate is a treat to enjoy every so often but often they are unaware of just how much chocolate they consume daily. I remember attending a Fat Loss Education Course for trainers in Canada back in 2013. Eoin Lacey, the presenter, used the analogy of a tube of Pringles crisps (chips for the North Americans) to describe people's self-sabotaging habits. 'Once you pop you can't stop' was the catchphrase Pringles used and they were right. The crisps were laced with so many chemicals that made them taste so good, you'd have the packet eaten before you knew it.

Changing habits without addressing the underlying layers is, in my opinion, almost impossible. It is the same as swimming against the tide in the sea. You place a whole lot of energy into changing that habit but the underlying current will eventually overpower you and force you in its direction. This is because of subconscious self-sabotaging habits; the currents of the higher levels in the human performance pyramid overpower even the best of intentions. The distress caused by an imbalanced biological state, combined with a fixed mindset and your conditioning to the negative habit, will always override any conscious decision you make to change. You eventually self-sabotage your new habits and return to old ones if you don't address all the underlying hierarchical levels of human performance.

PERFORMANCE

Men lie, women lie, numbers don't lie

FLOYD MAYWEATHER

Performance is perhaps the most apparent insight as to whether you are on track in life. Most elite athletes and businesspeople understand the value of tracking and analysing performance measures as a means of checking in to see if they are on course or not. 'What gets measured, gets managed,' was the famous saying by business consultant Peter Drucker. In elite performance, it is the outcome goals and the key performance measures which are tracked and improved upon. Ultimately these are the success barometer of all your effort and they keep you on track to attain your overall vision.

For example, an Olympic cycle for an athlete is four years long. During the cycle, the athlete aims to improve on their weak points and further enhance strengths with the overall vision of winning the Olympics at the end of it. Every competition entered has a purpose to serve. Every block of training within the cycle has goals, and every training session aims to improve a specific quality.

Ultimately, health and breath training are no different to training for the Olympics. Since health is the foundation stone to performance and breathing the keystone to health, it is obvious to me that we are starting from more humble beginnings, but the process should be the same. It is for this reason that I love the Buteyko breathing method.

Doctor Buteyko discovered the first breathing method, which put numbers on the quality of someone's breathing and health status. His breathing score, known as the control pause (nowadays referred to as the BOLT score), measures the physiological quality of your respiratory system. The main issue with the BOLT score is that it is a subjective measure of the breath. It times your awareness of your first urges to breathe. This awareness can create issues for people because many people don't know what it is they are timing, or can't sense it, so they misjudge the test. Although it has issues with the theory supporting the measure and its validity and reliability with stringent research protocols, I have found the BOLT score still proves to be a quality approximation to the health of my clients' breathing system in practice. More recently, however, the Art of Breath borrowed an objective measure of the breath from the freediving community and applied it to health. Instead of recording your awareness of your need to breathe, the Art of Breath measures the length of your maximum exhale from start to finish in seconds. Time is the same for us all so these scores may be more reliable and valid than the BOLT. The research on the absolute accuracy of these measures is sparse but time will tell. In practice, all of the scores work well at placing a baseline number on our breathing system. With numbers on our breathing, we are now able to assess the efficiency of our breathing system at rest and the effectiveness of our training. Ultimately, I feel there will always be an issue with 'measuring' the breathing system. I doubt we will develop a single measurement of our breath because it is influenced by so many critical underlying factors. Time will tell.

Once we become aware of our breathing patterns and in tune with our own body, we can begin to let go of analysing our progress and, instead, focus on the overall feeling of wellbeing that arises from breath training. Awareness of our breath efficiency in any given moment, combined with our feelings, is the primary indicator of health and resilience in the human biological system.

MEANING

> *Life is without meaning. You bring the meaning to it.*
> *The meaning of life is whatever you ascribe it to be.*
> *Being alive is the meaning*
>
> JOSEPH CAMPBELL

Feeling a deep sense of love is an innate response to living a meaningful life. Enjoying food, admiring a sunset, achieving in sport, being in a loving relationship, and earning status. These are all experiences and pursuits which feel good on the surface but may not transfer into the depths of ourselves. The deeper feelings of love and appreciation can be attained by anybody, despite your circumstances in life. In his book, *Man's Search for Meaning*, Viktor Frankl described how meaning can be found in anybody's life through activity, passivity or suffering (Frankl 2006). He should know; he was not only a psychiatrist, but also a prisoner for many years in the Auschwitz concentration camp during World War Two. In his book he explained the common traits between survivors of such dreadful atrocities and his patients in later years. He said that your ability to find meaning in your life is more important than anything that happens to you. That meaning is usually based on something you want to create from the experience, supporting a loved one or finding peace in the suffering. Each of these meanings requires faith, hope and a desire for a better future. A vision is the movie you play in your mind of the future you want to create. Creating a vision with meaning motivates you to change your habits, thoughts, feelings, and emotions for life. You see life as you would like to live it. Frankl quoted Nietzsche's famous saying, 'He who has a why to live can bear almost any how.'

Creating your meaningful why vividly is the ultimate stage of the human performance pyramid. It lies outside the pyramid in the sense that it is not a process of human life but a representation of what we want to become. A tree grows toward the sun but it never actually touches it. Through its ambitions to reach the sun, the tree grows deep roots, a strong trunk, and beautiful flowers. It is nourished by nature and it nourishes natures. So it is with your vision for life. A vision pulls you up to become a better person. It helps you to grow healthy, strong and flexible. It nourishes you and shows you how to share your talents with the world.

Your vision is an image which conveys the meaning of your life. It is the story or picture of the person you want to become for reasons that are deeply entrenched in you. You become that which you actively want to be in your life. A vision must be meaningful to you. You must feel it deeply and connect to it wholly. It embodies every aspect of your life, and it is in alignment with the health of your biological body. It is not a fantasy of the life you would love but aren't prepared to work for; rather, it portrays your life's meaning despite how difficult life might be for you. Your identity, values, habits and behaviours all centre round a meaningful vision. Not only do people suffer and become sick because they have suffered stress and trauma in their past, but it also happens because they live an inauthentic life, out of alignment with their future. Frankl called it 'existential frustration'. He believed that we develop neurotic behaviour because we have no meaning in our life. This type of experience is becoming more prevalent for young people nowadays for two reasons. The first is the need/desire to emulate the lives of social media celebrities, superstar athletes, actors and personalities. Secondly, they achieve greatness in one area of their life at the expense of all other areas.

The pervasiveness of celebrity culture on the lives of our young people leads them to live a vicarious life instead of finding meaning and purpose in their own. Celebrities are on our phones, our news feeds, the internet, our TV and radio. It's hard to get away from because the platform algorithms in our technology show us more of what we have already looked at. The more we look at the life of a celebrity on tech, the more tech shows us their life. We dress the way they do, eat the same, talk the same and try to live our lives as if we were them. If it is perceived that a celebrity finds fame, fortune or meaning through flaunting themselves on the internet, then why can't we find the same results and the same benefits in our lives? We seek meaning in emulating them or knocking their way of life. It is very easy nowadays to lose track of time and sense of yourself with the internet in our world. The other difficulty for young people is the cost of success in one area of their life, usually their career, for every other aspect. Their identity becomes so intertwined in their career that they lose sight of being a human and the other aspects of human life. If they lose their career, who are they?

There are almost a trillion people on the planet today. No matter what field of expertise you choose in your career, there are hundreds, if not thousands, of equally talented people. Sport, music, tech, business, art, banking, teaching, research, they're all the same – lots of people competing to become successful. The good thing today versus thirty years ago is that at least you can choose the area you love and make a success of it, because there is an audience out there who want to experience your talents. In my parent's era and the start of mine, it was unheard of to earn a living from sport, music or dance, for example. I still remember when Andy Cole became the most expensive soccer player in England for the princely sum of £7,000,000 in 1995. In 2018, soccer transfer fees reached £150 million. Financial stability and status are the gold standards for success in the modern world. To achieve this aim, you must pour every part of your being into your talent to become successful. The Chinese Olympic teams are known to recruit talented kids from the age of four. Russia and the USA are the same. One of my clients told me recently that it is common for the children of the elite in the USA to work 16-hour days. At eight years of age, they are chasing the American dream. They rise at 6 am and hit their pillows at 10 pm. They practise before breakfast, then commute to school. School is followed by after-school tutoring, then more practice and finally home. Ready for bed to start another day on the road to success. Fun, creativity, play, and free time do not exist naturally anymore; rather, it is built in and scheduled in their day. This norm for the USA elite is fast becoming more prevalent in Ireland and the rest of the Western world.

I see it in the worlds of Irish dance, GAA and judo. Even amateur sports, like Gaelic Games and Irish dancing, require children to train ten-plus hours per week to get anywhere near the top of their sport. Because of the societal pressure and quantity of people in the world, kids are expected to work, take extra private lessons, and then perform their own practice on top of that for years on end to make it. All of this effort does not even guarantee success. You need to have a lot of luck, good breaks, and kind people on your side too. The net effect of the pursuit of success is burn-out. Mentally, the kids and young adults get fed up with the rat race and lose interest in their passions. Physically they are plagued with injury, illness and mental disease issues because their body can no longer take the suffering.

Those who don't make it due to injury, illness, or bad breaks are ill-prepared for the mental shift from their little world to the big bad world of life. Of those who make it, they are retired in their forties or fifties due to burn-out. And the question then becomes, now what? Where is the meaning of life now?

Regardless of your age, talent or experience, with a lack of purpose and meaning in life, you become bored. With boredom, impulses appear to relieve you from that boredom – affairs of the heart, food, alcohol and thrill-seeking activities. More recently there has been a trend of people using forms of self-induced flagellation under the guise of health. Ultra-running, extended fasts and bodybuilding are some of these pursuits I see people do daily. They think it is a healthy pursuit because it is 'exercise'; they get a buzz from it or they think they will be perceived as awesome for doing it. In reality they are searching for meaning in the suffering of the event. But as Frankl said, 'to suffer unnecessarily is masochistic rather than heroic'. Having multiple sexual partners, affairs, drug-taking, and thrill-seeking are similar self-sabotaging pursuits. On a conscious level, we are seeking to feel good. Deeper down, though, we are seeking meaning in our life. The cost of thrill-seeking your way to meaning is reflected in the tatters of your life, psyche, and human body over time. As you seek bigger thrills to get the same feeling of satisfaction in life you find you lose energy and verve for living. Your body bears the brunt of the cost of thrill-seeking. Sleep gets disturbed, energy levels dip and wane throughout the day, the nervous system adapts, breathing and posture patterns change, and hormones become imbalanced internally. In time, you develop pain and disease as you seek out bigger and better thrills to feel more satisfied in a life you don't really want anyway.

Creating a vision and finding meaning in your life is hard and it can take a very long time. It takes faith, courage and persistence to stay the course until you find what you really love. With good habits, a growth mindset and a healthy biological system, it can be done. The Japanese call a meaningful vision of a long and happy life your *Ikigai* (García and Miralles 2017). They say your path to Ikigai is hidden deep within you. Just like logotherapy, meaning in your Ikigai is discovered through the insights gleaned from the experiences of your pastimes, career, relationships and life. These insights are combined with simple acts of healthy living to make for a long and happy life.

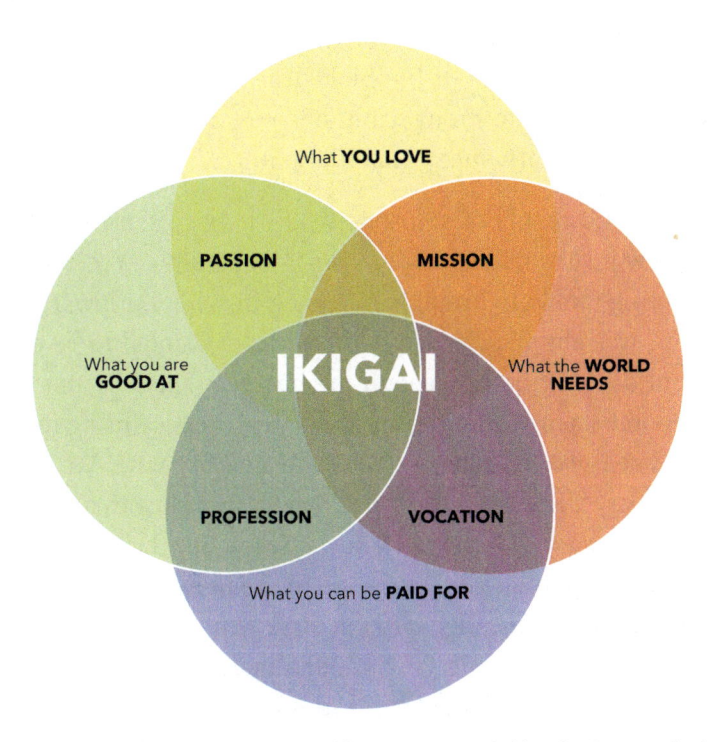

Ikigai – a meaningful vision of your life as determined by the inter-relationship between the different areas of life

Your life's path to date has brought you through some experiences (by chance or on purpose) to reveal deeper layers of yourself to you. Through the insights from these life experiences you discover what you dislike and you learn what brings you joy and satisfaction. From this vantage point you develop the knowledge, skills and experience to master the things you love. Then you begin to share those insights with the world through services or products you render. They say that you won't have to work a day in your life when you find the things you love. I'm not so sure about that, but I do know that when you connect to the deepest parts of yourself and find things you love to do, be and have, then your life bears a whole new meaning. Some people find their meaning early and easily. Others spend a lifetime searching for it and some people don't even know to look for it. When meaning is combined with acts of healthy living the result is a long and happy life. The acts include things like breathing, getting outdoors, challenging your body physically, resting, eating well, and sharing with people – all of the biological inputs and thought processes required to create strong habits and perform well in life. Sounds like the human performance pyramid, right?

Take me as an example of someone who has been searching for my Ikigai. I grew up in a middle-upper-class Irish family as a second child. I had a strong family upbringing. I was ok in school, I loved playing sport and I was chronically sick with asthma. I wanted to be an elite athlete but couldn't be because of my health. I followed the money into computer science and lost my way in my career during my early twenties, but I was also lucky enough to find my wife. We married young and have three beautiful girls. I cured my ill health and entered the fitness industry. For years I knew I wanted to be in fitness but couldn't find my niche. I did every job in the industry, from cleaning toilets, gym instruction, lifeguarding, swim teaching, group exercise fitness, supervisor, manager and general manager. Eventually, after eight years, I decided to become a personal trainer. Ten years into my career, with a master's level education, I was earning less than I did in a part-time waiting job as a teenager. I hired a life coach, read feverishly and modelled high performers to find out how I could make this work for me. I began to focus on becoming the best trainer I could be. I worked with some amazing organisations and clients in my time; but I always felt like I didn't fully connect with most of my clients and the environments I worked in. This meant it was hard for me to get busy and support my family financially. I continued to dig deeper. Through all of my experiences, I began to realise the type of environment I wanted to work in and I found the common threads in my favourite and most successful clients. They were simply people like me who wanted to live a great life, and be strong, fit and healthy, but usually, their health was a limiting factor in their life (just like when I started out). I found my way back to the breathing techniques I used to cure my asthma originally. I became curious about other breathing techniques, and I wanted to know how they all worked. That journey led me on a path of discovering the effects of breathing on health, life, and sports performance. At the same time, I found my way outdoors into nature more. I began using cold water immersion and challenging my physical body in ways I couldn't imagine just a few years before. I have connected to deeper levels of my being, nature and life. I found like-minded communities of people along the way. My family supports me, and I support them on their journeys. I have one or two friends, and I love my life. I am writing this book and discovering more about the type of trainer and man I want to become as a result of going with the flow and searching for meaning in my life. Life still presents me with challenges and there are times when I feel like packing it all in, but I know better now. I know that the hard times contain the greatest treasures in life. In those times I usually return to my vision and start finding ways to feel good again.

Living from the heart is the pathway to leading a meaningful life (Childre, Martin and Beech 2000). Feelings, in other words, guide us on a journey to discover what is right and wrong. In order to listen to our heart, we need to have clear messages sent between our heart, our head and the rest of our body. Did you ever take a left turn when you know you should have turned right, only to have something bad

PART 1   **THE INTERCONNECTION OF LIFE, STRESS AND THE BREATH**

happen to you? Did you ever eat some poor-quality food that tasted good, and feel rotten a few hours later? How about staying up past your bedtime when you're tired, only to have no energy the next day? Or following along with a gang of people when you know they're up to no good and then getting into trouble for your antics? Have you ever had a life-changing moment, like a car accident, being fired from work, a break-up or a failure in a pastime? When you look back on these situations can you see that there were signals telling you to take a different direction the whole time? Can you see those signals usually came as a feeling? Feelings you ignored that could have led to a happier ending? I remember when I was finding my confidence as a young man, I had to have difficult conversations with my dad. Every time I went to have one of those conversations, my throat would seize up and I'd get a terrible pain in my chest. In the beginning, I shied away from many conversations because of these feelings. Each time I shied away it became more difficult to speak the next time. I was extremely motivated to speak up, though, so I kept on plucking up the courage to speak. Over many years I eventually said everything I needed to say. The more I spoke with my dad, the more confident I grew and the easier it became to speak with him. To this day, when I need to have a difficult conversation with someone I still get those horrible feelings. The difference is now I know they are a sign to speak up, rather than retreat into my shell. Your heart feeling is the voice of your spirit during those moments. The reason I call it a heart feeling is to separate the voice of your monkey mind from that of your spirit. Generally, this heart voice comes as feelings in the body; the heart is the organ of love, as we all know. By listening to your heart, you glean insights into your life and derive meaning from it. It can be easier said than done. This is where I learned that breathing comes into the mix. Breathing makes the whole process of becoming healthy and finding meaning in life much easier.

BREATHING TETHERS EVERY LAYER OF THE HUMAN PERFORMANCE PYRAMID TOGETHER

We think doing nothing and just breathing is a waste of time when more often than not it's actually the most beneficial thing you could do for yourself

MARTHA MOUSSALLY, INNATE-STRENGTH CLIENT

Breathing is used to heal past traumas, delay fatigue, help you to focus and concentrate, improve physical performance, and it can even help to heal mental health issues. It enables you to quench the noise of the monkey mind and listen to your heart with clarity. When breathing is subtle, it calms the internal biological system, massages the heart and gut, relaxes the posture, opens the rational mind and helps you think creatively. Breathing is the foundation of biological health; it also gifts us that space in the moment to listen to the heart, comprehend our actions, and it tethers the mind to your vision. I know all this because this is what the breath has done for me. I have also witnessed it perform similar miracles for many others. When you become tuned to

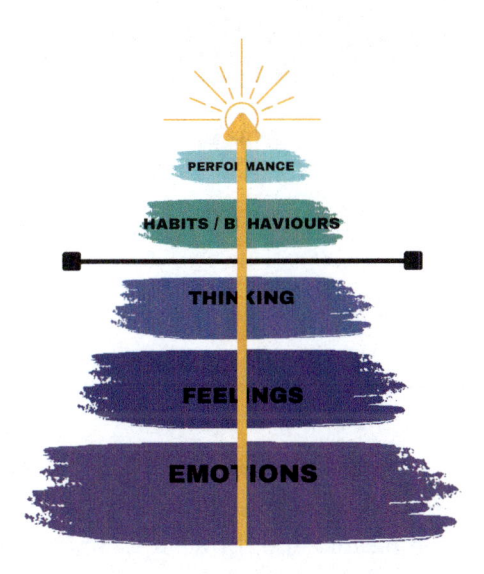

Breathing slices through the Human Performance Pyramid

your breath you quickly realise that, without your breath, you have but one dream; with your breath you can fulfil a thousand dreams.

WHICH KNIFE TO USE?

Breathing is unlike any other process in the human body for its adaptability and potential in the healing process. In his online *Breathing Fundamentals Course*, Dan Brulé, a breath teacher for over forty years, describes the concept of 'breathing to heal beautifully' (Brulé 2018).

Brulé has a model for the human being, similar to the human performance pyramid. Everything you are, as we know you today, conscious and subconscious, physically, mentally, emotionally, and spiritually, stands and lives at the top of the pyramid. Each subsequent layer of consciousness is tethered by the preceding layer, much like the human performance pyramid. At the top of Brulé's pyramid are the outward physical traits, our performance and behavioural habits. The next layer down is our thoughts and mindset. Feelings are the final layer of the pyramid.

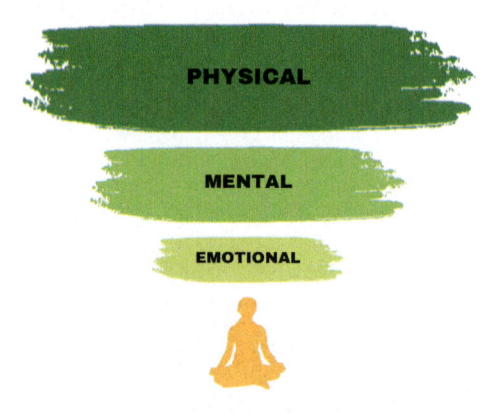

Dan Brulé's model depicting the layers of human consciousness

Although Brulé's pyramid looks like the HPP, it differs in its purpose. His pyramid is inverted in shape. Instead of reaching up to find a meaningful purpose in your life, Brulé's pyramid points down into the core of your being, into your spirit, to discover 'the real you'. This is the timeless part of you connected to nature, every person, every being, the universe and God. It is the same part of you that I called your 'heart voice' earlier on. From experiencing this perspective of your being, Brulé believes you can model your life with more clarity. In this sense, Brulé is more interested in cutting through the rubbish in life (behaviours/mindset/emotions), becoming aware of a more complete version of yourself (spirit), and then using this new perspective to go back and change all the layers of your life.

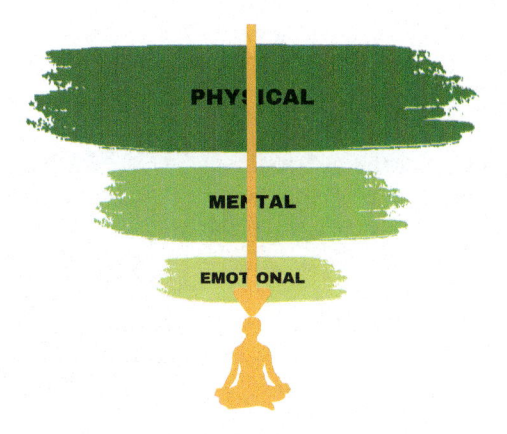

Brulé's preference is to cut through the rubbish of life and directly touch your spirit layer

I think there is great value to be gained in combining both models to form a framework for changing your life. The HPP outlines the need for change at every layer of your being, and Dan's model shows you how. The process of experiencing, understanding, finding meaning and choosing the life we want is referred to by Trevor Oswalt as 'the playing field' in his song 'Choices', when he explains the yogic ideas of karma and dharma. As Oswalt puts it, the playing field is another way to describe your life path or your dharma. It is the life you are given, including the parents you were born to and the external forces which impact your life, such as war, political change, weather and factors outside your control. Karma is 'choice'; it is the decisions you make with the hand you've been dealt in life and their consequences. The result of choices that make up the playing field is what's called the learning process. The HPP is an illustrative model for explaining the learning process. It shows you the areas of health and performance which you have choices over; the impacts those choices have on the functioning of your body and mind and the motivation for changing how you live. 'You cannot choose your genetics but you can choose how they are expressed' is a phrase I heard used often in the science of epigenetics.

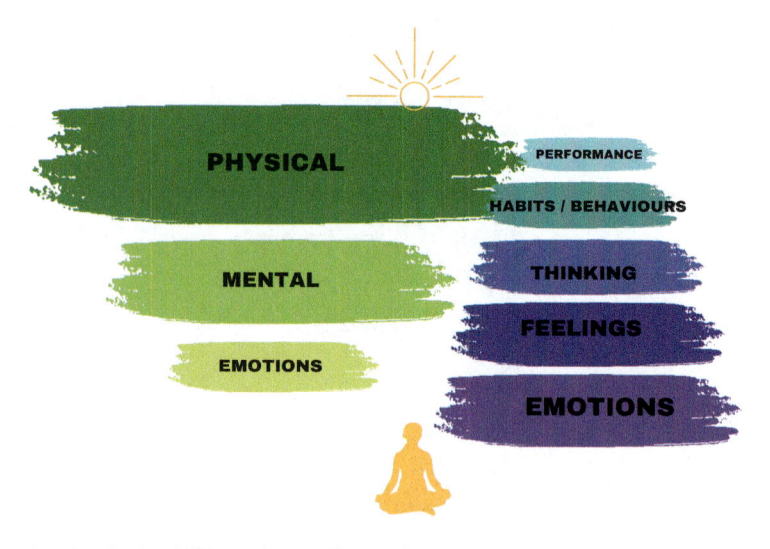

PHYSICAL	PERFORMANCE
	HABITS / BEHAVIOURS
MENTAL	THINKING
	FEELINGS
EMOTIONS	EMOTIONS

Merging both the HPP and Brulé's models help you understand your body, mind, and life at a deep level. Through the HPP, you can understand your biology and navigate your life better. Meanwhile, Brulé's model shows you the layers of human experience, from the shallow physical through to the deeper-spiritual.

If the HPP is a model that contains both the playing field and the entire playbook of life, Brulé's pyramid contains the best plays in the play book. He explains the two pathways that help you to hear your 'heart voice' more clearly. Once this voice is heard, you find it much easier to make better decisions and live a more fulfilled life.

During his *Advanced Fundamental Course,* Brulé explains that breathing is the process which slices through every layer of his model to find your heart voice. It can entrain your whole biological system into a unified rhythm. Through this rhythm, the body has the potential to heal itself, and it becomes easier to find meaning in life.

The process of changing your life, becoming healthier and performing better in life, begins by changing your physiology – and those inputs which impact your physical body. Most therapies are aimed at one of the upper layers of us or at a few, as Brulé explains in his course. Massage therapy is physical; talk therapy is mental; Emotional Freedom Techniques are obviously emotional. In particular, the simple acts of breathing efficiently, moving your body regularly and getting out into nature have the most profound effect on your whole life, more than science will ever reveal. As you breathe well, you bring sensation back into the body where it was once lost. You animate the physical sensations of the world, wake up the muscles, and feel what's going on inside. You can return sensation, proprioceptive awareness, and interoceptive awareness to the body through breathing. This has a compound effect on every subsequent layer in the HPP. With efficient breathing, it becomes easier to work on a growth mindset. With a growth mindset you enhance the effects of breathing and become open to changing your life more permanently. You find a way to ingrain new habits and begin to perform better in life, as measured by your chosen outcomes. Through the practices of changing your body and mind, combined with the awareness it brings, you find meaning in the other areas of your life and become future-focused. You find things you like doing and things you are good at doing. You notice the gaps in the world and see that you have a talent or skillset that benefits the world. That impact maybe on a small scale or a large one; it does not matter. You have found meaning through your life's passions, practices and being. You focus on making the most of that understanding by refining your life with a vision.

Breathing is the common physical thread that binds all other therapies and practices together. Psychologists use it to entrain the mind, physical therapists use it to relax and unwind the body, trainers coach it to gain strength and endurance, meditation is based on the breath and the breath is an integral part of yoga. Breathing is one of the most versatile and powerful tools we have to change our lives. Just as a knife can be used to succinctly peel an onion one layer at a time, or it can be used to slice through butter, so the breath peels through your biology one layer at a time, or it can slice through the whole system to the very core of your being.

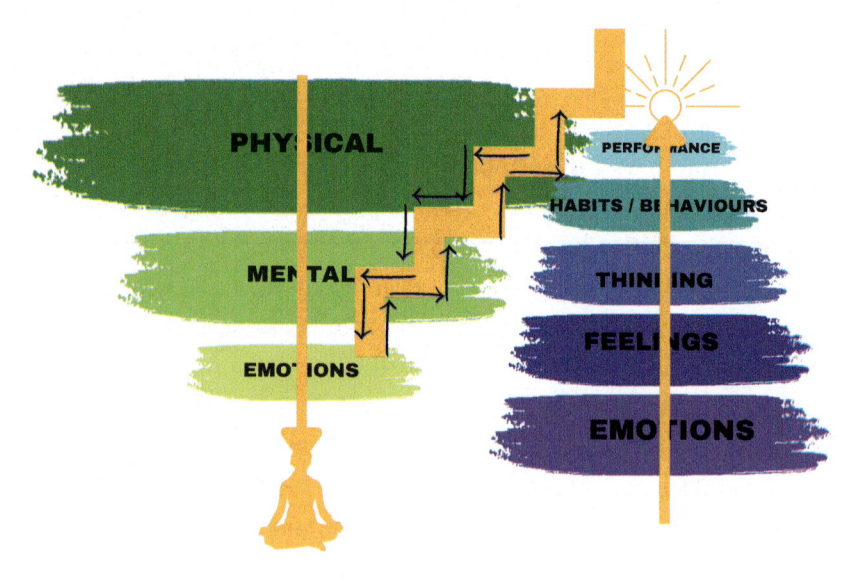

PHYSICAL — PERFORMANCE

HABITS / BEHAVIOURS

MENTAL — THINKING

FEELINGS

EMOTIONS — EMOTIONS

Breathing can be used directly or gradually to find deeper meaning in your life.

The mechanics of breathing is a fundamental must when training your breath. After that, you have two ways to approach breath training. The first is through breath-resilience techniques. The second is through rhythmical breathwork techniques. There is technically no right way or wrong way to restore your breathing; however, I do believe there are efficient ways and safe approaches to breath training. The next part of the book shows you the three main ways the breath adapts to long-term stress in our life. It then links these adaptations with specific dis-ease conditions for humans. Part two finishes by showing you the characteristics of a quality breath, both at rest and when used for a purpose.

PART 2

BREATHE-ABILITY

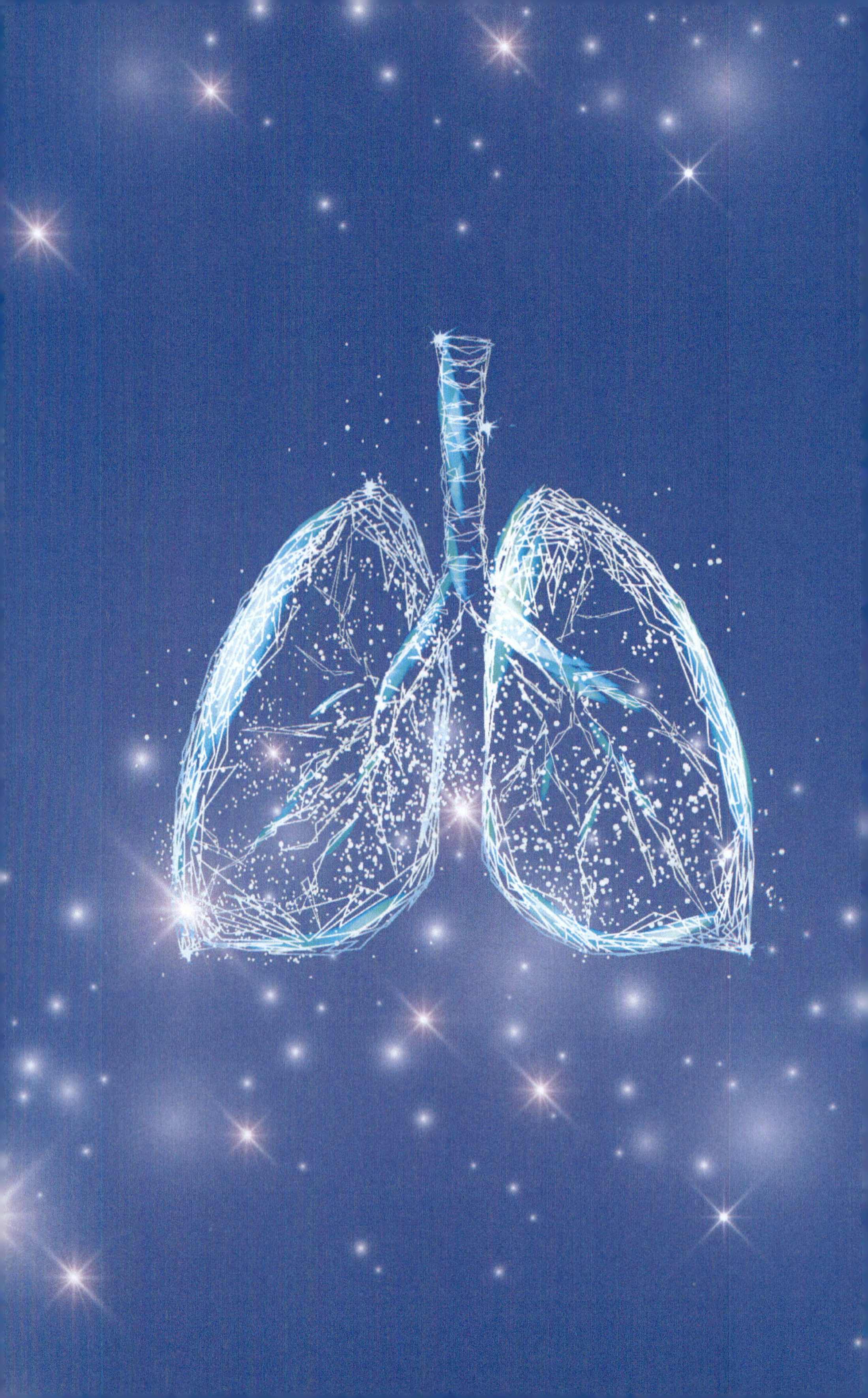

7
THE WAY THE BREATH WORKS

Breathing is an act performed by you both consciously and subconsciously. Conscious breathing is the top-down approach to changing your breath for a specific purpose. In this approach, we use our rational brain to change the way we breathe, which affects the deeper layers of the brain. Conscious breathing techniques are used to restore the subconscious breath to its natural centre, or they can be used to enhance performance in life. Subconscious breathing, on the other hand, is a bottom-up approach in the brain. It is the auto-regulated part of the breath we use when we're doing other things, like working or playing sport. The purpose of subconscious breathing is to regulate the flow of air and its gases (primarily oxygen and carbon dioxide) through the body as efficiently as possible. The body breathes to bring oxygen to the cells of your body. The cells, in turn, use this oxygen to create energy, to help us to live, survive, and thrive. The body always strives to perform this process and others as efficiently as possible. The fluctuating pressures of oxygen and carbon dioxide in response to life signals the brain to breathe. The brain then co-ordinates all inputs in an allostatic (whole-body) response by sending messages of its own back to the body.

The body breathes by inhaling and exhaling air, regulating oxygen and carbon dioxide gas pressures, and then the process starts all over again. The nose, mouth, nervous, musculoskeletal and respiratory systems are the primary systems involved in regulating gas pressure. These systems are supported by the cardiovascular system and they are influenced by the rest of the body. I refer to all elements of breathing collectively as the 'breathing system'. The breathing system observes the whole body-mind from the perspective that breathing is the central focus. It views the act of breathing beyond the respiratory system to include all systems in the body involved with breathing. I consider the regulation of the breathing system through the lens of neurobiology, neuroanatomy, biomechanics, respiratory physiology, psychology, spirituality and common sense. This is a very unique perspective on breathing. Usually, people (even highly experienced breathing coaches, doctors and practitioners) consider breathing solely from one area – respiratory or neurology or psychology or spirituality.

GAS PRESSURE REGULATION

In physics, air and gas flow from areas of high pressure to low pressure. Our brain senses the changes in these pressures throughout the system and alerts the body to breathe accordingly. There are six key points in the breathing cycle where pressure is regulated:

1. Our nose and mouth pull air from the environment into our body, filling our lungs with air. The throat provides a second stop-gap in this mechanism to use the breath for specialised functions
2. The alveoli in our lungs extract oxygen out of the air and send it to our blood
3. From the blood, the oxygen is sent to the various cells of the body
4. Carbon dioxide is one of the by-products built up in the cell from metabolic work (mainly from heat, food and exercise metabolism). As carbon dioxide levels rise, it is transferred into the blood
5. The blood whisks carbon dioxide back to the lungs
6. From the lungs it is sent back out into the environment through the nose or mouth with the rest of the air

These six points of pressure regulation can be condensed to three important processes, which the brain regulates in subconscious breathing. We can also manipulate these processes through conscious breathing practice to change our breathing patterns and state of being.

Pressure is regulated first of all through the upper airways. The upper airways consist of the nose, mouth, pharynx (throat down to the voice box), and larynx (containing the voice box). The upper airways regulate air pressure the same way a faucet regulates water pressure. A fully open upper airway allows air to flow naturally into the body through the nose and out of the body through the same route at rest. The airways can be closed fully, stopping air flow and locking pressure into the body. Finally, you can control the pressure at will by closing the upper airways partially. A full lock is commonly known as a breath-hold.

In general, the size of the vent you use (nose and mouth) is vital for the amount of air you pull into and release from the body. The smaller the vent you use to pull air in, the harder the body needs to work at drawing the air in. The secondary and tertiary breathing muscles work especially hard when the primary muscles are stiff (diaphragm and intercostals), you have a high sensitivity to carbon dioxide, or the anatomy of your nose, jaw and throat are narrow. I should note that naturally, at rest, the body only needs to breathe through one nostril when working efficiently. One nostril is a very small vent, two nostrils are a little larger and the mouth can be shaped from tiny to large to change the pressure gradient of air entering and exiting the body. The choice of vent can be manipulated subconsciously and consciously to perform different functions for the body. The body automatically switches which nostril to breathe through every ninety minutes to four hours. It naturally opens up the second nostril when the body demands more air exchange due to an increased metabolic demand (i.e. there's more pressure internally from stress, digestion, exercise or immune responses). Similarly, internal pressure on the system can be released through the mouth as needed through yawning, sighing, and panting. This is useful when we want to relax more, cope with the demand on our body or even train harder. When you are training really hard or your body is under chronic stress it automatically switches to mouth breathing. Mouth breathing allows for the greatest air flow into and out of the body. It is very important for the short-term release of high loads of pressure but, as you will see later, mouth breathing at rest is detrimental to long-term health and performance when it is ingrained as the go-to breathing vent.

The mouth, together with the vocal chords in the larynx, can be squeezed and shaped for specialised functions such as eliminating irritants, communicating effectively, and expressing emotions. We can sneeze, cough, and hiccup by controlling pressure at the vent and larynx levels of the upper airways to eliminate irritants/toxins from our airways. We talk, shout, cry, laugh, and sing by combining our voice with our mouth to communicate and express emotions. We hum by vibrating the vocal chords and breathing through either vent to relax and enjoy the sounds of the breath. The intentional partial closing of the airways and fully closed upper airways are also known as occlusive techniques.

There are three ways you can perform a breath-hold with the upper airways:

1. You can pinch the nose and close the mouth
2. You move the tongue to the back of the throat and block the pharynx (common in obstructive sleep apnoea)
3. You can close the vocal chords over the glottis in the larynx

These breath-holds can be combined with the diaphragm and the pelvic floor to create greater pressure in the body for a given purpose. In his online course, *Freediving 102*, the world champion free diver, William Trubridge, teaches full body-lock breathing techniques to train free divers to hold their breath longer and stay more relaxed. Using a nose clip to block the nasal passages, his locks combine a light contraction of the pelvic floor, diaphragm, throat, tongue and mouth in unison. Similarly, you can manage the flow of air using a partial occlusive technique by constricting the exhale with the tongue and lips. All of these functions are natural to the body and involve the exchange of pressure between the external and internal environment via the nose and/or mouth together with the larynx. This means there is no one 'correct' way to breathe. Breathing just through one vent is not right or wrong. Rather, we can choose to breathe as we wish. Problems arise when we are unable to use the breath as we wish because certain functions are unavailable to us.

The partial pressure of oxygen is the second major pressure point for gas exchange in the body. The body's primary concern is oxygen exhange at the lung-blood level. There are two processes here of note. The first is the ventilation-perfusion ratio, or the rate of air exchange between air and blood in the lungs. The second is the Haldane effect, which describes how oxygen and carbon dioxide displace each other in the blood at the lung-blood level. The ventilation-perfusion ratio is of the most importance to us from a practical perspective. Naturally, there is a better blood supply to the lower portion of the lungs and better air supply to the top portion. However, if you are mainly a chest breather, you ventilate or breathe air more into the top portions of the lungs. This leaves the lower lobes with less air flow. In this case the ventilation-perfusion ratio is unbalanced, and you fail to get a quality gas exchange at the lung-blood level of breathing. The same imbalance occurs when you don't inflate your lungs fully on a regular basis. Exercise and higher intensity exercise naturally open up the lungs so you use more of its capacity, but if you don't use it you lose it. In this case, your ability to exchange air and blood flow to the outer portions of the lungs decreases. Breathing tempo techniques are a much gentler and more specific form of training for improving access to your full breathing capacity. The Haldane effect is the second part of the gas exchange puzzle at the lung-blood level. It describes how high or low oxygen content affects the rate of gas exchange at the lung-blood level. The Haldane effect is nothing you need to be concerned about when living normally at sea-level, but it becomes important at altitude, in the depths of the ocean, or if you have any damage to the structures of the cardio-respiratory systems (such as in emphysema or COPD).

Carbon dioxide pressure is the final pressure point in the system and perhaps the most important to your subconscious breath regulation. It is important for the exchange of gases at a cellular-blood level. Carbon dioxide, heat, lactate, and hydrogen are the by-products of cellular metabolism. The Bohr effect explains that a rise in pressure from either or all of these metabolites pushes carbon dioxide into the blood from the cell. The transfer of carbon dioxide into the blood also helps oxygen diffuse from the blood into the cell for further metabolism to occur.

Fluctuations in gas pressure at these three sites are signalled to the brain through various mechanisms in the body. The key players in the sensory system are central chemoreceptors, followed by peripheral chemoreceptors, joint, muscle, lung, pressure, pain, temperature, and irritant receptors. The information they send to the brain is combined with other information to then develop a co-ordinated breathing action. Your perception of safety or threat in the present moment, your perceived state of centre, and information from other organs in your body are three powerful pieces of information analysed by the brain to co-ordinate the allostatic breathing cycle. In this sense, breathing is not just governed by the respiratory system and the brain; rather, it is the result of the co-ordinated assessment of your life by your brain with a focus on your respiratory system. Having said that, of all the signals to the brain that govern breathing, the fluctuations in carbon dioxide are the most important. 'The most important factor in the control of ventilation [breathing] under normal conditions is the PCO_2 [partial pressure of carbon dioxide] of the arterial blood' (West, 2016). Adapted breathing patterns, then, occur when one or more aspects of breathing are acting from a state of perceived centre. This means you can't access parts of the breath to perform functions as you would like. The breath itself has changed from a natural, resting, caveman-like breath to a 'stressed breath' (lowered or heightened). It can be excessively fast or slow, large, or small; you may hold your breath, control your exhale, or be unable to take in a full breath. The adapted breathing pattern may be stuck in your chest or your belly. It may represent an aroused biological state or a suppressed state of being. From an observer's perspective, you can see adaptations in the breath mechanically and/or physiologically. I identify a perceived breathing centre simply as a change in carbon dioxide sensitivity (over-sensitive or under-sensitive) and/or as a negative change in the length/tension ratio in the breathing muscles. When any of these processes are ingrained into your breathing habitually, people usually present with a myriad of other adaptations in the body and brain. Emotions are suppressed, leading to emotional imbalances, and the immune system becomes over-worked and is perceived as weakened, chronic general inflammation, chronic disease states, mental ill-health issues, recurring injury, and an inability to perform your best are some of the common

EXERCISE VIDEO ANALYSIS

Before we begin, take a video of yourself breathing.

Lie down on your back. Place the camera side-on to you so you can see your whole torso, and your head and press record.

Inhale. Fill your belly, and your whole rib cage with air.

Then 'let go' of the exhale.

Repeat. Take 5-10 deep, full breaths.

Take a moment, roll onto your side, and sit up gently.

If you feel dizzy, simply stop, take a moment, roll onto your side, and sit up gently.

Take a notebook and jot down what you see in your breath before you move on. We'll analyse this video of your breath later in the chapter.

symptoms of adaptations when breathing from a perceived centre. Let's look at these adapted patterns and the symptoms they commonly manifest in my coaching experience. I'll begin with the mechanical adaptations, then move onto the physiological adaptations.

THE MECHANICAL BREATHING ADAPTATIONS

> *Breathing the first pattern lays the foundation for all the other succeeding patterns. Wherever the breathing is blocked in the body, future patterns will be blocked; wherever the breathing is free, the future patterns will develop efficiently.*
>
> **BONNIE BANBRIDGE COHEN**

Jill Miller is the founder of *Yoga Tune Up*, and another international expert on breathing. She is perhaps best known for her mapping of anatomy and breathing. In an interview, Jill introduced me to the concept of 'breathing zones', whereby the mechanics of breathing can be broken into three main zones. In her practice, Jill noticed that people were performing breathing techniques without realising the compounding effects of muscle recruitment on their breathing pattern. No matter what technique they chose, if the person used adapted breathing mechanics with the technique, it added to their chronic stress load, instead of reducing it. Jill teaches and familiarises her clients 'to be able to map all of the muscles of respiration and the interfaces of connection via the non-feeling respiratory diaphragm.' Through her research, Jill discovered that the diaphragm contains only nine muscle spindles, all located in the crura of the diaphragm. The lack of muscle spindles to contract and move makes it very difficult for you to feel where your diaphragm is in your living body. For this reason, Jill says the diaphragm has no sense of itself, which can be very frustrating when you're trying to breathe better. Feeling the diaphragm is achieved by approximation. By feeling the neighbouring tissues move, you can get a better sense of a moving diaphragm. With a better-moving diaphragm, you are in a prime position to reap the rewards of any breathing technique. Thus, the mechanics of breathing can be broken down into three zones.

Zone 1 breathing is deep into the belly, where you use the diaphragm and the lower ribs to breathe. It looks like you are breathing with your belly but, in reality, your belly moves as you inhale with your diaphragm and lower ribs. You could also change this breath pattern to breathe more laterally. In this case you'll still be using Zone 1 – your lower ribs flare but your belly doesn't rise. Zone 1 is mainly used with a subtle breath at rest, throughout the day and during periods of low-intensity exercise. Breathing higher up into the rib cage is *Zone 2* breathing. It is usually performed with Zone 1 breathing so that the breath looks like a wave through the body. Zone 2 is a 360° breath; as you change your posture from standing to lying on your side to all-fours, you should be able to access and breathe into all aspects of the rib cage. For example, if I lie on my left side and use a full exhale, I'll notice that my left rib cage rises and falls more than any other area of my body. Zone 2 breathing is important for suppleness in the body, quality movement patterns, and moderate and high-intensity exercise. You can also take a large breath into Zone 1 and 2 to calm the body with a large breath. *Zone 3* breathing is anything above your collar bone (supra-clavicular area, including the neck, face, tongue and mouth). Zone 3 breathing is used for specialised techniques and expressing the breath with your voice. Talking, shouting, humming, singing, crying, and laughing are some of the practical functions involving Zone 3 breathing. Extreme exercise and expressions of emotions such as fear use Zone 3 breathing in many cases. Your nose and mouth are used as vents with any zone of breathing. For the most part, nose breathing is associated with Zone 1 and 2 breathing, whilst the mouth is associated with Zone 3 breathing.

Up until my interview with Jill, I didn't realise that a part of the reason why quality breathing patterns are so rare is that you can't actually feel the diaphragm directly. The zones of breathing help people see, feel and recognise a quality breathing pattern versus an inefficient

PART 2   BREATH-ABILITY

ASSESSING YOUR BREATH WITH THE BREATH OF FREEDOM

Lie on your back, with your knees bent. Breathe ten deep and full breaths. As you breathe, ask yourself the following questions:

When Inhaling:

- Does your belly rise?
- Does your rib cage rise?
- Is there a smooth wave of belly to chest?

When Exhaling:

- Does the exhale 'let go'?
- Are the mouth, jaw and neck muscles relaxed on exhale?

You should have full access to the breath of freedom. As you inhale, your breath moves into Zone 1 first (belly), then Zone 2 fills (ribs rise 360°). Finally, all tension in the body is released with the exhale, particularly around Zone 3 (mouth, jaw, tongue, neck).

If you can do this breath, you now have the mechanical foundations to use your breath for performance in life and sport.

SCAN ME

one. The mechanical adaptions to breathing are then found within each of these zones or in the way the zones are used together.

In 2017, I travelled to the north of Ireland to visit a colleague, Oliver Cummings. Oliver is a fantastic sports preparation coach and trainer, one of the best in Ireland. He was hosting a Level 1 Raggi Method course, together with another great friend and mentor, Dr. Eric Serrano. The Raggi Method is a ten-level physical therapy and training course put together by the famous Italian physiotherapist and chiropractor Prof. Danielli Raggi. During the course, the Raggi instructors, Alex Mauri and Pasquale Silvestri, explained the critical role of the diaphragm in the posture and the strength of the kinetic chain. For the first time, I saw pictures of the diaphragm from cadaver studies and from many angles. It enlightened me on the role of breathing mechanics in posture, strength, gut health, cardiovascular health and mental health. It also provided me with tools to quickly restore Zone 1, diaphragmatic breathing.

At the same time as taking the course, I started working with an online client for breathing. Nick was his name. Nick presented with symptoms of sleep-disordered breathing, low energy, allergies, chronic fatigue and heart arrhythmia. His timeline of ailments was:

- 16 years ago – moved country
- 15 years ago – developed allergies
- 14 years ago – developed the heart arrhythmia
- Since then – poor sleep, chronic fatigue, and worsening of all health symptoms
- During that time, the medics performed three interventions on Nick to restore his heart rhythms. They essentially stopped his heart in the hope it would restart again normally (*this is a typical medical intervention for heart arrhythmia)

I was originally supposed to teach Nick the Buteyko method for his allergies, but as we reviewed his health history, it became apparent to me that he was in dire need of restoring his breathing mechanics.

PART 2 BREATH-ABILITY

With the all-clear from the instructors of the Raggi Method and Dr. Serrano, I taught Nick how to restore his diaphragm. Within two weeks, Nick's major symptoms had all but vanished. By the end of our training, his heart rhythm had normalised, his allergies were gone, he was sleeping better and he had the energy to go about his day. It was an unbelievable turnaround for Nick and another critical turning point for me in my understanding of the breath. Now I knew breathing had several roles to play in the body and I was beginning to really understand the effects of adapted breathing on every system in the body – lungs, heart, gut, posture and brain. I also understood that when we correct the breathing rhythm, it has an exponential knock-on effect on life and sports performance. For these reasons and more, breathing is the lynchpin of all systems in the body.

Four mechanical breathing adaptations to life affect the three zones of breathing. Each of these breathing adaptations can be experienced individually, or you may find your normal breathing pattern has a combination of them all. From a breathing perspective, the result of these adaptations is a long-term adapted breathing pattern – a lowered breath or a heightened breath, with a natural centre breath lying in the middle of these two extremes. We can develop any stage of these adapted breathing patterns depending on our life, its stimuli and how we perceive it.

Once the adaptation to a stress has occurred and you've ingrained the new breathing pattern into your system, your body re-orients itself around this new pattern. It becomes the new perceived centre. Areas that once worked fine 'fall asleep', or you lose your ability to feel the body interoceptively and proprioceptively. The video analysis exercise helps you to see patterns you cannot feel. Your whole biological system responds to the mechanical breathing adaptations allostatically; the chemistry of how we process oxygen changes; our posture finds its perceived centre; our ability to think clearly and concentrate is affected and eventually, it can lead to the modern human condition. The four mechanical breathing adaptions to life are: a retracted diaphragm, an immovable chest, a controlled exhale, and mouth breathing. Review the video of your breath analysis and consider what you see in light of these adaptations.

1. A RETRACTED DIAPHRAGM

Breathing into your chest, tight tissues, or pain in the body during this technique is an adapted Zone 2 breathing, where you can't access your Zone 1 breath easily. This type of breathing pattern classically presents as reverse or paradoxical breathing, where the chest inflates on a full breath but the belly does not. Think of a retracted diaphragm; it is like taking a pair of jeans out of a dryer. When we put on the jeans, they are stiff, and it is difficult to squat in them. This is the same for a retracted diaphragm. When we haven't moved the diaphragm for a while, for whatever reason, it can become difficult to move it naturally. Even if we try to breathe into it, we will find it difficult to move. We end up pushing out the abdominals and forcing movement, but a diaphragm should move naturally. I'll show you how to train the diaphragm in the training program. First let's understand what the diaphragm is and common reasons for it retracting.

ADAPTED ZONE 2 BREATHING

Review the video of yourself breathing from the last section.

- Does your belly expand and rise as you inhale?
- Moving on from the video:
- Are the muscle tissues stiff and hard if you stick your fingertips under your bottom ribs?
- Is there any pain as you hook your fingers under your ribs?

Give it a try but be gentle; if you experience sharp pains in the immediate area or in the abdomen, then reduce the pressure with your fingers.

PART 2 BREATH-ABILITY

The diaphragm is a very thin (2-4 mm), dome-shaped or jellyfish-like muscle that separates the chest from the abdomen. The tentacle-like crura of the diaphragm attach to the lumbar spine at L1- L3. Its medial border attaches onto the xiphoid process at the tip of the sternum and its lateral portions connect with the last six ribs. The diaphragm is one link in many chains of muscles running from the foot to the head. It has a special role to play in posture, movement, generating force in the body, and supporting almost every other system in the human body. Some of the main functions and connections of the diaphragm are:

1. It is the primary breathing muscle (together with the intercostals)
2. It is the only muscle that sits horizontally across the whole width of the body. This means that all vertical and spiral chains of muscles connecting the lower to upper body pass through it
3. It is connected to the spine and rib cage, providing posture and supporting movement throughout the body
4. It is part of a chain of muscles connecting the floor of the mouth, jaw, neck, chest, abdominal muscles and pelvic floor together. The rest of the chain moves with the diaphragm as one unit
5. It massages the heart and all abdominal organs with each excursion
6. The main arteries, veins and oesophagus (pipe connecting mouth to stomach) pass through the diaphragm. Movement of the diaphragm creates a peristaltic effect, or massaging effect, on these structures to help the flow of blood and food through the body
7. The vagus nerve passes through the diaphragm. This is the main nerve connecting heart, lungs and abdominal organs to the muscles of the inner ear, eyes, face, jaw and throat to the brain. It is important for relaying signals between the face and body, the body, face and brain. It plays a role in providing a safe and nurturing environment as well as promoting rest and digestion in the body
8. The phrenic nerve is a second cranial nerve linked to the diaphragm. It innervates the diaphragm. It also relays signals between

the heart, liver, gall bladder, throat, head, jaw, eyes, tongue, inner ear, and brain
9. It has a role to play in regulating the cardiovascular and lymph systems

When life affects the diaphragm, it retracts. The reduction in movement can have a wide and deep impact on the quality of your life. The diaphragm can lose function due to direct and indirect insults, such as injury to the ribcage (direct) or a respiratory virus (indirect). The knock-on effect of the retracted diaphragm can result in far-reaching consequences for the body. Some of the associated issues I have seen in my coaching practice with a retracted diaphragm include:

DIAPHRAGM INSULTS & CONSEQUENCES

Possible Insults on the Diaphragm

Underlying respiratory disease	Lack of exercise	Inability to express emotion
Virus, bacteria, or pathogen affecting the lungs, and the diaphragm in turn	Mouth breathing during childhood development, at rest, during sleep, and aerobic exercise	Feelings of not being good enough
		Highly reactive person
Injury to the lower ribs, stomach, neck, or lower spine	Bracing abs incessantly from training	Prone to anxiety and panic
		History of trauma
Injury or dysfunction in the nose	Too much poor-quality food and alcohol	

Possible Consequences for a Retracted Diaphragm*

Reverse breathing pattern	Finds it difficult to stay warm in cold temperatures	Experiences phantom pains
Reduced ventilation-perfusion ratio		Contributes to fibromyalgia and chronic pain syndromes
	Finds it difficult to sleep at night	
Heightened breathing pattern symptoms	Sleep is not restful	Tends to be wired and experience life as an emotional roller coaster
Altered CO_2 sensitivity	Wakes up during the night regularly	

continued

Possible Consequences for a Retracted Diaphragm*

Mouth breathing	Needs to go to the toilet at night regularly	Contributes to racing and incessant thought patterns, anxiety, panic, and depression
Feelings of breathlessness	Pelvic floor issues, especially in females	Reduced ability to focus intensely
Inability to breathe full breaths	Hormone 'dysregulation', especially in females	Poor concentration level
Contribution to chronic sinus-respiratory disease (asthma, bronchitis, sinusitis etc.)	Weakened spine stability	Dry eyes
Recurring chest infections	Long-term lower back pain	Weakened immune function
Reduced breathing capacity	Reduced mid-back mobility and upper limb mobility	Contributes to GERD, bloating and digestive issues
Suffers with the second wind in sport	Adapted proprioception and balance abilities	Haemorrhoids and faecal elimination issues
Endurance is lower than potential	Contributes to recurring hamstring and lower body musculo-skeletal injuries	Adapted interoceptive signals
Recovery may be low		Adapted perception of safety and love
Finds it difficult to brace under load	Contributes to heart arrhythmia, high, or low blood pressure	Reduced ability to relate and communicate effectively to others
Hands and feet are often cold	Racing or lowered heart rate	

*A retracted diaphragm may not be solely responsible for these consequences but can play a significant role in these body adaptations. My experience is supported by (neuro) anatomical associations, the experience of other practitioners and some research.

2. THE INFLEXIBLE RIBCAGE

Believe it or not, some people breathe mainly into their stomach and lower ribs, with little movement in their chest. The ribs don't rise and fall so well, they don't flare out to the side and if you were lying on your belly, it would be hard to feel any air move into your mid-back. Can you see it in your own breath? This is a less well-known but important adaptation of breathing. It is a Zone 1 breath with no ability to access Zone 2 breathing. Just like with a retracted diaphragm, when we inhale into our chest, we may find it moves very little or not at all in this adaptation. Usually, I find an inflexible ribcage to be an exaggerated adaptation to the retracted diaphragm, but sometimes it can be inflexible all on its own. The inflexible ribcage is an external 360° view of rib cage movement during breathing. We are looking at the mobility of all joints, bones, cartilage, muscles and fascia throughout the thoracic region, excluding the diaphragm and the lower three ribs.

Twelve ribs, and their attachments, form the basis of the ribcage around the thorax. Each rib attaches to a corresponding thoracic vertebra on the spine, and to the sternum via cartilage at the front. This is known as the costal arc. There are more than eighty joints in total in the rib cage, making it a very flexible structure, much like the spine, hand or foot. The bones, and more so, the cartilage, are very flexible in the rib cage. The costal arc of the individual ribs and the rib cage expands in all directions with each inhalation, and shrinks during exhalation. The spine then serves as a solid base of support for the ribs and links between different body regions for breathing. It connects the chains of fascia from the feet, lower limbs, pelvic floor and abdominal areas through the diaphragm and ribcage to the hands and head. Its movement, especially at the thoracic region, should complement the movement of respiration and the ribcage.

During spinal extension, the sternum rises and the thorax is moved into an inhalation position. During flexion, the spine rounds, the sternum drops, and the thorax moves into exhalation. During side-bending, the ribs close on the concave side of the spine, and open on the convex

PART 2   BREATH-ABILITY

BREATHING EXERCISE TO HELP RESTORE ZONE 2 BREATHING

Take a rolled-up yoga mat or a pillow. Lie on your side. Place a hand on the upper side ribs and breathe full breaths. Can you feel the breath flow into your upper ribs?

Then change sides and feel the same.

Next, move into an all-fours position on your hands and knees. Curl your body over like you are squashing your head to your pelvic floor. Breathe into your mid-back (the bra-strap area for females). Can you feel it move?

Breathing into the sides of your ribs and into your back is all a part of good quality Zone 2 breathing.

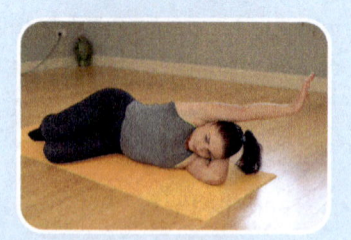

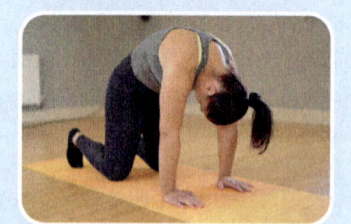

SCAN ME   SCAN ME

> **BREATHING EXERCISE ZONE 3 AWARENESS**
>
> Look into a mirror and observe your breath.
>
> Open your mouth wide and inhale big breaths. What do you notice?
>
> Can you feel tension in the mouth and jaw as the muscles are stretched open?
>
> Do you feel the neck muscles working and the upper chest filling?
>
> Can you feel how shallow the breath is?
>
> Does your throat become dry?
>
> Does the breath irritate you?
>
> This is Zone 3 breathing in its fullest expression.

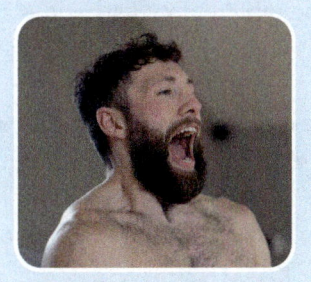

side. During spinal rotation in the thoracic region, the ribs and lungs are twisted in opposite directions. These are the standard combinations of movement and breathing throughout this region of the body. You can, of course, change the breathing pattern with movement to open up areas of the ribs that may have been closed. Inhaling with a flexed spine and dropped sternum, for example, will restrict your ability to breathe deeply into your ribs (low down) but it will open up your breathing in the mid-back of the body. Movement of the head, shoulder blades, arms, pelvis, and lower limbs, will impact your breathing too. This is something for you to play around with after you have mastered the basics of breathing and moving your spine/rib cage. There are so many little nuances and variations to breathing and movement affecting this area that it is too much to write about in this book. For the same reason, I am not naming the muscles and explaining their relationship to breathing. Rather than view the body from an anatomist's perspective, I want you to see it from the observer's viewpoint. When there is little movement in the chest as you watch it breathing full breaths, the chest, and the ribcage are considered to be inflexible. The costal arc of the ribs doesn't move so well, the spine is more rigid, and the muscles in the region can't fully lengthen and contract. Breathing is dampened, and with it the ability to upregulate your nervous system. This has a particular effect on regulating emotions. The brain finds it difficult to assess the safety of a situation, create strong social bonds and communicate effectively with others. With this breathing pattern, a conflict between body and brain can arise where a person loses their personal power and sense of confidence. The table below lists some associated insults and consequences for an inflexible chest:

RIB CAGE EVENT + RESPONSE
Possible Reasons for an Inflexible Rib Cage at Rest
Injury to C-Spine, T-Spine, ribs, sternum, or associated structures
History of (childhood) trauma
Hormone imbalances from a transitionary period in life (i.e. puberty or mid-life), or an adapted hormonal system
Lack of purpose in one's life
Lack of meaningful activities in one's life
Feelings of shame or guilt
Suppressed emotions
Introverted personality type
Depressed state of mind

continued

Possible Consequences an Inflexible Rib Cage at Rest	
Reverse breathing pattern	Finds it difficult to brace under load
Retracted diaphragm is common	
CO_2 sensitive	Hands and feet are often cold
Common nasal dysfunctions, such as adenoids and polyps	Finds it difficult to stay warm in cold temperatures
Exacerbated respiratory diseases	
Allergies	Finds it difficult to cope in hot temperatures
Anxiety and panic attacks are common	Finds it difficult to sleep at night
Suffers with the second wind in sport	Sleep is not restful
Endurance may be affected	Wakes up during the night regularly
Recovery may be slow	

3. THE CONTROLLED EXHALE

The exhale should naturally flow from the inhale in a resting breath. It is innately relaxed, helping to promote further relaxation throughout the body and mind. I think of the exhale like a coil springing out from the contraction of the inhale. The exhale has special functions to produce sound, express emotion, communicate, expel air forcefully from the body (coughing, sneezing, hiccupping, panting and crying) and tighten the fascial chain to produce more mechanical force. This is a quality use of Zone 3 breathing. An adapted Zone 3 breath occurs when you subconsciously hold the top of the inhale to make it look like an apex or you constrict the resting exhale (partially or fully); you disturb the natural flow of the breath and relaxation in body and mind. The throat and jaw muscles are tightened with every exhale in your (approximately) 21,600 breaths per day, when they should be relaxed, released and 'let go'. These partial occlusions of the exhale can dramatically affect pain in your body and have significant consequences for your sense of safety, confidence, and ability to regulate and express emotions. A constricted exhale has such powerful effects on your body because of the location of the upper airways, their connections to other structures and their roles throughout the rest of the body.

The upper airways of the respiratory system are in the same area of the body as the C-spine, throat, neck, shoulders, jaw and head. All structures in this area have a direct role to play in respiratory anatomy. They are also connected together neuro-anatomically and mechanically through the body's fascia.

A controlled exhale is executed by constricting the vocal cords, and the neck muscles connecting the head to the shoulders. The upper chest, upper back and shoulder muscles are all involved in a constricted exhale (depending on the level of constriction). These muscles were designed as secondary and tertiary breathing muscles, not primary muscles. Over time, these constricted exhales re-wire our brain to continuously squeeze the upper chest, back, neck and jaw. Overusing these muscles in breathing can lead to migraines, jaw pain, grinding teeth, earaches, and neck, shoulder, and upper back pain.

The area of the C-spine and larynx is also particularly important for the effective communication of nerve impulses between body and brain. Both the vagus and phrenic nerves exit the spinal cord between C5-C7 in the neck to relay messages between the lungs, heart, abdominal organs and brain. These two nerves also combine neuro-anatomically with the other cranial nerves in the face and neck (eyes, jaw, throat, inner ear, tongue and facial muscles) to signal to the brain states of freeze, flight, rest and digest. When the signals are unclear the body moves to a perceived centre and typically presents as a heightened breathing pattern. The table on the next page lists some of the common causes and consequences of ingraining a controlled exhale into your resting breath pattern.

THE WAY THE BREATH WORKS

CONTROLLED EXHALE EVENT + RESPONSE

Possible Reasons for a Controlled Exhale at Rest

Chronic high levels of perceived stress which you can't cope with
Underlying respiratory diseases
Injury to the lower ribs or diaphragm
Injury or dysfunction in the nose
Uncontrollable outbursts of anger often
Tendency to greed and gluttony
Little emotional connection to your impact on other's lives
Desire to control life, especially those areas out of your control
High achiever tendencies
Goal-oriented
Highly analytical
Dominant personality

Possible Consequences of a Controlled Exhale at Rest✽

Sometimes has a reverse breathing pattern	Regular migraines
Possible retracted diaphragm	Always 'switched on'
Reduced breathing capacity	Energy fluctuates throughout the day
Respiratory disease is common	Finds it difficult to sleep at night
Performance anxiety is common	Sleep is not restful
Likely to suffer a panic attack in highly stressful situations	Wakes up during the night regularly
Regular pain in the upper back, shoulder, neck, and jaw	Exercises a lot
Reduced mobility in the upper limbs	Tries to push the body and the mind to its perceived limit

4. MOUTH BREATHING AT REST

Mouth breathing is acceptable as a short-term, caveman, response to acute stress. It helps to express emotion through the voice, communicate, and regulate our energy systems when pushed to the limits. Subconscious mouth breathing at rest is a different animal. It is an adapted breathing pattern of Zone 3 to a myriad of stressors over a long period of time. Our biological self will only mouth breathe at rest when it's under so much pressure that it needs to 'vent off' that pressure. If you mouth breathe as a child, it affects the development of your anatomy and your health for the rest of your life. According to some writers, dating back as far as 1882, mouth breathing at night is the last sign before developing major lifestyle diseases such as altered postures, sleep problems, mental illness problems, pain, disease, and early death. One thing I've noticed in the breathing and coaching industry is that people blame a lack of nose breathing for the resulting mouth breathing. I haven't found that to be the sole case in my coaching practice. Over the last twenty years, in particular, the mechanisms for developing mouth breathing and its impact on the rest of the body are being teased out by combining many areas of interest together. Breathing experts, myofunctional therapists, dentists, orthodontists, anthropologists, neuroanatomists, neurobiologists, psychologists, sleep specialists, medical doctors and authors have all contributed to the body of knowledge of how mouth breathing manifests and its resulting consequences for the body. Of all the adaptations to breathing, mouth breathing at rest has perhaps the most powerful negative impact on the rest of your health and performance.

BREATHING EXERCISE NOTICE THE DIFFERENCE BETWEEN NOSE AND MOUTH BREATHING

Breathe through your nose for one minute. What do you notice?

- Is your mouth dry or damp?
- Do you breathe Zone 1, 2, or 3?
- Is there a lot of tension in your muscles or are they relaxed?
- Do you feel relaxed or anxious?

Now, open your mouth wide and breathe through it for one minute. What do you notice now? Is there a difference?

Unlike the nose, there is no filter or humidifier for air when inhaling through your mouth. All that polluted, dirty air from car fumes, cigarettes, paint fumes, industry and burning fossil fuels is inhaled straight into your lungs. In 1882, George Catlin likened it to drinking dirty pond water. The lungs also do not have much of a filtration system for air and so they easily become clogged up. Coughing, sneezing, allergies, adenoids, rhinitis and sinusitis are common complaints of mouth breathers. If you develop mouth breathing as a child it can lead to reduced airway size, craniofacial changes, forward head posture and crooked teeth. Mouth breathing tends to lead to a reverse breathing pattern. The ventilation-perfusion ratio decreases and oxygen is less easily absorbed into the blood stream. The diaphragm commonly retracts with mouth breathing, leading to its own problems. And finally, carbon dioxide is expelled out of your body with less stringent controls. Carbon dioxide sensitivity increases and oxygen is delivered to your cells less efficiently. With the body working harder to get oxygen in your cells to make energy, your whole body suffers the consequences.

Mouth breathing at rest is known as a stressful breathing pattern. The dry mouth is a sign of a sympathetically driven nervous system that alerts the body to action. The mouth, jaw and neck muscles are used much more in mouth breathing. This creates tension in this area, but also through the kinetic chains of the entire body. If you were to ingrain a variation of this pattern into your normal life, you would be ingraining a stressed state for the body, mind and spirit by default.

Combine this inefficient breathing pattern with the rest of your modern lifestyle. High-calorie, nutrient-deficient foods, GMO, synthetic foods and alcohol provide a huge additional load to the body's work rate. This is before we mention lack of meaningful activities in life, lack of purpose, trauma, highly stressful careers, commuting, Wi-Fi, technology, lack of exercise, overheating and a sedentary indoor way of living. Each of these common lifestyle ingredients impacts our breath. Together they overload our system resulting in mouth breathing; it is the natural way our body copes with modern life. Chronic pain, anxiety, nasal dysfunction, respiratory disease, gut issues, sleep problems, cardiovascular disease and immune dysfunctions are all expected consequences for people who chronically mouth breathe at rest. Here's a quick rundown of the common insults leading to mouth breathing and the effects of mouth breathing on the rest of your body:

MOUTH BREATHING EVENT + RESPONSE	
Possible Reasons for Mouth Breathing at Rest	
Bottle-fed as a baby	Unresolved injury to the body, especially the C-spine, and nose
Eating soft foods	
Too many calories from food	Structural problems with the nose
Food quality is poor	History of trauma
Food allergies and intolerances	A-type personality – always on the go
Poor sleep habits	Nervousness, anxiety, and panic
Lack of exercise, and too much mindless intense exercise	Inability to cope with fear
Alcohol, drugs, and smoking	Inability to cope with high stress levels
Living in a city	May be a high achiever or someone with great potential who is an underachiever
Air pollution	
Genetic susceptibility to a respiratory disease	
	Appears super confident, but may actually lack confidence
	'Poor me' attitude – everything happens against them, not for them
	Continuously sick

MOUTH BREATHING EVENT + RESPONSE
Possible Consequences of Mouth Breathing at Rest

Reverse breathing pattern	Needs to go to the toilet at night regularly
Retracted diaphragm is common	Bed wetting in children is common
CO_2 sensitive	Usually has crooked teeth, narrowed airways, and forward head posture if mouth breathing at rest as a child
Common nasal dysfunctions, such as adenoids and polyps	
Exacerbated respiratory diseases	Chronic pain throughout the body
Allergies	Pain sensitive
Anxiety and panic attacks are common	TMJ, neck, shoulder, and upper back pain
Suffers with the second wind in sport	Migraines
Endurance may be affected	Menstrual cycle, and pelvic floor issues for women
Recovery may be slow	E.D. is common for men
Finds it difficult to brace under load	Lack of sex drive
Hands and feet are often cold	Reduced ability to have a successful pregnancy
Finds it difficult to stay warm in cold temperatures	
Finds it difficult to cope in hot temperatures	Cardiovascular issues as you age
	Gut issues
Finds it difficult to sleep at night	Low immune function
Sleep is not restful	Reduced ability to focus
Wakes up during the night regularly	Poor concentration levels
	Finds it hard to retain information

THE PHYSIOLOGICAL BREATHING ADAPTATIONS

> *The theory of life, in brief, is such that carbon dioxide is the basic nutrition of every life form of Earth – if it disappears there will be no life on Earth. It acts as the main regulator of all functions in the organism; it is the main internal environment of the organism; it is the vitamin of all vitamins*
>
> DR. K.P. BUTEYKO

BREATHING EXERCISE

Provided it is safe to do so – you are not pregnant, you don't have epilepsy and you're not driving a car or operating heavy machinery – perform twenty big and fast mouth breaths and see what happens to you.

Big and fast breathing blows off carbon dioxide from your lungs. If you perform it for long enough you can change the pH of your blood, generate adrenaline, and prepare your body for action.

Quite often, your heart rate shoots up, you become dizzy and perhaps you develop some tingling sensations in the body when you breathe big and fast for a period of time, with no action being taken. The temperature of your hands may change and you get an over-riding sense of lightness and energy in you. This is the result of more carbon dioxide being dumped from your body by your big and fast breathing together with the change of pH and increased secretion of the stress hormone epinephrine (adrenaline). But with no action being taken, you create a false alarm for the body. Just like the boy who cried wolf in the children's tale, there is a cost to asking your body to be on alert when you are not going to use it. In the tale, the people stopped listening to the boy. In your breath, your brain dampens its response to a rise in CO_2. The long-term repercussion for the boy in the tale was

> that the people of the village never came to help him when a wolf did come and eat his sheep. In the case of breathing, your brain becomes hypersensitive to CO_2 and when you need to buffer the CO_2 during times of action, stress, panic and fear, you won't be able to handle it.

At its core, breathing is a physiological process. The job of the respiratory system is to inhale air, filter it, send oxygen to the cells that require it and then expel carbon dioxide through the various pressure-exchanging processes. The internal physiological process of exchanging oxygen and carbon dioxide is fundamental to the health and wellbeing of the human body, just as much as digestion or movement. Most people think the primary function of breathing is to take more oxygen into our system. This is not entirely accurate. True, we need oxygen in our cells for metabolism, but the primary stimulus to breathe is not a lack of oxygen, rather, too much carbon dioxide.

Air contains 21% oxygen at sea level and with any given breath we only extract 3-3.5% oxygen from that air. When working hard during exercise, we extract 6-7% oxygen. It's not much, right? We also know that we can get oxygen from our lungs and into our blood very easily. A simple home pulse-oximeter monitor will tell us our blood is almost always fully saturated at 96-98% oxygen. This means we have plenty of oxygen in our blood. If we didn't, then we would usually have an underlying virus, or respiratory disease, or we would have moved to altitude. Other than that, we almost always have enough oxygen in our blood. The issue with breathing arises when we can't get enough oxygen from our blood to our cells. And here is where carbon dioxide comes into play.

Carbon dioxide (CO_2) is a by-product of cellular metabolism. Any time a cell has work to do in your body, it produces CO_2 along with water, heat, lactate and hydrogen ion. A rise in CO_2 is our first stimulus to breathe because a build-up of too much CO_2 is sensed as harmful to the body. High CO_2 levels elevate the acidity of the blood. Blood acidity measured by pH is a very tightly regulated homeostatic process and so the brain wants to reduce acidity quickly. It does this by detecting small changes in CO_2 and then exhaling excess CO_2.

However, having enough CO_2 is also vital important to your system. Dissolved CO_2 helps the delivery of oxygen to the cells. Without enough dissolved CO_2 in the blood, oxygen can't get to our cells and our metabolism begins to suffer. A balance of CO_2 is what is required.

Think of CO_2 as a chaperone to oxygen

Carbon dioxide is not just a waste product. Excess CO_2 is, however, our primary stimulus to breathe. It's the rise in CO_2 which signals the brain to signal to the diaphragm to contract. It's a rise in CO_2 that elicits pain signals in the body's skin and tissues of the body. It's CO_2 (with heat) that helps deliver oxygen to the cells for metabolic work to occur. It's CO_2 that plants use in their lifecycle to provide us with oxygen for our lives to be sustained. Like lactate, heat and difficult-to-digest foods, CO_2 is not a bad thing; it is not solely a waste product; rather, excess quantities are harmful to us, and adequate quantities are necessary to sustain our life and perform better in sport.

Physiologically, we need enough CO_2 for three reasons:

1. Dissolved CO_2 delivers more oxygen to the cells
2. CO_2 regulates blood pH
3. Normal amounts of CO_2 in the brain dampen neuron excitability

THE HIGH SIDE OF BREATHING

Hyperventilation is a breathing pattern disorder defined as 'breathing more than our metabolic needs'. It is a long-term, subconscious breathing pattern – a habit. Its effects on our system are different to the specialised supra-ventilation techniques of breathing. Normal breathing is considered to be a volume of five to six litres of air per minute, or twelve to fifteen breaths per minute (bpm). Chronic hyperventilation for the general population would, therefore, be considered to be breathing more than fifteen breaths per minute. Having said that, some texts cite a breath rate of more than 25 bpm and others 30 bpm as hyperventilation. The exaggerated breathing depth and rate associated with hyperventilation syndrome eliminates CO_2 at a faster pace, resulting in low blood CO_2, a rise in blood pH, and respiratory alkalosis. Many patients present with multiple symptoms. However, medical tests and physical examination may reveal nothing out of the ordinary.

Chronic hyperventilation is linked with many adapted states in the body and disease states. In the 1800s, Da Costa associated over one hundred ailments with chronic hyperventilation. In the 1950s, Dr. Buteyko identified one hundred and fifty-plus diseases connected to over-breathing. Researchers have repeatedly shown that long-term hyperventilation has negative consequences for your body and mind. Here is a table of some of the ailments associated with chronic hyperventilation.

Respiratory	Musculo-skeletal	Neurological	Cardiac	Psychic
Breathlessness	Pain / fatigue	Dizziness	Chest pain	Impaired thinking
Pseudo-asthma		Headaches	Arrhythmia	
Dry cough	↑ Lactate	Fainting	Palpitations	Panic
Sighing	Myalgia	Tingling	Erratic heart rate	Sweating
Yawning	↑ Muscle tone	Hallucinations		Anxiety
'Air hunger'		Sleep disturbance	↑ BP	Urination
Upper chest breathing	Cramps		Light-headedness	Diarrhoea
	Weakness	Bad dreams		Constipation
Snoring	Chronic exhaustion	Giddiness		Depression
Chest tightness		Irritability		
		Apprehension		

Adapted from the book: Recognizing and Treating Breathing Disorders. A Multidisciplinary Approach. D. Bradley & C. Gilbert (2014)

PART 2   BREATH-ABILITY

As you can see, these are system-wide allostatic effects from the habit of over-breathing, affecting both body and mind. It effects the respiratory, cardiovascular, neurological, psychic, and muscular systems. Remember, there is no separation in us. When one system is adapted, all systems adapt. It just so happens that breathing plays a pivotal role in the centre of our biological system and so when it develops adapted habits, our whole system adjusts to compensate for it.

BREATHING EXERCISE

Begin in a standing posture. Inhale air fully into your body. As you fill your lungs, don't exhale fully, instead, keep 'topped up' with air by exhaling a little and pumping more air in.

As you lead with your breath, follow with your body.

You'll notice yourself assuming a very tall, erect and over-arched posture.

The hands and arms rotate outwards and you become like an over-extended ballerina.

Now think of those words – 'over-extended', 'topped up' – and then think of their meaning.

If you are posturally over-extended, what might that also mean for your psyche and your lifestyle?

Are you over-reaching in life, active the whole time, always switched on?

Remember, your breath reflects your reality and your reality is reflected in your breath.

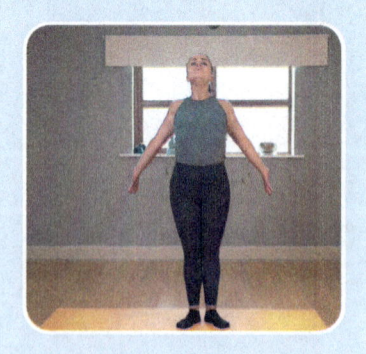

THE HYPERVENTILATION THEORY

If we develop the habit of chronically over-breathing and the levels of CO_2 chronically drop below 5%, the brain lowers the threshold for breathing; it signals the diaphragm to breathe in more air with a lower threshold. In laboratories this is known as CO_2 sensitivity or as lowering the CO_2 threshold in training circles. Release of oxygen from haemoglobin and its diffusion across the blood cell barrier becomes difficult. It gives us the feeling of needing more air but in reality, we have enough air, we have enough oxygen in the system; but we do not have enough dissolved CO_2 in the system. A few things happen in the system due to chronically lowered CO_2. The first is that the renal system is called upon to perform more work and balance the pH of the blood. The second is that the body lowers the CO_2 threshold. The brain becomes more sensitive to a rise in CO_2 levels and responds by maintaining lower levels of CO_2 in the system. A cycle of chronic, low-level hyperventilation becomes set into the brain. Dr. Buteyko hypothesised that hyperventilation resulted in a plethora of diseases, including asthma, hypertension, diabetes, anxiety, sleep-disordered breathing, panic, and over a hundred more disorders. This cycle has several implications for sports people too.

JUST A THEORY

One of the shortfalls of the hyperventilation theory is that the mechanisms of how it relates to disease states are unproven – it is still a theory. A few researchers have tested the idea and found it doesn't hold up to the rigors of scientific testing. Doctors, in general, don't seem to like the theory. And yet, at the same time, practitioners who use methods based on it can get phenomenal results with their clients. Doctors and researchers in completely different fields have discovered the effects of hyperventilation specific to their own field: Da Costa, Dr. Claude Lum, and Dr. Buteyko, to name the most notable researchers.

During the 1950s, Dr. Buteyko was one of the key medical doctors to piece together the mechanisms of the hyperventilation theory. His whole method is built on the hyperventilation theory. By reducing our breathing with relaxation, performing some breath holding techniques and including decent posture, we can re-train our body to breathe calmly and symptoms reduce or are eliminated entirely. Dr. Buteyko used his method to cure his own fatal diagnosis of high blood pressure. He also used it to treat diabetes, asthma and many other diseases of hyperventilation in others. During the 1990s and early 2000s there were three clinical trials in the West on the effects of the Buteyko Method on asthma. The results of all three clinical trials support the effects of this method. All of them showed a significant reduction in asthma medication. The method was recommended by the Russian, British, Australian and New Zealand healthcare systems as an adjunct training program for people with asthma as a result of these trials. However, there is still little appetite and awareness for it amongst general practitioners.

At the end of the day, Dr. Buteyko's method works. It produced significant results in three clinical trials, and has been reported anecdotally to work for thousands of other people internationally. It has worked for me. However, it is not for everybody. I have taught the method to hundreds of clients over the last six years and I must say in that time, I've found at least 60%-70% of people do not apply the method as recommended. When asked why clients don't follow the recommendations, it usually comes down to one of two things:

1. They don't like the techniques – it brings up feelings of anxiety and panic, and so these clients stop almost immediately
2. Clients train hard and gain great results, but then they get comfortable, life gets in the way, they reduce the training, and stop altogether before they've improved their breathing system enough to re-pattern a natural breathing state

The lack of long-term application for many clients set me off on the path of discovering other techniques in breathing and finding out how

I can help people best. Even today, I believe the tenets of the Buteyko method are on point: create a habit of calm nasal breathing at rest and promote quality movement of the breath. In the intervening years, I've found the method of Dr. Buteyko might not be suitable for everyone, and I have also found that there are other, more effective ways which deliver results to many types of people. Many roads lead to Rome, as they say. The most notable discovery I've made in my coaching career is that hyperventilation plays a major role in adapted breathing patterns. However, it is not the only factor. All aspects of adapted breathing need to be re-centred for the person to breathe freely and bring calm to their biological system. From that point, we can use specialised breathing techniques to perform at our best in life and sport.

THE LOW SIDE OF BREATHING

The opposite of breathing more than normal is to breathe less than normal, or hypoventilation. There are hypoventilation techniques, and there are hypoventilation patterns, just as with the hyperventilation side of the continuum.

Generally, hypoventilation breathing techniques are deemed to be beneficial for everybody. They are the most researched form of breathing technique and the most prevalent. Any form of breath-holding techniques or reduced breathing technique is a form of hypoventilation. As a breathing pattern, this is thought to be just as detrimental to health, especially in people suffering from cardio-metabolic syndrome, a host of diseases such as obstructive sleep apnoea, insulin resistance, glucose intolerance, high blood pressure, and central obesity. In 2021, Sikter proposed his theory that social defeat combined with hypercapnia (high CO_2) can cause changes in people's behaviours and habits that can lead to chronic disease. Social defeat is an insult arising from chronic stress or trauma. It is a different stress response to the more commonly known fight and flight system, which I've spoken so much about. This is the other side of the stress coin. This type of stress involves a parasympathetic nervous system phenomenon. It relates to our safety, love and meaning in life. Children may be susceptible to it with parental attachment difficulties or if they suffer a trauma early in life. It occurs in adults when a person accepts life's hardships as they are, and gives up hope for a better life. Hypercapnia is the result of breathing less and regular subconscious breath-holding. Combining this spiritual defeat with hypercapnia changes people's behaviour, posture and breathing. This is a similar human condition to the low autonomic arousal and lowered breathing patterns we saw earlier in the Red-Light-Reflex. According to Sikter (2017) this is a significant problem for the Western world. The proportion of people who chronically hypoventilate significantly increases beyond the age of 50, reaching almost half the population by 60 years of age. In 2022, he

BREATHING EXERCISE

Begin in a standing posture.

Just like a balloon deflating from the release of air, exhale all the air out of your body. Follow the breath with the movement of your body. Your body will eventually curl over into the foetal position.

Inhale small breaths and exhale fully each time, without strain.

After 2 minutes, notice how you feel in this bent-over posture and breathing pattern.

It's depressing, right?

A deflated breath is also a deflated psyche. Long-term suppression of emotions and breathing can be seen in your posture and breathing patterns.

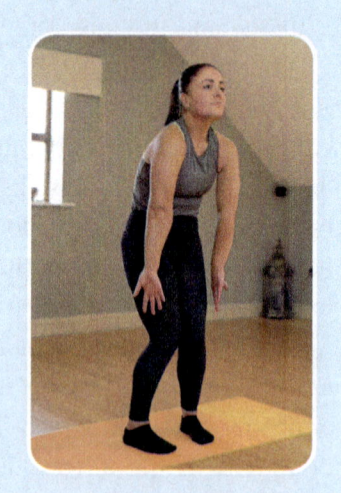

proposed that hypoventilation is the beginning of sleep apnoea. Sleep apnoea then leads to the host of cardiovascular and metabolic diseases which have plagued our modern lives.

According to Sikter (2021), there is no tested solution to this theory yet. Sikter again proposes that a diet rich in alkaline foods, an increase in exercise and a reduction in partial pressure arterial CO_2 (PCO_2) may improve the condition: all the normal recommendations for a 'healthy lifestyle'. To reduce PCO_2, he suggests taking bicarbonate of soda and controlling the regulation of CO_2 but, he says this is impossible to manage safely. From a mechanistic perspective I can see how he would think so. However, rebalancing PCO_2 is possible with breath training. Breathing is the primary regulator of PCO_2. Where breath-holding techniques and reduced breathing may not work for this type of person initially, supra-ventilating for short periods of time may bring the breathing system back into balance and with it the PCO_2. This is where a broader knowledge and experience with breathing becomes effective. As a coach, it is insufficient to know just one method in breathing; instead we have to dive into the principles of breathing and

HYPOVENTILATION

Likely Causes of Hypoventilation	Consequences of Hypoventilation
Trauma at any stage in life, especially as a child	Postural changes
Attachment issues with caregiver as a child	Low autonomic arousal
Low autonomic arousal	Loss of drive for life
Burnout resulting in depressive states	Feelings of hopelessness
States of mental ill-health	Mental ill-health including but not limited to anxiety, panic, and depression
Lack of meaning in life	
Loss including loved ones, animals, career, identity	

come up with a broader perspective on life. With the breath training, it may also be important to enhance those other qualities of a healthy lifestyle, such as safety, finding meaning in life, exercise, healthy nutrition, and the rest.

> ### GEM #3 THE MAJOR ROLES OF BREATHING
>
> Balancing oxygen and carbon dioxide gases for quality cellular health and energy; massaging the organs of the thorax for quality cardiac and gut health; providing strength to the kinetic chain; and supporting the brain in the processes of concentration and mental-emotional processing are the four major roles of breathing in the body.
>
> Breathing mechanics, physiology, and the mental-emotional sides of breathing are all important factors to consider when restoring your breath. If you decide not to address any one area, then you will never be able to fully utilise your breath.

CONNECTING THE BREATH WITH SPECIFIC DISEASE 8

Without a doubt, genetic factors play a role in the diseases we develop, and people with different genetic profiles are affected differently by lifestyle. There is nothing we can do about our genes. Our lifestyle, however, we have almost complete control over. Change your lifestyle, and you can change your life. And breathing is the most fundamental aspect of lifestyle change.

Adapted breathing impacts everything. If you are not breathing naturally, it will have negative implications for each and every system of your body. The most common consequences are on posture, pain, physiology, anatomy, sleep, emotional states, cardiovascular system, sexual desire, obesity, and the gastrointestinal and immune systems. In this section, I will dive into each of those systems and show you how an adapted breathing pattern can negatively impact that system. As you read this section, remember that breathing and lifestyle are multi-directional factors in your health. I say that breathing impacts the lifestyle/disease state; I could as easily say it the other way around too. Which came first – the chicken or the egg? Who knows? But what we do know is that when you change your breathing, you influence the lifestyle and disease state. You move yourself back towards the natural centre and put yourself in a position to perform in life and sport at your best. After addressing your breathing, your next step may be to address another area of life to benefit your system as a whole. Eventually, you meet with the success you seek.

BREATHING, POSTURE AND MOVEMENT

Respiration and physical activity are a unified process

VLADIMIR VASILIEV

EXERCISE

Lie on your back.

Inhale slowly and fully. Arch your lower back, open your legs, spread your toes, rotate your arms out, splay your fingers and tuck your chin. This is one, single, expanded movement of the human body.

Exhale, flatten your back, close your knees, squeeze your feet, rotate your arms in, close your fists and lift your chin. This is a second, contracted whole-body movement of the body.

Play with these positions five or six times each to feel them. Then perform other whole-body movements like squatting, rotating or hanging and feel how the breath moves with the body.

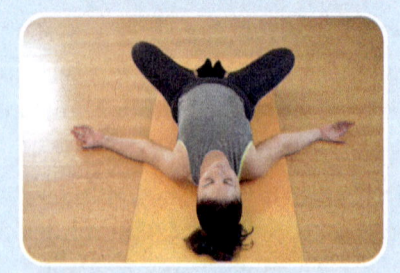

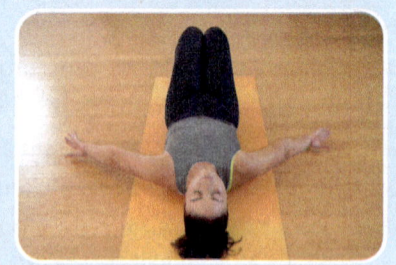

Breathing is movement. They are inseparable. We, the professionals in the industry, just separate them to help us understand each aspect, but we always have to remember to re-integrate the whole. On average we breathe 12-15 times per minute, 810 times per hour, 19,440 times per day or 7 million times per year. Each time we breathe, we inhale and we exhale. Inhalation is performed primarily by a concentric contraction of the diaphragm coupled with movement from the intercostal muscles. Exhalation is the recoil of those muscles during periods of rest and low activity. During exertion, the muscles of the abdominals, upper chest, neck and shoulders are the primary movers. During exertion the diaphragm eccentrically contracts; the abdominals and the muscles of the abdominal region concentrically contract on an exhale. Together with this movement, the breathing muscles also play a role in moving the spine, creating posture and moving the human body. With every breath, the body moves and with seven million breaths a year, this results in a lot of movement. When the breathing system is adapted, it has powerful effects on the rest of the body. Breathings impact on movement may be viewed from different perspectives. Here I will focus on the broad mechanical and physiological impacts on movement.

THE MECHANICAL IMPACTS OF ADAPTED BREATHING

EXERCISE

Begin in a seated posture.

Exhale, and continue to exhale until you can't any more.

As you exhale allow the rest of your body to follow. Squeeze the muscles and move the body naturally with the forced exhale. Where does the body go?

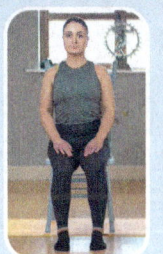

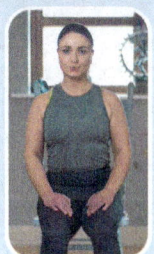

Do you see a pattern? The exhale folds the body over, internally rotates and pronates everything. From the head to the hands and the toes; this is the Red-Light-Reflex we described earlier. When you exaggerate the Red-Light-Reflex to its final point, it looks like you're in a very protected, closed-down, foetal position. The significance is that your normal exhale moves every joint in your body a few degrees in this direction every single time.

The abdominals shorten and tighten. The hip flexors take over much of the work of the abs. The quads tighten as do the tibialis anterior and peroneals. On the back of the body, the glutes tend to 'go to sleep'; the hamstrings and calves lengthen. The opposite is true for the inhale.

EXERCISE

From the same, seated posture above, inhale slowly and fully. Continue to inhale until you can't any more.

As you inhale, allow the rest of your body to follow, like the last exercise. Where does it go?

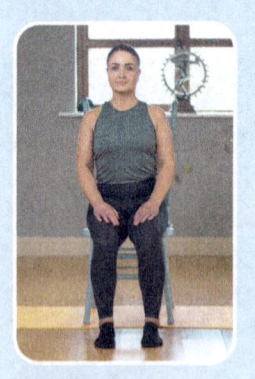

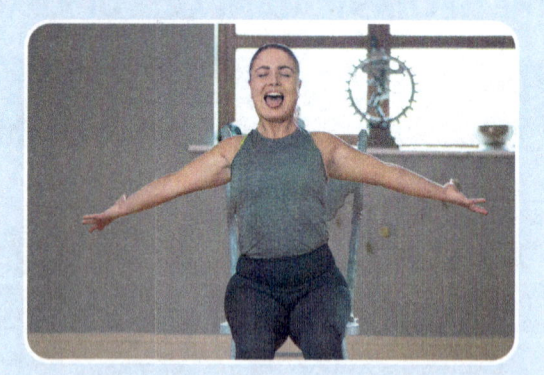

As the inhale becomes exaggerated, the front of the body opens up and externally rotates, while the back of the body shortens and tightens. This is the Green-Light-Reflex exaggerated. When either of these two breathing patterns becomes fixed in your subconscious you move away from your natural centre and develop a new normal. When you settle in this new normal state, issues begin to arise in the body and mind. These issues include but are not limited to:

- Headaches
- TMJ pain
- Grinding teeth
- Neck pain
- Shoulder pain
- Reduced thoracic mobility
- Low back pain
- Recurring hamstring strains
- Ankle instability
- Secondary pains and injuries due to an instable core

PHYSIOLOGICAL IMPACTS OF ADAPTED BREATHING ON MOVEMENT

Muscles move your body because the brain tells them to. The brain achieves this goal by sending signals through the nervous system to the muscles. These signals are combined with nutrients, oxygen and enzymes to help a muscle contract and move you. Breathing, and especially CO_2, has a few roles to play in this process.

1. CO_2 and Nitric Oxide signal the airways and blood vessels to dilate or constrict, depending on their levels in the body. Breathing controls these levels. Natural breathing dilates airways and blood vessels and helps to carry more oxygen and nutrients to the muscle cells
2. CO_2 has a role to play in muscle contraction via calcium. Calcium is required for the action potential of the nervous system to contract a muscle; it depends on a balanced blood pH. CO_2 is one of the primary regulators of blood pH. When too much CO_2 is exhaled, the blood becomes alkaline. Alkaline blood causes free calcium to bind more strongly with albumin. This reduces the amount of free

calcium available to contract a muscle and the result is the physiological inability of a muscle to contract

Adapted breathing patterns and a higher sensitivity to CO_2 have multiple effects on movement. Some of the negative physiological implications for breathing on movement are:

- Constricted airways and blood vessels
- Impaired respiratory function
- Reduced blood flow, oxygen and nutrient supply to muscles
- Free calcium bound to albumin reducing the ability for a muscle to contract
- Tetany and muscle spasms due to low free calcium
- Decreased power output
- Poor blood supply to extremities with implications for warming up, the need for a second wind, endurance and recovery

BREATHING EFFECTS ON FATIGUE AND PAIN

Breathing always wins

Fatigue is a term used to describe a lack of energy or an overall feeling of tiredness. Usually an overburdened lifestyle, combined with a lack of sleep, is the main reason for fatigue. However, there are many nuanced factors to fatigue, including: a lack of meaning in life, being over-worked, over-trained, over- or under-stressed, 'burning the candle at both ends', and undernourished, and adapted breathing patterns. It is thought that 20% of car crashes in the US are caused by fatigue and it is a contributory factor in one in five car crashes in Ireland. Fatigue is the primary reason why your skills and tactical thinking breaks down at work and in physical performance. The extreme end of fatigue is burnout. Burnout is a global epidemic, accounting for 37% of all work-related ill-health cases and 45% of working days lost. About 600,000 Chinese workers die every year from burnout. The problem is so widespread that they even gave it a name: *guolaosi*. It translates as 'death by overwork'. In Japan, they coined the term *karoshi*, meaning 'death by work'. One in five workers in Japan die due to burnout.

I like to think of fatigue, burnout and feeling energised as a continuum. Burnout is one extreme end. Fatigue is a state leading to burnout, and feeling energised is the opposite end of the continuum. The more things you put in place to uplift your body, spirit, and mind, then the more energised you become. When people think of increasing energy, they think of improving nutrition and sleep by default. But that's not the full story. Energy is produced as Adenosine Tri Phosphate (ATP) in the body. To build energy we need a quality environment for the cell, nutrients from food and oxygen from your breathing. Building energy is the sum of your lifestyle. Quality breathing patterns, exercise, sleep, food, meaning in life, expression of creativity, love, faith, support, and kindness, all contribute to good quality energy.

Chronic pain is defined as 'pain lasting more than three months'. More than 35% of Irish people, 43% of UK people, and 20% of the US population suffer from chronic pain. Lower back pain is the most common sub-type of pain. Pain limits work activities, pastimes, socialising, and physical performance; and it has detrimental effects on your mental health. On average, a person in chronic pain will spend €5,665 annually on their pain (PRIME Study, 2010). The mechanisms of pain are still being teased out in research. It can be a continuous dull ache, such as with arthritis, or it can be intermittent, as with migraines. We now know that your perception of pain plays a major role, as does your overall physiological state. A chronically heightened autonomic nervous system, extreme postural adaptions and your thoughts regarding the pain significantly contribute contributions to the duration and intensity of the pain experience. The most common solutions to chronic pain are painkillers, exercise, and psychological approaches.

Long-term pain and fatigue are often synonymous. Carrying pain with you for weeks, months and even years is extremely draining. Fatigue, on the other hand, often results in long-term pain. Beneath both conditions lies the balance in the human body. Both fatigue and pain are associated with adapted states of the human body and mind. Breathing, as we know, often becomes adapted with these results. We can use a maximal exertion test to discover for ourselves the connection between adapted states, fatigue and pain. Maximal physical exertion provides an excellent Petri dish for experiencing the long-term effects of fatigue and pain in a very vivid manner. The test also demonstrates the acute responses of breathing and mindset to fatigue and pain. Luckily for you, this is not a test you have to perform, as you have most likely experienced these feelings before. You just may not have connected them.

> **BREATHING EXERCISE**
>
> Depending on your fitness level, go for a twenty-minute walk or run.
>
> Over the course of the exercise, I want you to increase your pace gradually until you come to a point of exhaustion. Notice the changes in your body and brain as you move.
>
> What do you notice?
>
> How did your breathing change?
>
> Did your thoughts meander?
>
> Did your thoughts patterns change? From positive to negative, negative to positive, or remain neutral?

In the beginning, everything will seem a little hard. The body is cold and stiff and it can be difficult to get air into and out of the lungs. Your mind doesn't want to run and thoughts abound to get you not to run! Once started, the body warms up quickly and those thoughts subside. The airways begin to open; you may even notice that you began by breathing through one nostril and now you feel the second nostril opening. Blood moves more freely and heat begins to rise in your body. The muscles feel easier to move, they lengthen and contract more smoothly; your stride appears effortless. After a few minutes you'll settle into a rhythm in your run. Your body has adapted to the new state. As you build speed and time in your run, you'll notice your breathing becoming bigger and eventually you'll begin to sweat. This process will continue until you reach a point where you're pushing your body hard. Now you feel your legs burning, your heart pounding and your breath heaving. You feel the sweat dripping off you until it too can run dry. Eventually, the pain in the legs can become unbearable. The breath loses its rhythm and the negative thoughts return to your mind – you can't do this, turn around, it's not good for you etc. etc. In the end, your body is screaming and your desire to run wanes. Then you stop.

This run is an active physical example of how energy, fatigue and pain can work in your body. Initially, we focus our mind on the task, we ignore the monkey-mind and all its tricks and begin. This acceleration phase is difficult and some people don't make it. Like casting a boat out to sea, you have to pull away from the breaking waves on shore first before you find your rhythm. Once our biological system is up and running, it falls into a nice rhythm. As we begin to push our limits, our body and mind sends signals to us that they are being pressurised. Our breathing changes, thoughts kick off in our head, and pain builds in our legs. Some people are sensitive to these processes, untrained, so to speak. At the first sign of pain and fatigue, their biological system screams at them to stop, and they do. Meanwhile, those trained to accept higher levels of fatigue and pain continue. No matter what distance you run, how good a runner you are or how hard you push yourself, everybody can find a similar breaking point for themselves. When pushed to the limits, everybody gets overwhelmed by negative thoughts, fatigue, and pain; it's the body's way of keeping you alive.

The most fundamental process that connects body-mind-spirit to thoughts-feelings of fatigue-pain is breathing. It is the basic conscious process we have to regulate energy, change the sensation of pain and focus our thoughts. It can work for the person going for a run or it can work for the person in a dis-eased state like fibromyalgia or chronic fatigue syndrome. Fibromyalgia is a terrible condition, affecting 2-13% of the population; interestingly, almost 90% of patients are female. It is classified as a pain syndrome, characterised by generalised pain and tenderness throughout the body. A variety of factors are involved in this condition, such as: the person's attitude, personal history, co-morbidities and sociodemographic characteristics. Lifestyle and the person's perception of stress are key elements in reducing fibromyalgia symptoms. Chronic Fatigue Syndrome (CFS) is not unlike fibromyalgia, and again, it affects more women than men – four out of five patients are women. Muscle pain is the primary diagnostic criteria for fibromyalgia, and general fatigue in CFS. The rest of the symptoms tend to overlap between the two conditions, pain, viral-like symptoms, depression, sleep disorder, and impaired function. CFS affects 11-35% of the population internationally, depending on the national criteria for the syndrome. Common to both pain and fatigue syndromes are the underlying perceptions of stress, lifestyle, genetics, and co-morbidities.

MECHANICAL COMPONENTS OF BREATHING WITH PAIN AND FATIGUE

The diaphragm requires movement to maintain its blood supply. During maximal exercise, 15% of the total cost of oxygen is directed to inspiratory muscles (mainly the diaphragm and intercostals), and as exercise continues the respiratory muscles demand more of the total body oxygen consumption. The work of breathing during maximal exercise results in marked changes in locomotor muscle blood flow, cardiac output and both whole-body and active-limb oxygen uptakes. It is believed this blood flow is redirected to the respiratory muscles to maintain breathing, proper regulation of blood gases, and pH and overall balance in the system. 'Breathing always wins'; the body prioritises breathing above all other processes. When exercising at high intensity for long durations, the body steals blood from other muscles to ensure the respiratory system continues to function correctly. This concept is referred to as 'blood stealing' by Alison McConnell in her book, *Breathe Strong, Perform Better*.

In my coaching experience, I have found similar effects of blood stealing for athletes and non-athletes alike. Clients with mechanically adapted breathing patterns tend to become breathless, fatigue quicker, develop a higher pain sensitivity; their posture adapts, and their ability to exercise decreases. This is even more apparent in my clients who present with respiratory diseases like COPD and asthma and chronic stress and pain syndromes like fibromyalgia. With retracted breathing muscles, blood stealing, and continued exertion on the breathing muscles, the maintenance of blood gases is impaired, the person's pH eventually becomes dysregulated, and the physiological impacts of adapted breathing ingrain pain and fatigue into the system. From a physiological point of view, sensitivity to carbon dioxide has a multi-faceted impact on energy and pain:

- Sensitivity to CO_2 reduces the ability of oxygen to enter the cell to produce lots of energy. This hypoxic environment (low oxygen) can be felt locally, in one area, or systemically in non-localised pain
- Sensitivity to CO_2 requires other organs to maintain the homeostatic range of blood pH. Over time this elicits a decreased parasympathetic tone and increased sympathetic response of the nervous system. This is the arousal state. Oxygen supply, blood sugars and internal organ resources are re-routed to maintain this arousal state. The long-term re-routing of resources can lead to fatigue, pain and disease
- An increase in CO_2 sensitivity leads to chronically contracted muscles, muscle spasms and pain in non-specific localised areas
- Reliance on the anaerobic energy pathway produces a lot of CO_2 and H^+; H^+ acidifies the blood and creates a pain response
- Breathing is connected to attention in the brain. As your breathing

pattern changes, so too does your ability to focus your attention on a task
- CO_2 is a signalling molecule for a fear response in the brain
- Adapted breathing patterns (like mouth breathing or reverse breathing) reflect an adapted physiological and psychological response to life or a higher sensitivity to fatigue and pain
- Breathing is a lynchpin for the up-regulation or down-regulation of all systems in your body. Your heart rate, blood pressure, temperature regulation, hormones, movement, nervous system arousal and brain waves are affected by breathing. You can regulate all these processes to produce more energy, focus, and attention with your breath. This can delay fatigue, dull the pain response, and quell the negative thoughts in your head

The pathways above mostly describe how adapted breathing patterns help to create fatigue and pain. When we naturalise our breath, all of these symptoms can disappear. We produce energy more easily and we become more resilient to fatigue and pain. From that point on, we can also use our breath to enhance our ability to produce more energy, delay fatigue and withstand more pain. We can use our breath to focus our mind and body on a task for longer and get more out of our lives. This is in essence what the Wim Hof method does. Through Wim's specialised breathing techniques, it has been shown that you can create a feeling of more energy in the body, delay fatigue and withstand more pain. The research has also shown that these techniques, together with cold exposure training (CET), have far-reaching consequences for pain tolerance and the regulation of your immune system. 'You are your own alchemist,' as Wim says. Through breathing, you have the ability to create energy, delay fatigue, focus better, create a higher pain threshold, improve your immune system, and perform better in life and sport.

We can put this theory to the test right now, if you like!

BREATHING EXERCISE

This exercise is not for pregnant women or people with epilepsy. Only perform this technique in a safe environment. Never perform it before you get into water, in water itself, or whilst driving. If this technique makes you feel dizzy, please stop.

1. Perform as many push-ups as you possibly can. Count them. Really push your limits. If you don't think you can perform at least 12, then make the push-ups easier by putting your knees on the floor.
2. Sit on the floor or lie down with knees bent. Perform 40-60 full and big breaths. Use your mouth to breathe.
3. After your final exhale, hold your breath.
4. Turn over and perform push-ups again, with your breath held. Count them.
5. When you need to breathe, inhale and keep doing push-ups.
6. Perform as many as you possibly can – really push yourself once again.
7. Continue breathe and performing push-ups for as long as you can.

Did you get more push-ups the second time around, fewer or the same number?

I put this very same idea of breathing and fatigue to the test with clients on multiple occasions. In one of these instances, I had participants perform the exact protocol you have just tried. Out of seventeen people, eleven improved their push-ups the second time around, with one person even attaining a 110% improvement. Two participants achieved the same number of push-ups and four people performed worse. On average, the group improved their push-ups by 25%. Pretty impressive for just a few minutes of breathing, right?

Ideally, one should be able to get more push-ups the second time around. Why? Because breathing is linked to fatigue, pain and concentration in the body. As you exhale carbon dioxide, you give yourself a running head start on fatigue; you dull the pain response in your skin and you focus your mind onto your breath and away from pain. However, not everybody is successful here, and it can take some training. If you got the same number or fewer push-ups the second time around, it could mean several things:

- Your muscles are very unconditioned to push-ups and hadn't recovered
- You didn't perform enough breaths in the technique
- You can't mechanically move air in and out of your body effectively . . . yet!

BREATHING EFFECTS ON YOUR HOLLYWOOD SMILE

I had a conversation with a friend recently about breathing and the role it plays in teeth alignment. She laughed at me. She also told me that not everybody wanted the Hollywood smile and asked what was wrong with diversity? 'Absolutely nothing,' I told her, but a Hollywood smile is not just about good looks, it is also about health; health of your airways, health of your mouth-biome, and improved gut function. In the natural world, straight teeth are representative of a strong jaw-line, quality head posture, a large airway, and broad nasal passages. For modern humans, things are different; you can now have straight teeth with a pointed jaw-line, forward head posture, narrow airways and small nasal passages. We can do this because we take a short-cut to obtaining that Hollywood smile by extracting teeth as a first port of call, then aligning them with braces.

For the duration of my lifetime at least, modern orthodontics in Ireland has promoted teeth extraction and braces as the solution to crooked teeth. It costs parents thousands of euros, per year and still, you can wind up with crooked teeth. Take me, for example: I had eleven teeth extractions as a teenager, I wore braces for four years and a retainer after that, and my teeth still became crooked again. When I returned to the orthodontist, he wanted to remove another four teeth and repeat the process; his reasoning for his approach and all of this work was that I had too many teeth for my mouth! It doesn't make sense, right? Why would God give me too many teeth? Did cavemen have too many teeth and if so, how did they ever cope?

As far as we know, cavemen didn't have too many teeth, and they didn't have orthodontists either! In fact, humans are known to have had perfectly straight teeth up until about 200 years ago. Around this time, our diets and way of living changed significantly. In the 1930s, dentist Dr. Weston Price wrote a seminal book on diseases of modern living. He spent his life researching the difference between native tribes and modern humans. Regardless of whether the tribe was vegan, vegetarian, omnivore, or carnivore, they were healthier than modern humans. Their jaws were strong, teeth were beautifully formed, airways were large and nasal passages were broad. Native tribes from around the globe had less disease, less pain, and less postural adaptations than modern humans. The habits common to all native tribes compared with modern humans were:

- Babies were breast-fed to the age of four, not bottle-fed
- Native tribes ate hard, less processed, local food
- Native tribes chewed their food

Another researcher, George Catlin, observed a difference in the health and lifestyles of native tribes spread around the Commonwealth and the people of London during the 1800s. He couldn't understand why one in five babies died in London from birth to the age of one and another one in ten children died before the age of ten. Moreover, he couldn't fathom why so many London children frequently had diseases of the mind and the body. By comparison, native children only died due to accidents in that same period and, in the early days, none developed modern diseases, like those in London. Over the course of the 1800s Catlin observed that the tribespeople were adapting to a more modern life. They began to develop disease and postural adaptations similar to those in London. Their teeth became crooked, and their jaws began to point. They developed postural adaptation through the whole body and they developed diseases of the mind. He concluded that white sugar, alcohol and over-heating were the key factors contributing to the facial structure and disease prevalence. However, the most significant factor he observed to influence health occurred when the person breathed through their mouth at night. He even named one of his books *Shut Your Mouth and Save Your Life*. Catlin observed that children who breathe through their mouth at night demonstrated the final biological adaptation before crooked teeth developed, jaws under-developed, and pain and disease became prevalent.

Since the early 1900s, our diet and lifestyle have only worsened. So too has the prevalence of crooked teeth, and facial and postural adaptations. We are no longer the physical specimens we once were. In 2020, Italian researchers reported that children are now being born without their wisdom teeth. This is a case of evolution at work; you lose it if you don't use it. We have choices to make. We can continue down our path, rip teeth out of our mouths, align the teeth and make them look like everything is ok; or we can address the underlying causes of our crooked teeth.

MODERN DAY APPROACHES TO ORTHODONTICS

In 2013, I emigrated to Canada. Here, my wife and I met a lady who became a good friend; Dr. Denise Aguilar is her name. Dr. Aguilar trained for seven years as a dentist in Honduras and then specialised for a further two in paediatric dentistry in Columbia. Throughout her training, Dr. Aguilar was taught a different approach to orthodontics than we are commonly exposed to here in Ireland.

One day I asked her about her education on jaw development and teeth formation. She told me that both airway health and jaw development are critical in the formation of the Hollywood smile. She went on to explain that many factors contribute to the development of the jaw and airways. These include:

- Breast feeding
- Length of time using a pacifier
- Hardness of food
- Tongue placement and movement of the tongue
- Chronic rhinitis
- Mouth breathing

It blew me away. I found it fascinating that paediatric orthodontists in a third-world country were being taught differently, and in my opinion more accurately, than orthodontists in Ireland. With further investigation, I can see this perspective is also becoming more prevalent here in Europe. Since the 1970s, Dr. Mews' work in the UK, for example, also promoted large airways and strong jaw development in the formation of healthy teeth. Unfortunately for him, the British Orthodontist Society didn't feel the same. However, recently Dr. Mews received a lifetime's achievement award from the AAMS for his dedication to his practice and approach. Here in Ireland, I managed to find one orthodontist working locally who takes a similar approach. A few books have been written in the USA to promote this approach to forming the Hollywood smile. Sandra Khan, a craniofacial anthropologist, and Paul Ehrlich, a science investigator, wrote a brilliant book, aptly named *Jaws*. Meanwhile, Dr. Michael Gleb and Dr. Howard Hindin described the same phenomenon from their perspective in *GASP, Airway Health: The Hidden Path to Wellness*. All of these experts have built on the work of Dr. Price and George Catlin. It is becoming increasingly clear that the Hollywood smile is built on a strong jaw line, large airways, and broad nasal passages.

BUILDING THE HOLLYWOOD SMILE

The pathway to achieving a Hollywood smile is becoming clearer. Babies need to be breast-fed for up to four years. Recent evidence shows that not only is breast feeding good for gut health, but it's also important in promoting nasal breathing. When babies are breast-fed, their noses are flattened on the mother's breast and broadened over time. Breastfeeding also helps strengthen the tongue, and the muscles of the jaw. When the baby breathes nasally, the tongue naturally rests on the roof of the mouth. The tongue exerts a colossal amount of pressure on the roof of the mouth and shapes the whole mouth and nasal cavity with that pressure. The airway is better developed with a better foundation of broad nostrils, a wide jaw, and a strong tongue and neck muscles. (As you read this section and develop this new awareness, please remember to be kind to yourself and your mammy, everybody does the best they can. Solutions are coming.)

Some modern mothers didn't know breast-feeding was so important to their child's development. Some mothers wanted to breast feed but couldn't physically do it as it drained them, and compromised their own health; some mothers didn't know the ramifications of bottle-feeding children. What's more, even if some mothers wanted to breast feed their children to the age of four, perhaps they couldn't because our society isn't set up to help mothers breast feed their children to that age. Social, career, and financial pressures all influence a mother's ability to breast-feed for that long.

After breast feeding, the development of the airway, jaw and nose continues into childhood. The importance of nasal breathing and chewing hard food is still vitally important to the development of the face and teeth. Most of your food needs to be hard, and it does not matter whether that is local raw vegetables and fruit or a variety of softly cooked meats and fish. As we chew more, we develop the jaw structure and the muscles of our face, tongue and neck. Nose breathing is equally important. With nose breathing, our tongue rests on the roof of our mouth. The pressure exerted on the roof of the mouth shapes the jaw and teeth as the child develops, and grows into adulthood.

BREATHING EXERCISE

Go to your fridge and find a raw carrot – if there's none in your fridge, then find another hard vegetable to eat.

Take a bite of the carrot, and eat it with just ten chews.

How did it taste and feel?

Is there much saliva in your mouth?

How is the tension in your jaw?

How is your breathing?

Now sit down and take another bite of the carrot. Chew the carrot a minimum of forty-three times, with a closed mouth. Pay attention to the flavours, your saliva, jaw, and breathing as you chew.

Was there a difference between the two bites?

Research shows that we should chew our food at least 43 times per mouthful! Until I read that research I don't know if I had ever had food in my mouth that long. I was more of a 'one bite and swallow' kind of guy. However, I now know that if you don't nasal breathe, and chew hard food throughout childhood, you are decreasing the likelihood of developing a Hollywood smile and increasing your need for orthodontic treatment. With an anatomically adapted face, jaw, airway, and nasal cavity, you are also setting yourself up for a lifetime of postural issues, and the likelihood of developing a multitude of diseases arising from adapted breathing patterns, posture, and physiological processes. Having said all of that, you can always improve your Hollywood smile, jaw shape, and airway size by changing your lifestyle, and that of your children from this point on. James Nestor described in his book *Breath* how he began to change his lifestyle habits as an adult in an effort to broaden his jaw, and increase his airway size. Through nose breathing, chewing hard gum, and some unique exercise techniques, he was able to achieve an incredible 20% increase in airway size. You can do the same even if you weren't breast-fed, didn't eat hard food, and mouth breathed for most of your life up to now.

Habits to instil for a Hollywood smile:

- Develop nasal breathing with the Innate-Strength Breath Training Programme
- Eat hard, natural, local foods
- Forks down at mealtimes between mouthfuls of food
- Chew hard chewing gum to build the jaw
- Perform tongue exercises to improve tongue mobility and strength
- Receive orthodontic treatment from a professional who uses this approach

BREATHING EFFECTS ON CARDIOVASCULAR DISEASE

Cardiovascular disease (CVD) is the collective name for all diseases directly associated with the heart and cardiovascular system, including heart disease, coronary artery disease, and myocardial, pulmonary and cerebral infarction. It is the leading cause of death in the world, responsible for 16% of all deaths. In the USA, CVD is responsible for 1 in every 2.8 deaths. In 2019, almost 523 million people suffered from some form of CVD, and more than 18.6 million people died from CVD that year. It has also been the leading cause of disease burden internationally for more than seventy years. Atherosclerosis is the process by which CVD occurs. Typically risk factors such as smoking, lack of physical activity, poor lifestyle choices, stress and genetics are associated with an increased risk of CVD. Breathing, as a cause and a part of the solution to CVD, tends to be overlooked in most cases. But if you were to breathe rapidly for a minute you would clearly see for yourself the connection between your breath and your heart, your heart health, and cardiovascular disease.

> ### EXERCISE
>
> Sit down for a minute then take your pulse. Count your heartbeats in one minute. Got it? (You could also use a HR monitor for this exercise.)
>
> Now close your eyes. Focus on your heart and increase your heart rate using the mind alone.
>
> Can you do it?

If you can, you must be a pretty well-trained meditator. Most people can't increase their heart rate with their mind alone, and it takes years of training to be able to perform this feat. But when you breathe fast, you can increase your heart rate; when you breathe slowly, you can slow your heart rate. Give that a try now.

> ### BREATHING EXERCISE
>
> Take 30 fast and big breaths. Watch your heart rate increase.
>
> Now slow your breaths and watch the inverse happen.

Why does this happen? Because your heart sits into your diaphragm. There is no separation between the diaphragm and the pericardium of the heart. As you breathe, your diaphragm moves down and up. With every excursion of the diaphragm, the heart is moved with it. The heart beats slower on an exhale and faster on an inhale. As you breathe more, the diaphragm moves more quickly, increasing the heart rate. This is just one of the many ways breathing influences cardiovascular health and you've experienced it for yourself right now.

Let's dive into a few of the other ways breathing impacts cardiovascular health:

1. Respiratory sinus arrhythmia

The anatomical position of the heart and diaphragm connects the breath and cardiovascular system in many ways, the most important of which is the synchronisation between the breath and heart rhythms. In an anatomy chart, there is no separation between the heart and diaphragm – the heart's pericardium (a sac containing the heart) sits into the diaphragm. The beating rhythm of your heart is known as the R-R interval. It is the rhythm monitored by an ECG, and gives rise to the heart rate variability (HRV) measurement. Ideally, there should be good variance in your R-R rhythm. If you've ever watched an episode of *E.R.* or a similar hospital-based TV show, you'll know that a patient who just died has a flat tone to their heart in their ECG while a healthy person has a good variation to their heart rhythm. A good quality HRV is indicative of a properly functioning nervous and cardiovascular system. It is fast becoming a standard measure of general stress for both elite athletes and the general population. Research shows that the intervals of time between the beats of your heart are synchronised with your breath. The interval is shortened with an inhale and extended with an exhale. A mismatch of timing between your breath and heart rhythm has negative consequences for the supply of oxygen, heart health and the effects of stress on the body.

2. All blood flow below the rib cage passes through the diaphragm

The diaphragm sits horizontally across the bottom of the rib cage. For any blood to flow from the heart to the abdominal organs it must pass through the diaphragm. The aorta, the main artery to the lower body, and the inferior vena cava (the primary vein) both pass through the diaphragm. If the diaphragm becomes retracted for any reason, it can exert pressure on both the vena cava and the aorta. This in turn increases blood pressure in the cardiovascular system. For similar reasons, a retracted diaphragm can also cause the heart to skip beats (heart arrhythmia), to have a peculiar heart rhythm and can lead to blood stealing, as described in the *Fatigue and Pain* section.

3. Big, fast and/or mouth breathing can induce a sympathetic nervous system response

An adapted breathing pattern can look like mouth breathing, big breathing, fast breathing, chest breathing, belly-only breathing or a combination of any of the above. Adapted breathing patterns can induce a chronic arousal state in the autonomic nervous system, the called flee or freeze response. The response can look like this:

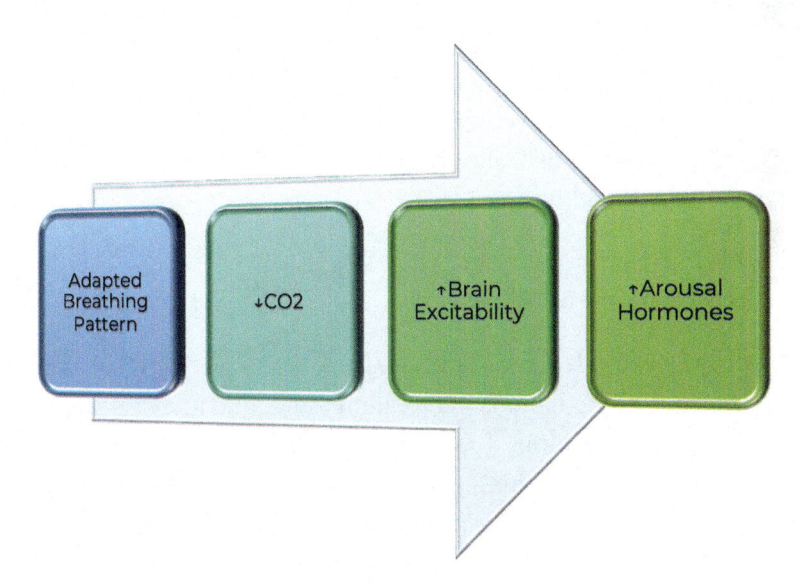

Adapted Breathing Pattern → ↓CO_2 → ↑Brain Excitability → ↑Arousal Hormones

Relationship between adapted breathing patterns and hormones

4. CO_2 and nitric oxide dilate blood vessels

The promotion of nasal breathing in combination with calm and light breathing increases the amount of nitric oxide produced in the paranasal sinuses, regulates CO_2 better, and improves the ventilation-perfusion ratio (V:P). Nasal breathing and natural breathing enhance paranasal nitric oxide secretion by up to fifteen times more than adapted breathing patterns. One of the primary roles of nitric oxide is to dilate airways and blood capillaries; it is one of the main ingredients in Viagra for this very purpose! Combined with a better regulation of CO_2, natural nasal breathing dilates both airways and blood vessels better.

In adapted breathing patterns, a low V:P creates a more difficult environment for oxygen to diffuse from the lungs into the bloodstream and CO_2 to diffuse from the blood back into the lungs. Blood circulates the lower lobes of the lungs more than the upper and air is circulated around the upper aspect of the lungs more than the lower. Combining nasal breathing with diaphragmatic breathing improves the V:P. Oxygen and blood mix through all the layers of the lungs, and produce a better diffusion of oxygen and carbon dioxide across the alveoli and blood barrier.

5. Blood Pressure and Breathing

The aorta and carotid arteries have pressure receptos, called baroreceptors. These sense fluctuations in blood pressure, and relay information to the brain on breathing. Changes in blood pressure (such as from CVD) can influence breathing patterns. An increase in blood pressure gives rise to a suppressed breathing pattern, and a decrease in blood pressure is linked with long-term hyperventilation.

When we combine all these processes together, it is clear that there are many relationships between the heart and breathing. It is also clear that any long-term changes to the breath can have direct consequences for the health of your cardiovascular system. When you breathe well, you can reduce the workload on the heart and cardiovascular system, thereby reducing the risk of heart disease.

ADAPTED BREATHING PATTERN EFFECTS ON SLEEP

Meditation, mindfulness, walking in nature, and even breathing are secondary practices to sleep when it comes to restoring the body. As the Dalai Lama put it, 'sleep is the best meditation'. Insomnia is the generic term given to all sleep disorders. Sleep-disordered breathing, snoring, and sleep apnoea all fall under the heading of insomnia. Insomnia is linked with an increased risk of CVD, depression, mental health issues, ADHD, anxiety, obesity, diabetes, and many more lifestyle diseases. Within one year, almost 30% of the population suffers from insomnia, and more than 10% of the adult population experiences chronic insomnia at some stage. Insomnia is so prevalent that it is now considered an epidemic in the USA, with a third of Americans regularly getting by on too little sleep. A lack of sleep is responsible for 109,000 road accidents annually in the USA, and costs the US economy $411 billion annually due to poor productivity and sick leave. As of 2012, three times as many high school students had troubled sleep compared to 1982. Twice as many said they went to their doctor for mental health issues.

During sleep, your internal organs work at cleaning out, and detoxifying the day's leftovers. In your brain, everything is either filed away in long-term storage cabinets or it is sent to the trash, to be forgotten. Sleep mainly has two phases: deep NREM and REM. It is said (and still debated) that the two main sleep phases are approximately 90 minutes' long. Both phases are important for restorative sleep, and you need a certain number of cycles between them per week for a good operating body, a healthy brain, energy production, and a strong immune system. Personally, I love my sleep. I can sleep anytime and anywhere. My wife tells me I inherited this wonderful trait from my family. I'm not so sure because I work on it pretty hard too! As a coach, the one problem I have with sleep is that we cannot induce sleep or directly improve the quality of sleep.

Try to get to sleep faster tonight and you'll see what I mean. Sleep is a passive lifestyle practice, and it's quality depends on everything else you do during the day, and the environment you create for sleep at night. It depends on your rhythms. Nowadays, it is said that sleep is determined by what you do in the first hour after you wake up. The rhythms that most affect sleep are: daylight, general daily activity, meal times, bed time and, you guessed it, breathing. Breathing has a many-fold effect on sleep. Adapted breathing patterns imbalance your hormones, make you thirsty, make you want to get up in the middle of the night and go for a pee, increase snoring, incite sleep apnoea, affect blood sugars, and can even decrease cognitive function due to their impacts on sleep.

MOUTH BREATHING AND SLEEP DISTURBANCES

This is becoming a common theme, right? When we form an adapted breathing habit, we lock our body into that chronically aroused state. In particular, mouth breathing plays a hugely damaging role on sleep disturbance. When we mouth breathe, we alter our posture, increase sympathetic tone, and decrease parasympathetic tone. In the case of sleep, either mouth breathing or an adapted posture can come first. No matter which comes first, they can both affect sleep terribly.

Pathway 1: Chronic mouth breathing during the day ingrains a long-term aroused state. This state changes your hormone balance and upsets the rhythm of your sleep. In particular, the balance and timing of cortisol and melatonin secretion is affected. This may make it more difficult to get to sleep, and it may wake you up during the night and bring you out of sleep early. The longer we are in this rhythm, the more difficult it is to change. It is the same for any habit, good or bad.

Pathway 2: Mouth breathing dehydrates the airways up to 40% more than nasal breathing. Dehydration combined with chronic sympathetic arousal decreases vasopressin and other substances. These substances should signal the body to store more water in cells. With less vasopressin in the body, the kidneys release water and trigger the need to urinate. Now we are thirsty and we need to pee!

Pathway 3: Mouth breathing in particular, combined with an adapted posture as we grow through childhood, leads to smaller nasal cavities, smaller airways, a weaker soft palate, a tongue too large for your jaw and it can result in snoring, sleep disturbances, and sleep apnoea.

Pathway 4: When you are sleeping and you lie on your back, gravity pulls the lower jaw down and opens the mouth, resulting in mouth breathing. These altered mechanics can reduce the size of the airway and even block it completely to produce a subconscious breath hold. Luckily, we are built to survive. After a period of time with our breath held, our brain will reflexively wake us up and make us take a breath. Although this is an amazing strategy, ingraining this sleep pattern into our system is terrible for our health. We call it obstructive sleep apnoea. Sleep apnoea is one of those dis-eases which leads to a whole host of other problems in our body and brain the longer we have it. Increased risk of heart disease, stroke, cancer, diabetes, ADHD, and cognitive function are just some of the major diseases of the body brought on by sleep apnoea.

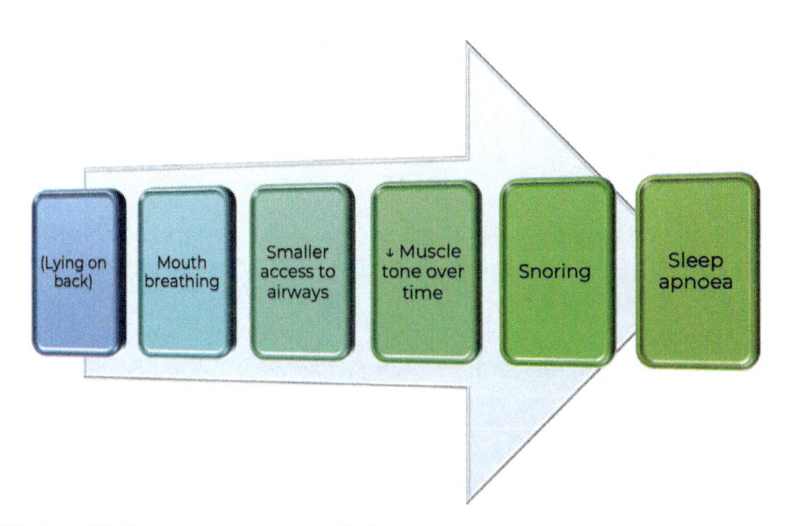

(Lying on back) → Mouth breathing → Smaller access to airways → ↓ Muscle tone over time → Snoring → Sleep apnoea

Relationship between posture and sleep apnoea

Pathway 5: Typically, as the sun goes down in the evening, melatonin begins to rise in the body and cortisol starts to fall. These two hormones have an inverse relationship. They both have a role to play in the onset of sleep. During the night, cortisol stays low and melatonin relatively high. In the morning, cortisol rises to wake you up as melatonin falls. Cortisol remains relatively high during the day, with a few dips here and there, while melatonin remains low. When we ingrain an altered breathing pattern into our system, particularly mouth breathing and reverse breathing habits, we shift our centre to a higher sympathetic tone. The aroused nervous system will secrete more cortisol as a part of this response. The increase in cortisol upsets the balance of cortisol and melatonin, and then sleep becomes affected. Over time, sleep worsens. This kicks off a vicious cycle where adapted sleep patterns further imbalance the cortisol-melatonin balance and it becomes more difficult to both get to sleep and remain asleep for a full night's restoration and recovery.

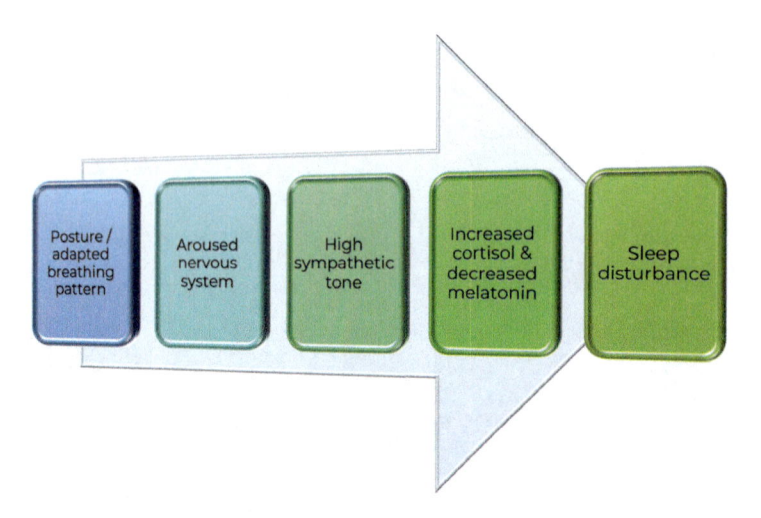

Posture / adapted breathing pattern → Aroused nervous system → High sympathetic tone → Increased cortisol & decreased melatonin → Sleep disturbance

Relationship between adapted breathing patterns, posture and poor sleep quality

If sleep is the king of restoration, then breathing is its queen; breathing is the path to help you relax your way into deeper, more restorative, sleep. Better breathing habits throughout the day improve the tone of your nervous system, balance energy levels, calm the mind and prepare your body for a good night's rest. Quality breathing habits at night enhance your overall sleep experience. A better sleep results in improved health and performance the next day, and the cycle continues.

EFFECTS ON INFLAMMATION AND THE IMMUNE SYSTEM

The immune system is our defence system. It protects us against pathogens and tries to clean up the damage caused to our biological system by our lifestyle. Pathogens are the instigators of diseases. They come in the form of viruses, bacteria, spores, parasites and other living organisms that want to enter our body and use our vital resources. Without the immune system's defence against pathogens and lifestyle, the body would struggle to survive. When functioning properly, the immune system can recognise and remember millions of different enemies, distinguishing them from the body's own healthy tissues. To prevent pathogens finding a way into our body and infecting us, the immune system offers three lines of defence: the external defence (first line), innate (second line) and adaptive (third line).

The role of the first line of defence against pathogens is to provide a barrier between the internal body and the external world. This reduces the likelihood of a pathogen or harmful substance gaining access to our body's resources, stealing from it or irritating it. The first line of defence includes the skin barrier, nasal cavity, ear wax, saliva in the mouth, stomach acid, and tears in the eyes. Although external defences do a good job of keeping out most external invaders, the body is still vulnerable.

Wounds in the forms of cuts and abrasions are common 'faults' in the skin barrier's defence. Polluted air in the environment, inhaled through the mouth, reaches the lungs unfiltered, and un-chewed processed food is more difficult for stomach acid to break down. These are three examples where foreign invaders can penetrate the first line of defence.

The innate immune system is said to be naturally present in our body since birth. It's constantly ready for action against foreign bodies. Its response is non-specific and it acts on any type of pathogen. It also has a role in the healing process by co-ordinating a sequence of events, collectively known as inflammation, to help close the wound and seal the fault in the first line of defence.

The more complex adaptive immune system targets pathogens specifically. A distinctive feature of this system is its capacity to remember a first encounter with a specific pathogen and to mobilise a speedy and targeted response to future infection by the same source. We develop the adaptive response after an infection, for example. The two aspects of the immune system we're going to focus on with respect to breathing are the first and second lines of defence; that is, the barrier and the inflammatory response.

BREATHING EXERCISE

There are no contraindications to this exercise but it is not very comfortable to do. Give it a try if you want a visceral experience of the nose's filtration system.

Go to your cupboard and find some ground black pepper. Pour some pepper onto the palm of your hand.

- Snort the pepper in through your nostrils and observe what happens.

Watch out for your nostrils opening/closing. Does anything change within the nose? Do you wheeze or cough? What happens to the rest of your body?

Recover for a minute.

- Suck the pepper rapidly in through your mouth and observe what happens.

Whenever I have people perform these exercises, I find that when they snort the pepper through their mouth, they end up coughing. By contrast, their eyes water, and their nose opens and becomes itchy when they snort the pepper in through the nose. The body coughs after sucking the pepper in through the mouth is because there is no filtration system in your mouth for air-filled pollution, toxins or particles. By comparison, the nose has a fantastic filtration system, so the body adjusts differently to snorting the pepper through the nostrils. The nose is the first line of defence for the lungs. It is designed to moisten, filter and prepare incoming air for the lungs. It has hairs, mucus, enzymes, nitric oxide, and antibodies on hand to purify incoming air and prepare the body to use that air. The nose protects against viruses, pollution, and noxious gases. It regulates CO_2 and nitric oxide to dilate or constrict both airways and blood vessels, as needed by the body's demands. Without the nose, we have no first line of defence for the lungs.

Particles deposited in the nose can be filtered in fifteen minutes, compared with 60-120 days for particles that reach the alveoli. Unfiltered, polluted air, containing pathogens and viruses, can easily enter the lungs, increasing the workload on the second and third lines of defence. In particular, the second, non-specific line of defence is activated, often resulting in a chronic inflammatory response. Remember, we breathe an average of 10,000 litres of air per day. When we mouth breathe, our breathing rate increases, and we inhale up to 30,000 litres. All of this unfiltered air aggravates the immune system, causing chronic inflammation.

Chronic inflammation arises from foreign bodies passing the first line of defence, the external barriers, and entering our body. Sources include unfiltered air, poorly digested food and pathogens entering through the skin, eye, and ear barriers. Negative thoughts and high levels of psycho-emotional stress can also produce chronic inflammation from within the body. Acutely, it presents as swelling, pain, redness, and heat. Most people can deal with acute inflammation, but chronic inflammation can really impede your quality of life. Chronic inflammation results in worsening symptoms such as headaches, fatigue, pain, and fever. If you think about it, the body is trying to repair itself, but foreign invaders are continually bombarding your body. With all of its resources going to deal with the invaders, it leaves very little energy for you to function well, and so the body becomes overworked and begins to break down. It places a demand on energy from the body and its resources and hence, a demand on the breathing system to supply and regulate that energy.

The net result of chronic inflammation and an over-active second line of defence is a host of dysfunctions and lifestyle diseases. Low sexual libido, poor endurance, energy slumps, and dips throughout the day are some of the stronger symptoms of chronic inflammation, and an adapted biological state. Asthma, bronchitis, rheumatoid arthritis, IBS, cardiovascular disease, obesity, diabetes, and deep depression are just some of the many conditions linked with chronic inflammation.

From a breathing perspective, here's what we can do to improve chronic inflammation:

- Restore nasal inhaling to filter, moisten, and prepare air for the lungs
- Restore nasal exhaling to regulate nitric oxide and CO_2 gases better
- Breathe through the nose during the day, night, and all aerobic exercise
- Restore a calm, gentle, daily breathing pattern
- Improve the condition of the diaphragm
- Use specific breathing patterns to regulate our body, brain, and emotions throughout the day – especially around stressful events
- Smell our food before eating it to prepare our system to digest, and absorb the food
- Use specialised breathing techniques to process and integrate traumas

All these tips are practised and trained in the Innate-Strength Breath Training Programme.

FREEING THE UNIFIED RESPIRATORY SYSTEM

The nose and lungs form a single, unified airway. This means that where inflammation is present, it can travel from the nose to the lungs and from the lungs to the nose

PATRICK MCKEOWN

Breathing big and fast for one minute can bring on dizziness, feelings of shortness of breath (dyspnoea), tingling fingers, ringing ears, dried airways, chills, coughing and a desire to breathe more. This is an old test used by doctors called the hyperventilation provocation test. It is not used as part of medical assessments much nowadays because it doesn't relate to a specific disease, but it does certainly give you a flavour of the body and brain's response to long-term adapted breathing patterns. Once the brain recognises that this is your new normal breathing pattern, it accommodates it. Physiologically speaking, your chemo- (CO_2), baro- (pressure) and mechano- (stretch) receptors are all sensitised, your ability to breathe fully into the lungs becomes restricted, your desire to breathe more increases and your arousal state is heightened. You find it more difficult to focus, your concentration becomes scattered, thoughts can be erratic and you can become more prone to feelings of anxiety, panic and fear. Depending on your genetic profile, inflammation can ensue in the nose and/or lung.

Some people with respiratory diseases are genetically pre-disposed to sensitive nasal passages and lungs, resulting in inflammation, congestion and adapted breathing patterns. Others have degraded the quality of the lung tissue over the course of their lifetime from habits like smoking, or inhaling air pollution, unfiltered, through the mouth. In the latter case, people are likely to develop one of many inflammatory and structural respiratory illnesses when they push their body and immune system to the brink. The final type of respiratory disease one can develop is that of the mind – specifically anxiety and panic disorders. I'll say more about them in the next section.

As a breathing coach, I classify many lifestyle-diseases with roots in the lungs, throat, and nose as respiratory diseases. This is not how the medical community define these diseases, but if you consider the nose, mouth, upper airways, throat, lower airways and lungs as a 'single unified airway', as Patrick McKeown describes it in his book *The Breathing Cure*, then you can see why I consider a breakdown in any part of the system as an aspect of the whole system. Considering I also coach breathing and health from a global whole-body perspective, you can appreciate why I don't get bogged down in the details of a disease so much, and I view it from a breathing perspective. Having said that, it is important to consider the unique characteristics of every disease and ensure the whole body is restored when you want to return to whole health and improved performance. Undoubtedly, each of these ailments requires care beyond breathing to fully restore the body to health. The diseases that fall into the respiratory category include:

- Asthma
- COPD, emphysema and bronchitis
- Enlarged adenoids and tonsillitis
- Allergic rhinitis (hay fever), sinusitis and nasal polyps
- Anxiety, panic and fear (*covered in the mental health section)

Asthma is a physical illness with genetic, emotional and psychological components to it. It is a 'chronic respiratory disease of unknown origin'. It is characterised by shortness of breath, hypersensitivity of the airways, wheezing and coughing. The typical symptoms of asthma include an inability to breathe, air hunger and tightness in the chest. Breathing during an asthma attack is characteristically wheezy as the airways constrict and the air whistles through the narrow passage way. The wheeze is usually accompanied by lung inflammation and an accumulation of mucus in the airway. 7% of the US population suffers from asthma; 1 in 13 adults and 1 in 10 children in Ireland have asthma. Every four minutes a person is admitted to hospital for asthma. It costs an individual €1,242 and the state €472 million per year. There are 5.4 million people in the UK living with asthma and, on average, three people a day die in the UK due to asthma.

The onset of asthma can occur at any stage of life. I believe I started showing symptoms aged four, during a holiday to the Canary Islands. The dry, desert air of the Canaries irritated my airways and I displayed symptoms for the first time. My dad also has asthma, his symptoms worsened significantly when he lost his job and couldn't find employment for several years after the world-wide economic crash in 2008. I have three daughters, two of whom have been told they have asthma. Their symptoms developed after different circumstances; one was born with her umbilical cord wrapped around her throat and displayed symptoms almost from the beginning of life, and the other developed symptoms after a viral infection later on in childhood.

Severe asthma is associated with allergic rhinitis, also known as hay fever. The risk of allergic rhinitis is higher in those who have had allergic asthma in childhood. According to the World Allergy Organization, allergic rhinitis is the most common form of non-infectious rhinitis, affecting 10-30% of adults and up to 40% of children. It is an inflammatory-mediated disease. It can occur due to pollens, dust mites or by a specific allergic environment. Nasal congestion, due to inflammation, is the most common and problematic symptom of allergic rhinitis. Sinusitis has very similar symptoms to allergic rhinitis; the difference is in onset. Allergic rhinitis manifests after breathing in something you are allergic to whilst sinusitis is a general inflammation in the lining of the nose. Nasal polyps are another effect of an over-active immune system. This time the immune reaction is a soft-tissue growth in the nasal cavity. Nasal polyps occur in sinusitis conditions lasting more than 12 weeks. They arise due to chronic inflammation and are often associated with asthma, allergies, recurring infection, drug sensitivity and certain immune disorders. Once the nose becomes blocked in any of these conditions, the person resorts to mouth breathing. After that, sleep is affected and the health of the whole system becomes adapted.

Adenoids are small patches of tissue located at the back of the throat and beneath the nasal passage. They are similar to tonsils, and they're located right above them. Both adenoids and tonsils form part of the immune system. The adenoids' role is to trap bacteria and viruses that enter the body through the nose. Enlarged adenoids frequently occur in children. They are the result of an immune reaction and inflammatory response. Symptoms include difficulty swallowing, glue ear, sleep problems, headaches, tiredness, difficulty breathing through the nose, sleep apnoea, and tender lymph nodes in the neck. Tonsillitis is a similar condition affecting the tonsils. The symptoms are also similar but more specific to the throat and neck than the nose.

Emphysema is a subset of a larger group of diseases known as COPD. These structural lung conditions cause shortness of breath and an inadequate supply of oxygen to the cells. The leading cause of COPD and emphysema is smoking. In 2015, 3.17 million deaths globally were attributed to COPD. The average life expectancy of a person with emphysema and/or COPD is just five years. COPD and emphysema are irreversible, life-limiting diseases. The leading causes of emphysema are smoke, air pollution, chemical fumes and dust. Tiredness, fatigue and shortness of breath are common symptoms. In people with emphysema the alveoli are damaged. Over time they weaken and collapse, creating larger air spaces in the lungs. The larger air spaces reduce the surface area of the lungs and impact the exchange of oxygen and carbon dioxide between the alveoli and the bloodstream (known as the ventilation:perfusion ratio). A poor ratio results in less oxygen availability for metabolism in the body's cells. Most people with emphysema also have chronic bronchitis. Bronchitis is an inflammation of the (bronchial) tubes, which carry air into and out of the body. It can be acute or chronic. It is associated with less serious lung infections, asthma, and more serious conditions like emphysema. The inflammation in bronchitis leads to a persistent cough and wheezing. Together, emphysema and bronchitis make up the condition of Chronic Obstructive Pulmonary Disorder (COPD).

These respiratory diseases, like most others, have a multifactorial lifestyle basis. In other words, many things in our lifestyle have brought us to our knees, for example food quality, air pollution, psycho-social stress, exercise, and viruses. The diseases are usually a combination of genetics, lifestyle and specific immune responses. However, because these diseases directly affect parts of the respiratory system, improved breathing habits can help them more than most people realise. This is why most of the research in the Buteyko method has concentrated on asthma as opposed to heart disease or diabetes. Even though the Buteyko method is an excellent fit for helping improve the health of these people, it is a clearer fit with asthma. Adapted mouth breathing patterns, in particular, are the primary breathing culprit to eliciting symptoms in these diseases. During childhood development, mouth breathing patterns ingrain smaller airways, an arousal state of the nervous system and a hyper-sensitive immune response to triggers of disease. Combine these developments with the lifestyle effects of mouth breathing (such as dehydration of the airways and inhaling unfiltered, unprepared, polluted air into the lungs). Add psychological factors such as sensitivity to fear, panic and anxiety on top of the development and lifestyle issues and you can begin to see how these symptoms develop in people over a lifetime. In some of the more serious cases the structural respiratory tissues are degenerated, and people regularly end up with diseases like COPD and emphysema.

EFFECTS ON THE BRAIN, MIND AND EMOTIONAL STATES

Quick or uneven breaths are an inevitable accompaniment of harmful emotions states: fear, lust, anger

PARAMAHANSA YOGANANDA

Breathing is inextricably linked to the body's mind, brain, and emotional states. There is no separation between the mind and the breath.

As the mind thinks, the body breathes; as the body breathes, the mind thinks. When you change the pattern of the breath it affects your thoughts, focus, and attention. In effect, a cascade of hormones is secreted to influence your emotions and how you feel. The reverse can also be true. Direct anatomical and physiological connections between the brain, and the breath facilitate the actions of the mind and breath as one. The general processes and influences between brain, breathing and mind can be mapped out through the simple inputs, throughput and outputs workflow. Please remember, this is an overly-simplified version to familiarise you with the link between brain, breathing and mind. It is not supposed to be a linear equation.

- The rhythmical breathing centres in the brain are located in the pons and medulla of the brain stem. The role of these centres is to influence both conscious breathing and subconscious breathing patterns
- The primary job of the brain in relation to breathing is to assess the inputs of breathing, interpret them and control the rhythm, rate and volume of breathing in response to life
- Chemoreceptors in the body and brain, mechanoreceptors in the lungs and thorax, the cerebral cortex and hypothalamus, all feed information into the brain to control the breathing rhythm. This input is stimulated by changes in CO_2, blood pH, hormonal changes relating to stress, body movement, O_2, thoughts, memory, perception, awareness, language, and consciousness
- Through these centres in the brain, the output breathing patterns influence sleep-wake cycles, arousal states, attention, hormone secretions, posture, pain, and attention

As you can see from the diagram on the next page, the brain accepts inputs from the body; it interprets them and then changes the rhythm of breathing to influence many processes in the biological system. Due to the frequency of breathing, as designed by God, it just so happens that it plays a pivotal role in influencing every other state

Changes in CO2, blood pH, hormones, movement, O2, thought, memory, perception, awareness, language → Chemoreceptors, mechano-receptors, cerebral cortex, hypothalamus → Respiratory centers in the brain interpret the information → Breathing patterns are altered together with.... → Sleep-wake patterns, arousal states, hormone secretions, posture, pain, attention

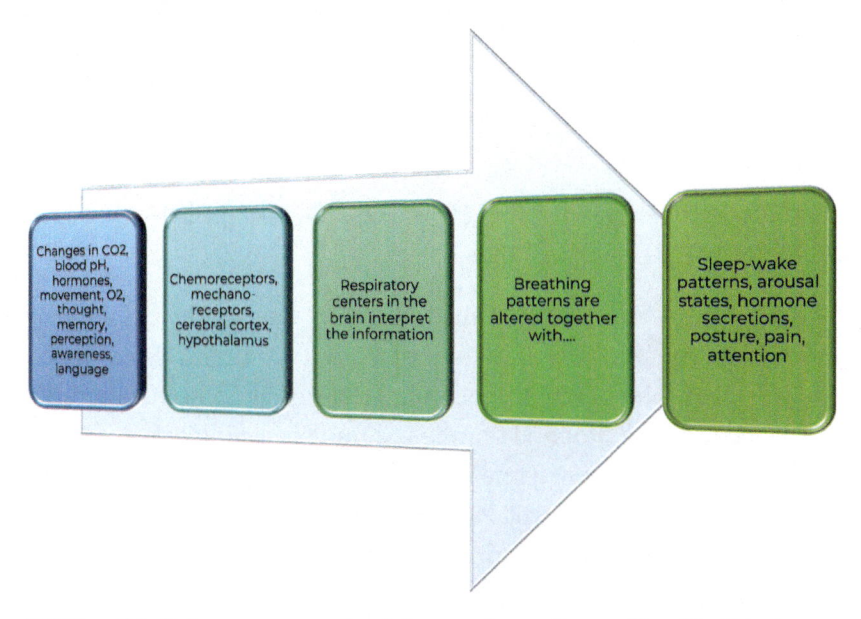

Relationship between neuro-physiology and symptoms of health disturbance

in the biological system – body and mind. So far in science, it has been shown that breathing influences the following states originally thought to be controlled by just the brain:

- States of consciousness (waking, sleep, non-ordinary)
- Focus, attention and concentration
- Fear, panic, and anxiety
- Calm relaxation

This means that breathing can be consciously changed to elicit one of these states on purpose; or a subconscious adapted breathing pattern may ingrain one of these patterns into your system. In particular, the knock-on effect of adapted breathing patterns can contribute to many negative mental dis-ease patterns. These include:

- An inability to focus on tasks for a period of time
- ADD, ADHD, and learning disabilities
- Stress, the fear cycle, panic cycle, and chronic anxiety

- Reduced capacity to express yourself
- Major depression
- Bi-polar disorder

FOCUS, CONCENTRATION, ADD, ADHD AND LEARNING DISABILITIES

Taking notice of something is called attention. Being able to hold your attention on something with all of your body and mind is described as concentration. The ability to hold all of your attention on something and concentrate for a period of time is a universal skill. Sports people needs to focus on their game, ignoring their opponent's jibes and distractions from the crowd. People working in the corporate sector require the skill of concentration to problem solve. Mothers, fathers, husbands and wives need to give their attention to their loved ones to communicate effectively, show and receive love. Unfortunately, modern life has become one big distraction for us on a daily basis. 40% of us check our phones on waking. Apparently, we check-in with them every 12 minutes throughout the day, and 20% of us interrupt meetings to check our emails. The cool thing about modern tech is that we can track our usage trends on it and find out for ourselves how much time we spend on it. You can download apps to your laptop to track time spent on email and surfing the net or you can check your phone directly. Why not take a moment to check your phone usage? Under your settings and digital wellbeing tab, you can see how much time you are spending on your various apps and how often you access them. All of these mini-disruptions throughout our day affect our concentration levels on an everyday basis and even perhaps in peak performance settings. For example, one research study I found revealed that 96% of participants performed worse in a 20-minute writing essay when interrupted at random intervals than when there were no interruptions. Similarly, we also know that long-term stuffy noses impede concentration levels by way of sleep disturbances. Researchers have found that if a child is snoring by the age of 8 and the problem is left untreated, there is an 80% chance that the child will develop a permanent reduction in mental capacity. In the same vein, almost 40% of people with sleep disorders develop ADHD, ADD, or a learning disability.

In 2017, a Canadian researcher named Mike Melnychuk (in an Irish University) discovered the exact area of the brain where your breath is connected directly to attention, called the locus coreleus (LC). In his research he noticed that attention changes with breathing patterns and breathing patterns change with focused attention. While writing this book, I contacted Mike to ask him a few questions about his research and dive a little deeper into the topic of breath and brain connection.

Mike told me a few really interesting things. There are two types of arousal: cortical (in the brain) and peripheral (in the body). The LC mainly controls cortical arousal and peripheral arousal is controlled by the adrenal glands. Specifically, cortical arousal is measured by fluctuations in nor-adrenaline in the brain and both adrenaline and nor-adrenaline in the body. These processes are very much intertwined. 'Body and brain levels of nor-adrenaline and adrenaline correlate,' as Mike told me. This means that breathing is linked to both nor-adrenaline and adrenaline levels throughout your entire system. During the interview, Mike told me about a study he came across in his research.

The study divided a group of female rock climbers into two groups. In one group the rock climbers were clipped on to safety ropes and hormones levels were evaluated. In the second group, they were unclipped. When the climbers were unclipped they experienced a 794% increase in nor-adrenaline compared to when they were safely clipped on. Obviously, that surge in nor-adrenaline needs to be controlled.

As any rock climber will tell you, when an energy surge like an 794% increase in nor-adrenaline is untethered and left to flow freely in the body, it can lead to fear, panic, mistakes and an increased risk of death when you are rock climbing. This energy surge needs to be tied into another process to help manage it. The surge can then be focused on the task at hand and used positively to help you make good decisions when climbing. Breathing is the obvious process to tie nor-adrenaline and focus it. We know this, because Mike's research showed us that breathing and cortical attention are naturally tied together at the LC in the brain. Mike himself said it to me like this. 'An almost 800% increase in noradrenaline requires something to control it, otherwise the body can go into freeze. Breathing helps you to do it . . . If you can bring your attention to breathing, it will bring you hyper-focus.' Sports psychologists worldwide also know this instinctively because breathing techniques are continuously recommended to athletes in an effort to alleviate performance anxiety and calm themselves in stressful periods. Thanks to Mike's work and researchers like him, we are now beginning to understand the underlying mechanisms that drive the power of this process and why it works so well.

STRESS, THE FEAR CYCLE, PANIC CYCLE AND CHRONIC ANXIETY

High long-term stress levels can rewire your brain and body to think and move from a perceived centre. If you spend more time in an adapted perceived centre, fear and additional stress have a greater potential to impact your body, mind, and spirit negatively. Fear is a feeling with physiological and psychological roots. In a natural centre, fear plays a very important role – to keep you safe from harm – but when we live from a perceived-centre state, fear can overtake our lives and cause us to close in on ourselves. We retreat from the world and live in a state of constant anxiety and worry. At a perceived centre you are also more susceptible to being tipped over the edge by the most benign of experiences. Often people break down because of 'the straw that breaks the camel's back', but the real issue is living in the long-term state of perceived centre. Anxiety, panic disorders and mental ill-health lie on the edge of that cliff. Feelings of tension, worried thoughts, hyperventilation, shortness of breath, dizziness, palpitations, fatigue, high blood pressure, headaches, and other physiological changes characterise anxiety disorders. Panic is the sudden uncontrollable attack of fear or anxiety, often caused by wildly incessant thoughts.

Anxiety Cycle Diagram

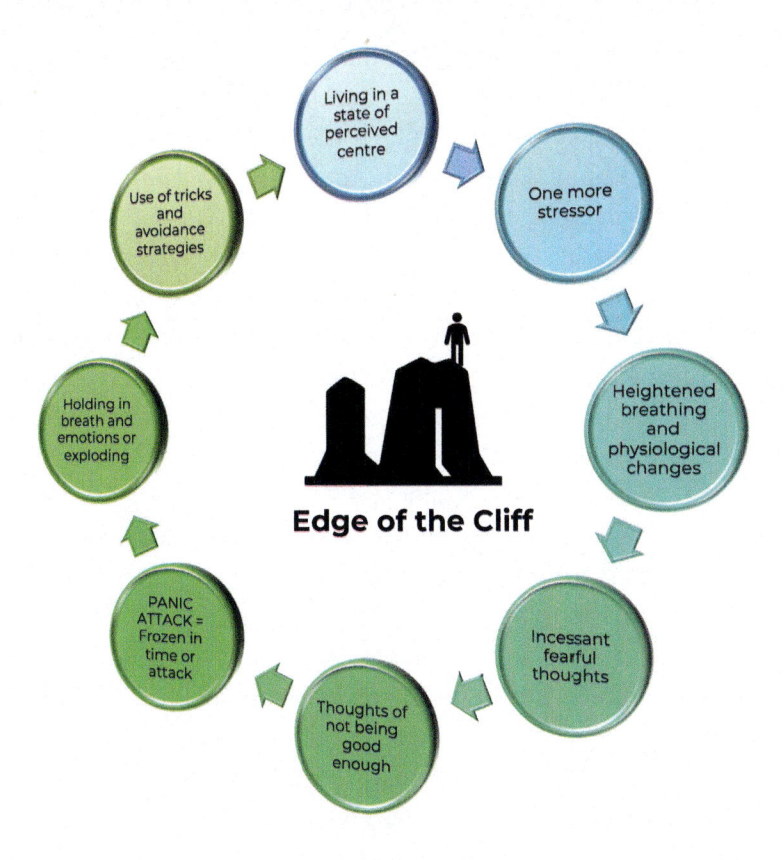

- Living in a state of perceived centre
- One more stressor
- Heightened breathing and physiological changes
- Incessant fearful thoughts
- Thoughts of not being good enough
- PANIC ATTACK = Frozen in time or attack
- Holding in breath and emotions or exploding
- Use of tricks and avoidance strategies

Edge of the Cliff

Most patients (83%) with anxiety disorders present to their physician with physical symptoms. This classification of disorder includes: general anxiety disorder (GAD), post-traumatic stress disorder (PTSD), phobias, obsessive-compulsive disorder (OCD) and social anxiety disorder (SAD). People with anxiety usually have intrusive thoughts and a fixed mindset. Mental ill-health co-morbidities often present with anxiety disorders, especially major depressive disorder. 85% of people with major depressive disorder present with anxiety symptoms. People with anxiety disorders are less likely to speak up for themselves in difficult situations and tend to avoid conflict. Their whole world can close in on them over time with seemingly no way to escape. They become shut off from society, their peers and even themselves. A lack of both proprioceptive and neuroceptive sensitivity is common with my clients with anxiety disorders. According to the National Institute of Health, it's estimated that 19% of the US population had an anxiety disorder in the last year and 31% of the US population experience an anxiety disorder at some stage in their life. It is estimated to cost the US economy $46 billion per year in mortality, lost productivity and other indirect costs. Lost productivity from anxiety and depression combined is thought to cost the US exchequer $1 trillion each year. It is interesting to note that anxiety disorders account for 30% of all mental illness costs and more than 50% of mental illness drug therapy is spent on medications for anxiety. Ireland has one of the highest rates of anxiety disorder and mental health disorders in the world. Almost 20% of young people in Ireland have a mental health disorder. As of 2017, there was a 26% increase in the number of referrals to child and adolescent mental health services. There were 8,000 people on the waiting list for primary care psychology service and more than 30% had been waiting in excess of 12 months. It is estimated that mental health costs Ireland €11 billion per year. To put this in context, the cost of obesity in Ireland in 2009 were estimated at €1.13 billion. According to the Minister for Health, Simon Harris, mental health costs are said to have a greater impact on our economy than Brexit. According to the WHO, annual government spending on mental health accounts for a meagre 2% of their budget. Ireland spends a mere 6% of their budget on mental health services per year. This is in comparison to a recommended 10% by Sláintecare, a German spend of 11%, and a UK spend of 13%.

Breathing has a critical role to play in both the physiological and psychological aspects of anxiety, panic and mental ill-health disorders. We already know its role in removing us from the edge of the cliff and resetting us to a more natural centre. But it also has a direct relationship with fear. The breath connects the body and brain directly in a variety of ways. The vagus nerve runs from the brain stem to the lungs and diaphragm; the phrenic nerve connects brainstem to diaphragm. Three brain centres control the breath, and CO_2 is the only gas to pass the blood-brain barrier. CO_2, in particular, has a role creating and proliferating fear, anxiety, and panic. Brian Mac Kenzie refers to it as the 'stress molecule'. In James Nestor's brilliant book *Breathe*, he writes about some research on the effects of CO_2 on fear and panic disorder by Dr. Feinstein in the USA. Typically, humans have a tolerance of 5-7% CO_2 in our blood. In his research, Dr. Feinstein gave bolus doses of 35% CO_2 to patients with a rare brain disorder. In this disorder, the amygdala in the brain doesn't work so well. Dr. Feinstein's patients had never experienced fear in over 30 years, despite innumerable traumas experienced by them over that time. Up until this seminal research, psychiatrists thought the amygdala was the structure responsible for fear, panic, and anxiety in the brain, and without them people would have no sensation of fear. When he administered inhaled CO_2 to them, the patients immediately experienced a panic attack from fear. Not psychological fear, but fear as a result of CO_2. Dr. Feinstein showed that CO_2 had a significant role in the development of the fear cycle, regardless of the amygdala. When you think about it, the only time we would sharply increase CO_2 levels is when we hold our breath, and the only reason for you to hold your breath for a significant period of time in nature is when you are dying due to asphyxiation or drowning. CO_2 is linked directly to fear because of its role as part of breathing in near-death experiences. It's interesting to observe that the other times we hold our breath are when we are really angry (and suppressing our emotions) or when we want to produce a lot of force. From my observations of people with adapted breathing patterns, they often subconsciously hold their breath or control their exhale because they hold a lot of anger inside them or do not have the confidence to express their emotions.

I am not saying that breathing is the cause of any of these dis-ease states, but I am saying that it contributes to the state of anxiety, panic, and mental ill-health and the power it has over you. As you change your adapted breathing pattern, these patterns can ease and sometimes even disappear entirely. In some cases, other work needs to be done to completely re-centre your body, mind and spirit. For me, panic, anxiety and mental ill-health result from an adapted lifestyle combined with genetics. This can be due to an acute traumatic event or long-term stressors promoting a perceived-centre. The opposite of these states of mental ill-health is mental strength. Mental strength starts in the body with the breath, and it is the peak state of mental and physical health. It is developed by restoring the breath to its natural centre, building health and then challenging yourself in meaningful pursuits. As one of my clients, Paul, wrote to tell me:

> *I continue to feel much calmer and capable for what life has in store for me. At times where I would usually get stressed, I now feel calm, peaceful and relaxed. It feels great now that I have hardwired those feelings into my daily life.*

MENTAL HEALTH BEGINS WITH PHYSICAL HEALTH AND PHYSICAL HEALTH BEGINS WITH THE BREATH

Breathing and movement are the core functions of our conscious human body. Without either of these processes, we die. When either of these processes doesn't work so well, we develop a range of diseases and pains. For example, exercise outperforms any drug for relieving mild-moderate depression, every time! When we use these processes of breathing and movement, train them and optimise them for performance, our whole system (body and mind) becomes healthy and works fantastically well.

Remember, CO_2 has two major influences on mental health. The first is that it is one of the primary signallers of the fear response. Fear, panic, anxiety and the 'need to breathe' operate on a continuum. Learning to breathe well influences the fear response and calms it.

CO_2 also has a role in getting O_2 to the cell to create energy. If your brain is sensitive to CO_2 then O_2 doesn't get to the cell and the body becomes inefficient at making energy. Decreasing energy, fatigue and poor working organs are all possible symptoms of high CO_2 sensitivity. This can have knock-on effects including depression and mental health issues. Breath training can improve cellular O_2, enhance energy levels and help lift the veil of depression.

EXPRESSING THE BREATH

Our breathing pattern expresses our inner situation

MAGDA PROSKAUER

Vocal communication is another vital function of breathing. Most people know this, but not many realise the importance of it. Whispering, humming, talking, singing, shouting, and roaring are expressions of the breath. Breathing is the foundation of all vocal communication. As air is exhaled out of the body, it passes through the larynx and the vocal cords in the throat. The larynx is a valve between the upper airways (mouth and nose) to the lower airways (lungs). Its primary job is to seal off the upper and lower airways to prevent foreign substances from entering the lungs. Its secondary functions are preventing air from escaping during maximal strength exercises and producing sound. As air passes the larynx, the air is spun and vibrated through the cords to produce vibrations and sound. The nasal passages, tongue and mouth provide tone and texture to the breath by shaping and 'finishing off' the sound being expressed. Most people, even some singers, think of sound coming from the voice-box alone, and forget the impact of quality breathing patterns on sound. Developing the foundations of a quality breath, then, is extremely important in the production of quality sound and communicating effectively. Adapted breathing patterns affect the voice on mechanical, physiological and psychological levels. It manifests as some simple behavioural habits as listed in the box overleaf. With a decreased ability to use the breath for breathing, the whole body and mind finds it difficult to live, let alone to express themselves.

Ineffective vocal communication is known as a speech impediment, the most common of which is a stutter (also known as a stammer). Stuttering affects about 1% of the population worldwide. It is a condition where the person just can't seem to get their words out. There is continued involuntary repetition of sound, particularly with consonants. It starts around three and a half years old, and sometimes

BREATHING ADAPTIONS AFFECTING VOCAL COMMUNICATION

Mechanical	Physiological	Psychological	Behavioural
Smaller airways and jaw	Higher sensitivity to CO_2	Increased risk of fear, panic and anxiety	The desire to be heard can lead to inhaling through the mouth, chronic hyperventilation, and 'rushing your speech' in everyday life
Less tone in the throat muscles	Feelings of breathlessness, and air hunger	Incessant thoughts	More words are spoken per breath
Less ability to access full lung capacity	Adapted ANS		In crucial conversations and moments of fear/anger, we close the larynx, and 'hold back' the speech, emotions, and the breath
Less ability to shape the voice			
Increased use of secondary breathing muscles			
Increased strain on the voice box			

continues into adulthood. Most literature indicates stress, genetics and abnormalities in speech motor control as a cause for the stutter, but Dave McGuire goes a step further. McGuire is the author of the book *Beyond Stuttering,* and the founder of the McGuire Programme. His programme has trained thousands of people with a stutter since the mid-1990s. His goal for his clients is to 'play to win' and attain 'articulate eloquence' with their speech. The McGuire Programme views stuttering from a sports psychology perspective. From this point of view stuttering is similar to choking in sport and it arises due to performance anxiety. Adapted breathing habits, incessant fearful and negative thinking, and holding back emotions are all elements of stuttering. We already know the vital importance of adapted breathing on voice, and physical and mental health, but breathing also plays a role in expressing emotions. Your emotions are expressed through your breath and voice, together with your muscles. Joy, love, happiness, anger, resentment, fear, guilt, rage and sadness are such emotions that you need to express. If you're in the habit of keeping these emotions locked inside, they tend to wreak havoc on your whole system. They are the long-term stresses trapped in our bodies, which we speak about so much. If you hold them in, your breath, voice, and movement patterns all adapt.

If you don't tell people what you are feeling regularly, those emotions become pent up inside, and you end up exploding like a volcano. My cousins call it the red mist. They used to wind me up as a teenager by teasing me. They could visibly see I was beginning to boil inside even though I wasn't saying anything to them. They called the moment I was just about to explode red mist. Like when Dr. Eric Banner turns into the Incredible Hulk or when a volcano is about to explode, the red mist descends when you lose control of your ability to regulate your feelings. The breath is held, pressure builds inside, my face turns red and I explode when I can't hold it back any longer! The red mist is not unique to me, though. It can be seen in almost any child of a young age. Many people know it as a temper tantrum. It is observed most commonly in children aged two to three years of age. This is a stage of development when a child knows what they want but they either can't communicate their desire effectively to their caregiver or they don't understand why they can't have it.

The red mist is a childish reaction to being teased, which is common to lots of people. By the time we reach adulthood, children have become experts at suppressing their anger and many more emotions. We hide our internal reactions much better. We stuff them down deep inside and only show people what we feel comfortable showing them. Unfortunately, we can't cheat physiology. Those emotions always escape. Most often, it's in the reprieve of food, alcohol, sex and drugs, but not always. Some people tend to get overwhelmed by the emotion, they break out and express their emotion uncontrollably or they break down in a puddle of tears. In a person with low awareness of this process it can take years and even decades to unlearn these patterns. Breath training and breathwork (sometimes combined with therapy) are highways to re-patterning and understanding your emotions.

BREATHING, FAT LOSS AND BLOOD SUGARS

Fat + Carbohydrate + Oxygen = Carbon Dioxide + Water
$(C_{55}H_{104}O_6 + C_6H_{12}O_6 + O_2 = CO_2 + H_2O)$

Overweight and obesity are progressive states in which you store excess energy as fat, which presents a health risk. The more fat you store, the higher the level of obesity and corresponding risk to your health. According to the World Health Organisation, four million people die each year due to being overweight or obese. Rates continue to grow internationally and childhood obesity has more than quadrupled since 1975. Worldwide, 1.9 billion adults were considered to be overweight in 2016. Soon, obesity is projected to cost Ireland €5.4 billion, the UK £9.7 billion, Canada $7.1 billion, Australia €11.8 billion, and the USA $210 billion per year. People with obesity can expect to also suffer from cardiovascular disease, diabetes, sleep apnoea, and an array of eating disorders and psychological problems. Losing the additional pounds on your waist is simple, but never easy. The saying 'eat less and move more' rings true for losing weight; at least initially. Calories in and calories out are the foundations of fat loss. The other two base components to weight loss are the quality of the processing plant (your gut and supporting organs) and human behaviour. The calories in and calories out formula should be more accurately written as calories in + calories processed efficiently + calories out/human behaviour = weight loss. It's a little more complex, I know, but then again, so are we as human beings. In general, the equation is simple; we know what to do lose weight but why we choose not to do it is a more complex topic. One part of the solution to motivating you in the right direction is to understand the fundamentals of what happens to fat when you lose it. I'll give you a clue; the answer is right under your nose.

When you lose weight, where does that fat go? Write down your answer, and let's see if you're smarter than 98% of the weight loss professionals. In 2013, an inquisitive physicist named Ruben Meerman asked a biochemist this simple question during his quest to lose some weight; the biochemist didn't know the answer. In April 2014, Mr. Meerman asked the same question to one hundred and fifty health professionals with a vested interest in weight loss. Fifty of them were doctors, fifty were dieticians and fifty were personal trainers. 98% of the professionals surveyed did not know how fat escapes the body. Mr. Meerman was perplexed; the answer had to be out there and there had to be a scientific rationale for it, surely. Do we wee it out, poo it out or sweat it out? The truth is, we breathe it out. 'You lose weight by exhaling it,' according to Meerman's book *Big Fat Myths* and the paper he published in the British Medical Journal with the biochemist Andrew Brown. Specifically, fat turns into 84% carbon dioxide and 16% water. The carbon dioxide is exhaled out of our body. The water is recycled and eventually eliminated by sweat, urine, faeces and any other fluid the human body produces. 'That makes lungs the major excretory organ for weight loss,' according to Meerman.

When we take energy from food into our body, it comes in the form of carbon, hydrogen and oxygen. Sugars are small chains of these atoms combined; fats are large chains. Both look like carbon, hydrogen and oxygen chains in their most simple form: $C_6H_{12}O_6$. Fats tend to have twelve-plus chains combined. Sugars have one to three chains of carbon, hydrogen and oxygen combined. Proteins and micronutrients are a little different; proteins have added nitrogen and are not considered primary fuel sources. I will simplify this conversation by leaving them out for this reason but check out Meerman's paper, his book or analyse any biochemistry book and you'll find your answers there. When sugars and fats are eaten, they are broken down by the body, together with the oxygen we inhale from air and water (aerobic metabolism). The off-shoot of aerobic metabolism is energy in the form of ATP, carbon dioxide, water, hydrogen, heat and lactate. We use ATP to live, move, think and perform. If there is not enough oxygen present in the cell to produce ATP, then hydrogen and carbon bond together with the remaining oxygen to form lactic acid. The lactic acid converts to lactate and it is recycled to provide a burst of energy, known as anaerobic metabolism.

Heat is a conduit for cellular metabolism. The body maintains a constant temperature of 37 degrees, which helps all fats to stay fluid. Increased heat in your system due to environmental temperatures, eating lots of food, or exercising, raises energy production efficiency. Too much heat and the whole process burns out; too little and everything comes to a standstill, more or less. I like to think of heat as akin to riding a bike on a flat, incline or decline. You can have a lovely rhythm to your pedalling on a flat surface, speed is ideal and you can cycle for a long time. When you cycle down a hill, your speed and cadence both increase, but, if the hill is too steep, you lose your rhythm and risk burning out. Climbing a hill has the opposite effect; everything slows in your body when you're cold, just as your speed and cadence slow when cycling uphill. When the hill becomes too steep, you're forced to stop moving at all. When your body becomes too cold, metabolism slows and all other systems are affected negatively.

ATP is not formed directly from food, oxygen and water, as most health professionals think. Instead, it is released from the breakdown of these nutrients. As Meerman describes it in his book, 'your body cannot turn atoms into energy.' Fat cannot simply disappear into thin air (well it can as a matter of fact) but it needs to be transformed into something else. If it's not converted to ATP, that leaves us with carbon dioxide, hydrogen and water. We can view these atoms as CO_2, H_2O and some remaining H^+ or, if we have enough of them together, they look like this: $C_6H_{12}O_6$. That's right, once we've used food, oxygen and water to produce energy, the leftovers look exactly the same. These atoms are then transported through our blood network and out of the body via our lungs. The chemical 'human weight loss equation' can be simplified as this:

$$C_{55}H_{104}O_6 + 78\,O_2 \rightarrow 55\,CO_2 + 52\,H_2O\;(+ Energy)$$

Fat + oxygen → carbon dioxide + water

All the carbon atoms in fat become carbon dioxide and all the hydrogen atoms become water. Oxygen is split between the two; 7% joins with the carbon to become carbon dioxide and 4% joins with hydrogen to become water. That means our fat and oxygen converts to 84% CO_2 and 16% H_2O. We exhale most of our fat and the rest is lost in the fluids we produce. Energy in the form of ATP is released as a result of this process.

DIABETES AND BLOOD SUGAR MANAGEMENT

The process of breaking down fat is an arduous task for the body. It is a large molecule and not a very good fuel source for immediate energy supply. The refined version of fat is carbohydrate. Carbohydrate comes in many forms. The simplest and most ready-to-use form for the human body is glucose, otherwise known as blood sugar. Its structure is: $C_6H_{12}O_6$. Again, it is made of just carbon, hydrogen and oxygen. The body has the capacity to store a little glucose in the muscles and liver; the rest is either in transit in the cardiovascular system or stored as fat. The amount of glucose in the blood is an extremely important marker for health. A continual low amount of blood sugar decreases physical power and strength and starves the brain of a vital fuel source. It also pressures the body by forcing it to make energy through more complex pathways. Too much blood sugar (that can't be managed by the system) is toxic for the body. Diabetes is the disease associated with dysregulated blood glucose. It is a long-term disorder of fat, carbohydrate and protein metabolism. Elevations of fasting blood sugar levels characterise diabetes and it greatly increases the risk of obesity, cardiovascular disease, renal disease and neuropathy.

There are two major categories of diabetes: types one and two. Type 1 diabetes most often occurs in children and adolescents. It accounts for 5-10% of all people with diabetes. Type 1 is an autoimmune disease that results in the pancreas's inability to produce insulin. Insulin acts like a doorman for blood sugar; it allows the flow of atoms into and out of cells. If insulin isn't being produced, blood glucose levels can rise dangerously high and result in many life-limiting disease complications. The same as if there was no doorman to a nightclub, crowds could come and go as they wish, causing mayhem. Why the body attacks the pancreas is unknown. Viral infection, food sensitivities and chemical damage, combined with genetics, are thought to be the main culprits. People with type 1 diabetes require daily insulin injections for life to manage the disease. The amount and type of insulin dosage depends on the individual and their lifestyle.

Type 2 diabetes historically had an onset after the age of 40 in overweight individuals, but today even children develop the disease due to the worldwide obesity epidemic. Initially, insulin levels are elevated in type 2 diabetes, indicating a loss of sensitivity to insulin by the body's cells. To return to our nightclub analogy, think of the body as having adequate security in a nightclub for a normal night. Imagine the club owners supplied the same amount of security for a celebratory night like New Year's Eve; what would happen? The crowd would be controlled until their numbers overpower the security. The crowd stops listening to the security. They bustle past them and ignore the rules. The club owner then calls in reinforcements. For a while, the crowd settles down again, but then the numbers coming to the door start to rise and they overpower the security once more. Type 2 diabetes works in a similar fashion. It can even progress to the point where insulin deficiency is present. In other words, there are no more reinforcements to call. Now you have a critical situation that looks just like type 1 diabetes and its symptoms (albeit for different reasons). Obesity is a major contributing factor to type 2 diabetes. Achieving an ideal body weight is often associated with restoring of normal blood glucose levels.

Jimmy is a client of mine. He developed that end-stage of type 2 diabetes earlier in life. He was about six stone overweight (roughly 14 kg or 90 lbs), had suspected sleep apnoea, and a host of other health problems and he even had to be put on insulin. It has taken Jimmy five years so far, but according to his specialist, he is the only person in Ireland to improve his symptoms so much that his doctor removed insulin completely from his medication. His bloods have reduced to pre-diabetic levels, he's lost five stone, sleeps better, and is on the road to becoming healthy once more. How did he do it? He changed his lifestyle.

The management of blood sugars isn't just important for diabetics. It's crucial for everybody. It's important for maintaining a healthy weight, for fat loss, and muscle gain. It's important for energy management, avoiding crashes during the day, regulating emotions, decision-making, focus, concentration, sleep quality and of course, your breathing. The links between breathing and blood sugar level are tenuous at best. Most of the research is focused on the root cause of diabetic complications. One theory in research is that tissue hypoxia may be the root cause of diabetic complications. In other words, there is a problem for diabetics in delivering oxygen to the cells (tissue hypoxia), and the outcome of this problem leads to many diabetic complications. An overactive sympathetic nervous system, alterations to the baro- and chemo- reflexes, and poor cardiovascular control, mediate these effects of diabetes. Slow breathing is known to improve all these mediators; it can directly improve tissue hypoxia itself and it may help reverse the symptoms of diabetes.

My personal training practice and research leads me to take a different viewpoint on breathing and blood sugars than the current research. My theories view diabetes as an adaptation to poor breathing patterns in combination with genetics and lifestyle habits, especially: nutrition, sleep, exercise, heat regulation and alcohol. For example, in sports physiology research, it is known that mouth breathing is associated with higher carbohydrate usage than fats in exercise. When people use more carbohydrate, their body responds accordingly by breaking fat down into blood sugar more readily. Athletes and nutritionists know this as being 'carb adapted'. At the same time, when we eat more carbohydrate, the brain is motivated to seek more carbohydrate. When people crave something, they tend to eat a lot of it. This increase in their overall calorie intake, and the sugar itself, now directly impacts blood sugars and their management. Alcohol, sleep, and a lack of environmental temperature diversity adds fuel to the flame. Mouth breathing then becomes a symptom as well as a contributory factor to diabetes. Now, not only does it affect blood sugar management, but it also contributes to the mediators of diabetic complications. It impacts the baro- and chemo-reflexes, promotes an overactive sympathetic nervous system and increases tissue hypoxia. In this sense, there is still much work to do to determine the extent of the impact of breathing on blood sugar management and diabetes.

BREATHING IN EXERCISE IS ABOUT OVERALL HEALTH, AWARENESS AND FEELING GOOD

Having read this whole section on the chemistry of weight loss, you would think all you need to do is to breathe more to lose weight, or eat less. Technically you are correct; eat less, breathe more and you will lose weight. In reality, breathing more alone will not solve your weight loss equation and it's not something I recommend to any of my weight loss personal training clients! Breathing bigger and faster occurs naturally because of a workout or an increase in metabolism, not instead of the workout. In the long term, breathing more than you need to has other consequential effects on your body and mind beyond any weight issues (see *Physiological and Mechanical Breathing Patterns*).

If you think about it, you breathe more in all exercise, right? Perhaps it is the increased breathing effect of any exercise that helps in the weight loss equation. Weight training, running, yoga, swimming and tai chi could all be as effective as each other for weight loss if they stimulate your system to work equally hard. The only way to exercise hard is to train yourself over time to gradually tolerate a higher exercise level. As you know by now, exercising hard with adapted breathing patterns results in one of two situations:

1. You physically can't tolerate the high training loads because your breathing system is too sensitive. Exercise-induced asthma, general anxiety disorder, performance anxiety, and low thresholds of exercise endurance are common
2. You can train hard and push your body but you are insensitive to how hard you can push it. This results in over-reaching, over-training and burnout. Injuries are common; general fatigue, recurring illness, depression and mental health issues often arise

This means that any exercise will do in the equation. I would say you just have to enjoy the exercise you choose for weight loss, so that you stick with it for a long time and gradually build up a tolerance to it. Improving your breathing patterns specifically helps you on your weight loss journey by:

- Starting more prepared
- Regulating your exercise intensity and volume more sensitively
- Delaying fatigue and increasing endurance
- Recovering quicker
- Enhancing the feeling of wellbeing and enjoyment in the exercise
- Improving the overall exercise experience because the body is breathing efficiently

BREATHING ENHANCES THE EXERCISE EXPERIENCE

At rest, nasal breathing is the ideal breathing vent, not only because it prepares the air coming into the body, but also because it regulates the flow of air on the way out of the body. When our system is at rest, our brain only opens one nostril fully at any one time. The nostril it opens depends on your position relative to gravity and the time of the day. The cycle alternates nostrils every one to four hours.

When our body comes under increasing metabolic pressure, our brain opens both nostrils to breathe. This is most noticeable when you warm up slowly during exercise, but it can also happen when we overeat, or overheat our body through environmental stress.

If we continue to increase our metabolism, our body will breathe more and more. It is responding to a signal to offload carbon dioxide and heat. As your body approaches its capacity to nasal breathe, it will automatically switch to exhaling through the mouth to cool your system. Mouth breathing cools and dries the airways. Panting is a more exaggerated form of mouth breathing. Both processes dump CO_2 and heat from your system as it overheats. Although I am yet to find out who encouraged the habit of breathing in through your nose and out of your mouth during exercise, I can understand why it is such a prevalent breathing cue throughout all exercise in the Western world. It does make sense in the weight-loss journey, since inhaling through the nose filters and prepares the air for the body and 84% of fat is expelled through the exhale. However, I see problems arise with endurance, recovery and health, as most people are already in an adapted breathing state before they even exercise, then nose-mouth breathing during exercise increases the overall burden on their breathing, and their health/performance suffers for it.

REGULATION OF HEAT IN THE BODY WHEN GENERATED THROUGH EXERCISE OR HEAT TRAINING

1. Nasal breathing through one nostril
2. Nasal breathing through both nostrils
3. Inhale through the nose and exhale through the mouth
4. Onset of sweating
5. Sweating profusely
6. All mouth breathing/sweating decreases

If inhaling through your nose and exhaling through your mouth is unsuccessful at cooling your body, if your body is retaining more heat than it can get rid of, then it needs another way to cool itself down. The body will further cool itself by sweating. Sweating is the third stage of your cooling system. It is a process the body uses to cool itself when it is working hard and beginning to overheat. Sweat is composed mostly of water, with some trace minerals, urea and lactic acid. If you have plenty of water in you and you are exercising, or in the sauna, as a means of increasing metabolism, sweating is a very efficient system to keep you cool. It's a good sign. Sweating, together with breathing, will help regulate CO_2 and heat in your system as you aim to improve your performance. When your body is really being pushed to its limits, it will again give you another sign. One of two things can happen: you will use your final breathing option, in and out of the mouth, or your system will stop sweating altogether. Either of these are clear signs that you are pushing your body to its limits. The other reasons you may be sweating are due to the temperature in the environment or over-consuming food. Sweating, in these cases, is not a positive sign and it may become a problem for your health if it is an ingrained habit. Sweating due to overeating is a sign you are overindulging in food. Simply put, you are eating too many calories for your body's needs. When we overeat and our bodies can no longer get rid of the excess carbon, hydrogen and water, then it is stored as fat in our body's fat cells. Excess storage of body fat, as we know, can have hugely detrimental effects on our breathing and health. Mouth breathing as an adapted breathing pattern, sleep-disordered breathing, type 2 diabetes, cardiovascular disease and obesity are just some of the major issues arising from excess heat due to overconsuming food on a regular basis. Sweating is a very visible sign that we are overheating, but it is not our system's first way to cool us. Instead, heat is regulated primarily through breathing and it is closely linked with carbon dioxide management.

DETRIMENTAL EFFECTS OF OVERCONSUMPTION

1. System is overheating due to overconsumption
2. Adapted breathing patterns become ingrained, particularly mouth breathing
3. Profuse sweating occurs throughout the day and night
4. Sleep-disordered breathing

5. Inability to regulate temperature naturally, leading to:
6. Possible sleep apnoea, type 2 diabetes, cardiovascular disease, thyroid issues and obesity

Sweating because of environmental heat stress can be just as detrimental to your health. Usually, we overheat ourselves in this manner by living our life indoors and wearing too many clothes outdoors. As a child, I remember my mam dressing me up in many layers of clothes and encouraging me to remain indoors when it was cold and raining outside. I was forever cold and it was not until I studied with Wim Hof (known as 'The Iceman') that I came to understand the detrimental effects of our lifestyle on our body's innate ability to regulate heat and keep us healthy.

Typically, we wrap our children up for fear of the cold and we avoid it at any cost. Research suggests we now spend more than 90% of our days indoors, between houses, cars and office, and I think that is generous. As I watch people walk the streets, they are wrapped up in hats, scarves, base layers and many layers of clothing. Even when we are outdoors, it feels like we are indoors. It is no wonder that people are also suffering with heat stress too. When our body remains in the same temperate environment for a time, it loses its innate ability to regulate heat. We stop nasal breathing, our cardiovascular and nervous systems weaken, our thyroid output decreases and we lose levels of active brown fat to keep us warm. With this reduced capacity to regulate temperature and remain warm, we suffer from the cold. Our body works overtime to maintain a basic function, and we see it reflected in cold hands, cold feet, an overburdened immune system and a more frequent susceptibility to colds and flus.

> **TOP TIPS FOR BREATHING IN EXERCISE AND ON YOUR WEIGHT LOSS JOURNEY:**
>
> 1. Train your breathing foundations for a better overall exercise experience
> 2. Find exercise you love
> 3. Become aware of how you breathe throughout exercise
> 4. Become aware of your breath in different temperatures
> 5. Lead your exercise with your breath
> 6. Push yourself with breath awareness
> 7. Eat less, breathe efficiently, move more

MAKING BABIES, SEX HORMONES, BREATHING AND HEALTH

If a murderer is chasing you and you are running for your life, do you think it would be a good time to stop, have sex, and make babies? The obvious answer is no; but that's what we often ask our bodies to do when we want to make a baby and we live from a perceived-centre state. All breathing adaptations due to a perceived centre have the potential to negatively affect your ability to make a baby, balance your sex hormones, and be healthy.

We do not 'have' babies; babies are made. The man's sperm must be fit and healthy enough to journey to the woman's egg. The woman's egg must accept the man's sperm and the woman's body requires enough nutrients in reserve (in addition to her own needs) to feed and grow the baby over nine months. A part of making a healthy baby is the plentiful supply of building blocks from both male and female, combined with as few little 'nasties' in there as possible which might upset the process. One of my mentors, Dr. Eric Serrano, playfully refers to babies as 'vampires'. They pull every last nutrient out of the mother's body even if that results in deficiencies for the mother. After they are born, babies are completely helpless until they reach maturity in their teenage years. During all this time, they still require complete care from their parents, from breast feeding to love, kindness, support, nurturing and developing their social, physical, mental, and spiritual capacities. Even when it's fully grown, the baby still 'bleeds the parents' bank account dry,' according to Dr. Serrano! Considering our bodies are already telling us they are 'stressed', is it really that difficult to see why it can be a problem for some couples to make babies? The WHO defines fertility as a 'medical condition characterised by the failure to achieve pregnancy within 12 months'.

More than 25 million EU citizens are affected by infertility. One in six couples experience some form of fertility problem at least once during their reproductive life. 20-30% of fertility issues are due to physiological causes in men; 20-35% to physiological causes in women, and 25-40% of cases are because of a problem in both partners. In up to 20% of cases, no cause was ever found (perhaps because of psychological, emotional or spiritual reasons: the research hasn't been done yet). Lifestyle factors are one of the most common explanations today. Living from a perceived-centre or stressed state is very much front and centre to the issue. 25-60% of infertile individuals report psychiatric symptoms and their symptoms of anxiety and depression are significantly higher than fertile controls. In one study it was disclosed that 56% of women and 32% of men reported significant symptoms of depression and 76% of women and 61% of men reported significant symptoms of anxiety. However, these statistics may only be the tip of the iceberg, when it comes to evaluating the impacts of stress on fertility; it is easy enough to 'fake-good' in self-reported research questionnaires.

MEN'S SEX HORMONE HEALTH

A lack of physical health in the father accounts for 30% of infertility issues in couples. Stress levels, heavy metals in the blood and general good health are essential factors for creating healthy and strong sperm in men. Breathing, to my knowledge, has no specific benefit to the production of sperm. It can indirectly benefit the father, though, by improving stress levels and general health.

WOMEN'S SEX HORMONE HEALTH

As a man, I obviously do not know what it's like to have a menstrual cycle and never will. I do have a wife, three girls and many female clients from whom I am observing and learning from the whole time. I have seen the impact of lifestyle and breathing on their bodies. From my experience, women tend to suffer more than they need to with their menstrual cycle. I've seen many women at the beginning of their health journey with extremely heavy and/or irregular menstrual cycles. As they rebalance their health, the pains associated with their cycle decrease, and the cycle normalises.

Irregular and excessively heavy cycles can dramatically impact women's lives. Worrying about when it will arrive, sometimes days of pain every month and being confined to bed are some of the common symptoms I hear women speak of. None of which sound very pleasant. Prolonged, excessively heavy periods and irregular cycles are associated with a variety of female reproductive conditions, as well as infertility. Premenstrual syndrome (PMS), cervical cancer, polycystic ovarian syndrome (PCOS), uterine fibroids and endometriosis are some of the more common reproductive conditions, specific to women, negatively affecting fertility. Endometriosis is the UK's second most common gynaecological condition after cervical cancer. In Australia, it impacts one in nine girls and women. Worldwide, 20-50% of infertile women have endometriosis, and rising to 71-87% of women with chronic pelvic pain.

All these conditions are drastically improved with better lifestyle choices. Often, when women re-centre their body and mind, their cycle balances out, pain is reduced, and they can function normally. In this light, I see women's health like a finely tuned violin. When the violin is in tune, it sounds divine, but when it is even slightly out of tune, it makes a terrible screeching noise. They are the noises we all hate to hear, but we must recognise that these are signals that the violin is out of tune. Women's bodies work the same way too. The noises a female body makes when it is out of tune with its natural centre are a painful/irregular menstrual cycle, fluctuating energy levels and a cycle that is out of rhythm. To re-tune her body, the woman needs to restore her natural rhythms. Lifestyle and breathing have a very important role in helping women listen to their bodies better and find their natural rhythms. Breathing is closely linked to women's health, both physiologically and mechanically. Mechanically speaking, the breathing muscles and pelvic floor move together synchronously. If there are any mechanical adaptations to the diaphragm, it has negative consequences on the pelvic floor muscles. Physiologically, CO_2 is tied to progesterone levels, affecting women's pain perception and PMS symptoms. Up to 40% of the female reproductive population experience symptoms of PMS regularly. PMS is associated with feelings of hopelessness, depression, lack of energy, mood swings and insomnia. The symptoms of PMS and hyperventilation syndrome are synonymous. When the luteal phase of the menstrual cycle ends, progesterone decreases, CO_2 levels normalise, and the symptoms disappear. When the brain is overly sensitive to CO_2, it can exacerbate the symptoms of PMS. It also means that women are more susceptible to feelings of air hunger and possible hyperventilation.

My observations of breathing's unique effects on women's health were confirmed to me by a friend and breath-worker colleague recently. Her name is Shereen Yusuf, and she specialises in breathing and women's health. Shereen identified four different ways women specifically are impacted by life and how breathing can help them. These unique impacts are:

1. The culture women are raised in
2. The societal demands on women
3. Birth control
4. Pain during natural hormonal changes

Shereen is a model of success by any modern standards for women. She has played semi-professional tennis, graduated as an engineer, and worked in oil and gas. These are all traditionally very male-dominated arenas and she's thrived in them, but it came at a cost to her and women like her. To reach the peak of these arenas, she acknowledged that society often didn't give her due credit, and it demanded ten times more of her to gain her status than it would have for a man. Often, there was no leader with female-dominant characteristics to adopt as a role model; rather, it was a very harsh, ego-centric and male-energy-oriented route that led to the achievement of her goals. But when she added breathwork to the mix, she found that she balanced the male and female energies and 'became more compassionate, more gentle and I evened out'. Similar to her own experience, when Shereen introduced breathwork to the women at work she found that the women's energy balanced. 'The way they carry themselves, their demeanour and self-worth, there is a shift; there is an absolute shift in your demeanour when you start doing breathwork as a woman.'

Shereen also found women's expectation to perform worsened during the pandemic. As families were forced to work from home, it was the women who were expected to home-school children as well as do their work. Meanwhile the men in the relationship, for whatever reason, just focused on their work. For these women, Shereen found breathwork to be an incredible tool to manage themselves better. They could better gauge their stress levels and find a gap in the day for themselves to manage life better. This shift in self-worth and balancing of energy may have its roots in the physiology of women. Breathing, as we know, is directly related to the female menstrual cycle. As Shereen said to me, 'Can you imagine a man having to account for pain, low energy and mood swings during a quarter of the month, every month? Can you imagine a man accounting for 1-3 days per month with low productivity, holiday leave and adjusting schedules due to his own body's needs?' Many women can't function because of an adapted menstrual cycle and what do we do as society? Sometimes we tell them to ignore it and get on with it. We usually tell them to take birth control and suppress it. This is what happened to Shereen. She got acne in her thirties, and her doctor told her to take birth control. Girls in their teens are told the same thing. What is the solution for women with almost any hormonal issue? Take birth control or something similar. They are essentially being told, 'It doesn't matter – you don't really need to have your period'. But it does matter and breathwork can help alleviate the pain and symptoms of an adapted menstrual cycle. For Shereen, 'Breathwork completely solved all of my pains. Don't get me wrong, it's not like your cramps don't happen, but I'll never forget the day I got my period while I was teaching in a workshop; I cried that day. I remember thinking so clearly: this is the first time in my life I didn't have to completely arrange my entire life around my period. It had become such a part of me and now I didn't have to think about when it was coming, adjusting my workshop schedule, asking whether I need to take pills to avert the period. Because in the past when I did Ironmans and I knew my period was coming, I couldn't change the date of the Ironman and I couldn't change the date of my period, so I took pills to avert my period so it wouldn't come during the time, because if it did I wouldn't be able to function'.

PREGNANCY

Pregnancy further intensifies the relationship between breathing and female health. Oxygen consumption and CO_2 sensitivity are increased and there is less room for the diaphragm to move, due to the increasing size of the uterus in the abdominal cavity.

Progesterone gradually increases six-fold through the course of pregnancy. It acts as a trigger for the primary breathing centre by increasing sensitivity to carbon dioxide. It also acts as a bronchodilator (opening the airways), and contributes to nasal congestion. Oestrogen gradually rises before or in parallel to progesterone. It prepares the way for progesterone by increasing the number and sensitivity of progesterone receptors in some of the brain's respiratory centres. Prostaglandins are hormone-like compounds. Some prostaglandins increase airway constriction whilst others have a bronchodilator effect. The enlarging uterus is the primary cause of lung volume and chest wall distension during pregnancy. The diaphragm is displaced upwards (up to 5 cm), shortening the chest height and ballooning the chest outwards. Total lung capacity remains the same but the elastic recoil after a natural exhale is decreased by up to 22% (functional residual capacity). The amount of air exhaled during a forced exhale is reduced by up to 40% (exhale reserve volume). The inhaled capacity remains the same to maintain a stable total lung volume. Secondary and tertiary breathing muscles are used (traditionally known as paradoxical or reverse breathing) to compensate for the reduced pliability of the diaphragm. During the first trimester, breathing volume per breath (minute volume) increases by up to 48% and is maintained throughout the pregnancy. Up to 70% of healthy pregnant women report breathlessness from the early onset of pregnancy. Breathlessness leads to hyperventilation, which can have a majorly disruptive chemical impact on common gestational diseases such as gestational diabetes, gestational sleep apnoea, and cardiovascular issues.

Restoring a calm, gentle breathing pattern is vital for women to regain their natural centre, reduce pain and rebalance their menstrual cycle. Pregnancy exacerbates any underlying breathing issue and may even cause a new issue to develop. Together with breath training, I recommend women restore their body as part of normal everyday training (in advance of pregnancy). Plenty of rest, nutrient support, community support and living a life filled with love and purpose are equally important components for a woman to rebalance her health and return to a natural-centre state. Each of these aspects has proven vital to help the women I have trained to restore their natural centre, rebalance their hormones, and have a natural rhythm to their menstrual cycle.

RECOMMENDED PRACTICES FOR WOMEN'S HEALTH SPECIFICALLY:

- Restore a calm, gentle and centred breath using the Innate-Strength Breath Training Programme
- Utilise more gentle movement and wellbeing practices, especially during low-energy periods
- Add heat to your body with liquids, foods, hot showers, saunas and clothing
- Improve nutrients through quality food and a good quality multi-vitamin
- Talk to other women and develop your human connections
- Find a way to live a life of purpose and meaning

When it comes to breath practices for pregnant women, please remember:

- Practice any technique that calms and slows the breath gently
- No breath-holding or big and fast breathing techniques as it may upset progesterone levels and affect the pregnancy inadvertently

BREATHE-ABILITY 9

Up until now, I've developed a picture of how our body and mind works as one biological system. I've shown how life impacts us biologically and how we adapt to life, from breathing, movement and autonomic nervous system perspectives. I've spoken mostly about adapted breathing patterns and how they affect your life. You now know that these patterns can have disastrous consequences both for your health and your performance. Ingraining one of these patterns into our system, and moving away from our centre, is one of our most insidious lifestyle habits. It is worse than over-consuming sugar and alcohol, staying up late at night, not exercising enough, and remaining indoors all day. Adapted breathing patterns are worse than any of those lifestyle habits because breathing has a more central role in the body. Everything that we do involves breathing, so when we change our subconscious breathing patterns, it affects every aspect of our life. Very often it becomes a hindrance to performance, and it increases fatigue, pain, and disease. From now on, we change the tune of what is happening from what has happened in the past to instil an adapted breathing pattern on the opposite end of the spectrum. The rest of this book will tell you about quality breathing patterns. In this chapter, I want to explain:

- What they are
- How they look
- Their benefits to you

A quality breathing pattern has two aspects: the first is that it reflects peace and relaxation in the body as the person is at rest, and the second is that it can be used on demand for expressing emotion and performing under pressure in life. I call the sum of these two patterns breathe-ability. The most important goal in breath training is to have high breathe-ability by ingraining a strong resting breath and a flexible conscious breath to be used on demand. The resting breath contributes to the overall balance in the biological system, or centre, as I have been calling it. It forms a key element in maintaining a high parasympathetic tone in the autonomic nervous system and it provides balance to the Green and Red-Light Reflexes of the somatic nervous system for developing good posture. I call a good quality resting breath a naturally-centred breath, because it reflects the state of a naturally centred and balanced person. A person with a naturally centred breath needs to utilise that breath as required by life. This leads us to the second aspect of breathe-ability: the *Deliberate Breath*.

A deliberate breath needs to be skilful and flexible in the expression of emotion, exercise and focused skill performance in high-pressure scenarios. With the deliberate breath, a person should be able to gain full access to all their lung capacity and express that capacity with their breath through their voice and body. They should be able to use that breath expression in the most high-pressured circumstances. Multi-million-dollar corporate deals, playing in highly competitive sport, front line responders, studying for exams or moderating an argument are some of the high-pressure situations different people find themselves in on a regular basis. No one situation is worthier than the next and all require a level of heightened breathing to help the person negotiate the terrain. Taking these two aspects of a quality breathing pattern, an image begins to emerge of what breathe-ability looks like at rest and then in performance.

CHARACTERISTICS OF THE NATURALLY-CENTRED BREATH

- The naturally-centred breath breathes as if it is not breathing at all
- It is subtle and imperceptible, quiet, calm and gentle, low in the body and slow
- With the naturally-centred breath, the air is pulled gently in through the nose, filtered, and prepared for use in the body. It flows effortlessly through the body, infusing the cells with oxygen-rich nutrients and eliminating excess waste products
- The naturally-centred breath massages the body, calms the mind, and relaxes the entire biological system
- As a breather requires the breath to perform in life and sport, the resting breath is consciously awakened to the needs of the breather to become a deliberate breath

CHARACTERISTICS OF A DELIBERATE BREATH

- The deliberate breath expands 360°. It shape-shifts as required and moulds itself to the person's needs
- The deliberate breath expresses and regulates emotions delicately, and it connects the breather more deeply to themselves, others, nature and God
- In any given moment, the deliberate breath is ready, at the flick of a switch, to move decisively into action. It provides balance and strength to the body, focuses the mind, and under the greatest of pressures, supports the execution of skills
- The deliberate breath can also be used to downregulate your entire system, and induce states of rest, relaxation and regeneration
- The deliberate breath can send you deeper into states of meditation, visualization and contemplation

THE TWO ASPECTS OF BREATHE-ABILITY	
Naturally Centred Breath	**Deliberate Breath**
Imperceptible/subtle	On-demand
Quiet	Expressing emotion through the exhale, the voice and movement
Calm	Ability to fully use the lungs
Gentle	Capitalise on breath holding to create pressure
Low into the belly	Controlling the exhale
Let go of the exhale	Use the mouth to vent fatigue
	Use the breath to create strength, power, force through the kinetic chain
	Change the breath pattern to focus the mind
	Find creative solutions to problems
	Change the breath pattern to connect more deeply with yourself, others, nature and God through meditation and visualisation

Together, the components of the two quality breathing patterns, the naturally-centred breath and the deliberate breath, form an overall picture of a quality breath. The next section will review the use of this quality breath (breathe-ability) in practice as applied to daily life and performance.

BREATHING DURING THE DAY

The naturally-centred breath is used as the optimal breathing pattern throughout the day. It is performed with the nose only. It is calm, quiet, low, and rhythmical. The exhale 'lets go' or has a recoil effect. It looks like a gentle ocean wave rolling onto shore on a calm summer's day. It rises gently out of the sea, rolls over at the top and washes out on the shore.

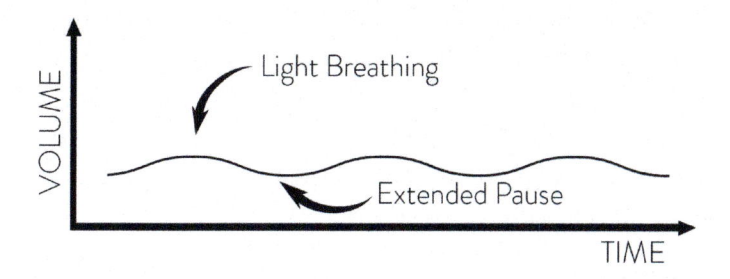

As you inhale through your nose, you breathe low or deep into the belly using the diaphragm. Belly breathing, is of course, an analogy used to symbolise diaphragmatic breathing. You don't actually breathe with your abdominal muscles at rest but, as the diaphragm is engaged, you notice the tummy protrudes a little; the lower ribs expand laterally and to the back. Due to the size of the hole, nasal breathing encourages the diaphragm to be used 50% more than mouth breathing. The diaphragm needs to pull the air deeply into the body to overcome gravity, as opposed to allowing it just to flow in through a large, open mouth, and so a nasal inhalation automatically creates a 'low' breath (the only exception to this rule is when our diaphragm is retracted, and I'll address that one in our training).

The naturally-centred breath is calm and quiet; it is not a big breath. You do not need to use your full lung capacity when you are resting during the day. You want efficiency in the breath. As your breathing becomes more subtle during the day, breath efficiency improves, cells receive more oxygenation, the body relaxes, and the mind calms. The main regulator of the naturally-centred breath is carbon dioxide. That is why a nasal exhale becomes so important. The nose is built to regulate carbon dioxide better than the mouth. As you nasal exhale, your brain senses carbon dioxide more efficiently, and it regulates a more rhythmical and calm subconscious breathing pattern.

With a gentler diaphragmatic inhale and a smoother breath rhythm, the exhale just falls out of the body, like the wave washing upon the shore. At rest, that is how the exhale should look; it is a recoil action or a spring. Activities during the day, such as eating and speaking, will obviously change the depth of breathing; nonetheless, it should contain all the characteristics of a quality breath.

Ideally, when eating, you should eat with your mouth closed. As you chew your food, you breathe through your nose. This encourages better tongue, jaw, head and neck posture. It builds stronger jaws, broader nasal cavities and bigger airways. It promotes better breathing habits and prepares the food better for digestion by your gut.

When speaking, you inhale through your nose and exhale through your mouth. The exhale is no longer a spring; it becomes an expression of the breath through the vocal cords. The throat muscles contract and change the shape of the breath to produce various sounds. This is all normal and natural for us. When speaking, you should articulate the voice slowly and clearly. When you need to inhale, check to make sure you inhale through your nose. Very often modern-day people rush their speech, inhale through their mouth, and begin to ingrain a heightened breathing pattern. Strain is placed on their neck, jaw and upper chest muscles to produce sound, posture alters, subconscious breathing adapts, and an aroused biological state ensues.

BREATHING TO EXPRESS EMOTION

The second part of voice control is using the breath and voice to express emotions: crying, laughing, anger, sorrow, frustration, joy, and happiness. All the emotions are expressed with a combination of breath, voice and body movement. Your exhale plays the most significant role in expressing emotion. The expression of the breath works just the same as any other expression of power in the body.

Bruce Lee, for example, described a punch a long time ago. In his description, he said that a punch should be relaxed until the very last moment before impact, then it tenses for the split second of impact, and returns to a nice, relaxed state.

The punch is a whole-body elastic movement; so is running and so is the voice's expression. At rest, the exhale of the breath is relaxed, the voice box and upper neck and chest muscles also maintain a low tone. When you want to express your emotion loud and clear, you upregulate the breath, voice, and body to work together in a coherent manner. After the expression, it automatically relaxes once more.

The issue for many people is that they constantly have a high tone of tension in their exhale, voice, and body. All the muscles are working when they should be resting, and when it comes to needing to use those muscles at the right time, they don't have much power to give. The emotion does not get expressed as the body needs. The body is left feeling unsatisfied with the outburst and there is residual emotion left over. Think of your exhale like a guitar string tuned to play beautiful music. If the string is overtightened, the notes played by the musician appear different to a perfectly tightened string. It is the same with the exhale. Over time, the tight muscles of the exhale and the lack of emotional expression results in a suppression of emotion, and an embodying of that emotion. To express that emotion, we need to train ourselves to let go of the exhale, in particular, and we need to build some capacity to breathe into the body.

BREATHING DURING SLEEP

Quality sleep is vitally important to the health of your body. Without it, you don't fully restore your system from the events of the day; you don't clear the clutter of our mind, you don't detoxify the body's organs from the pollutants you take in. Quality sleep is composed of two phases repeated several times during the night. A relaxed biological state is imperative for you to get to sleep easily and remain asleep during the night to enable all these processes to occur. Heightened breathing patterns, especially mouth breathing, reduce your ability to relax, it keeps you awake, and even wakes you up during the night. When you breathe well at night, you subconsciously create the environment for quality sleep to happen. You set a relaxed body state, and you enable the body to get on with its jobs while you enjoy your sleep. The result is a great night's sleep and rising awake and refreshed in the morning. Breathing well at night requires only two things, the first is a quality day-time breathing pattern, and the second is nose-only breathing at night.

It is much easier to address breathing during the day before you start to address breathing during sleep. If you try to address breathing during sleep first you may become anxious, and you may not be able to embed the habits long-term because of the daytime breathing patterns. There are always exceptions to the rule, of course! Encouraging nose breathing at night involves two things: good posture, and taping your mouth at night until you can nose breathe automatically. I'll speak about these practices in the lifestyle section of the training programme.

BREATHING TO CONNECT

People synchronise their rhythms with each other. That is why it is said you are the average of the five people you spend most time with; it is why the ovulation cycles of women who live together synchronise and it's why groups of people all have amazing experiences together. Synchronising rhythms is the way people and nature connect. When you are out of sync with nature and with the people you are around, you feel 'off'; you feel like something is wrong and you feel disconnected.

The way you synchronise with people and nature is through some elemental practices. Spending time in nature, swimming, walking, drumming, music, singing, chanting, dancing, taking on challenges, experiencing a traumatic event, focusing on achieving something special, and breathing are a few of those elemental rhythms innate to us all. When you immerse yourself in an environment with these elemental practices, you connect deeply with others. You just can't help but join in the beat of a strong rhythm. Everyone is attracted to a more powerful rhythm. That may be a slow, loud beat of a drum or a fast and light quick-step. In general, the faster the energy flows, the more you are attracted to falling in step with that rhythm. The same applies to every rhythm, including breathing.

When we breathe together, we connect more deeply together. This is what is being seen in breathing workshops all over the world. It doesn't matter whether you do the Wim Hof method, holotropic breathwork, box breathing, or meditation. If breathing was featured as a source of power in a movie, you could say that it is the one ring that binds everything together. The only thing that separates us is our perception that we are different. If you removed people's desire for difference in the world, you could strip back all these other practices and simply connect to breathing to bind us all together. Because there is such diversity in the world and such beauty in that diversity, we keep those other practices. But now you can make sense of those other elemental practices and enhance them by breathing the rhythm of the state you want to produce in that practice. Breathe bigger and faster to increase your state of autonomic arousal and that of the room. Breathe more subtly to induce calm and peace. Simply breathe together to connect more deeply with the ones you love.

Communicating, expressing emotion, and sharing are how we connect to other people. All these processes involve the breath. When you breathe well, you automatically connect better with people.

BREATHING UNDER HIGH MENTAL PRESSURE

Breathing is connected to states of arousal in the brain. It is also tied to focus, attention, and fear in the brain. The more calmly you breathe, the more relaxed you remain, and the more clearly you can think.

PART 2   BREATH-ABILITY

> *The first benefit that I noticed from these breath exercises was that I had more energy throughout the day and that I was starting to sleep more soundly. Whenever I was feeling tired, I would go for a walk and do a few breath holds and immediately feel that I had more energy to continue about my day. I also started to feel more in control at work and better able to regulate myself and my moods. I felt that as a result I was better able to work through problems again and I had a much clearer head to deal with problems. I also noticed that I was a lot calmer during the day and was better able to deal with difficult issues that arose at work and at home.*
>
> LIAM O MAHONY, INNATE-STRENGTH CLIENT

The naturally-centred breath is still the most apt breathing pattern to use in period of high mental stress. However, sometimes the pressure is too much for you, and you need to vent or let your system breathe. You can do this in advance to prepare for a high-pressure scenario and/or you can do it in the pressure cooker itself. According to Dr. Feldman, a prominent neurophysiologist in the study of breath and the brain, all you need to do is to interrupt the rut. In other words, you just need to change your breathing pattern any way you prefer – faster or slower, longer or shorter, it does not matter (at least not yet, according to research). You simply need to change the way you breathe to change the way you think. Breath awareness becomes the first key to changing your breath. Once you become aware of your pattern, you can perform any technique for as little as two minutes to change how you feel and to improve your thought pattern. I find a ten-breath coffee breathing technique very effective in preparing you for a pressure cooker scenario. Breathing in for four seconds and out for six seconds using the nose is perhaps one of the most powerful techniques to interrupt the rut amid a boardroom battle. Recently, Dr. Feldman and another neurophysiologist, named Dr. Huberman, promoted sighing as a great way reset the body, on the *Huberman Lab* podcast. According to Dr. Feldman, the body naturally sighs once

BREATHING EXERCISE PERFORM AN INTENTIONAL YAWN

Inhale fully through your mouth. As you inhale, open your mouth wide and stretch your whole jaw.

Stick out and wiggle your tongue, then bring your whole body into the stretch.

Repeat this intentional yawn five times.

Look out for the relaxation. The recoil of your exhale and the ease of your body after the stretch.

That's where the beauty of this technique lies.

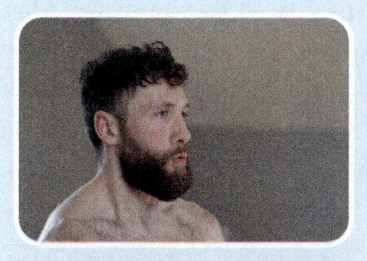

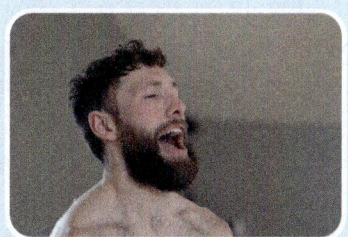

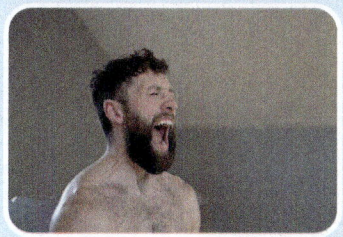

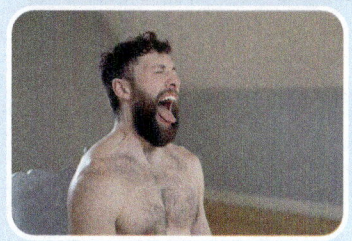

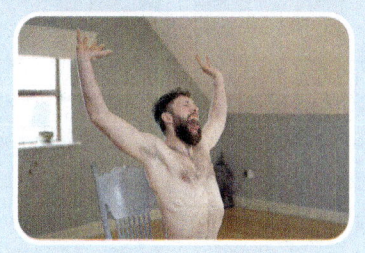

every five minutes. The benefit of this innate body action is to maintain alveoli function in the lungs by bringing movement and lubricant to these tiny air sacs. If the body did not sigh, Dr. Feldman said that we would lose lung function very fast and it could even result in death. Dr. Huberman believes you can capitalise on this innate action by consciously using it to help you relax. His research is unpublished yet, but he says that this conscious 'physiological sigh' is the fastest way to change the state of your system. It simply involves a double inhale followed by an exhale repeated multiple times. This conversation fascinated me because I similarly discussed yawning with Matt Nichol back in 2020. Matt is one of the best strength coaches in Canadian professional sport. He noticed that some of the NHL hockey professionals he coached would yawn right before a game, which perplexed him. While researching his observation, he found that yawning, like sighing, was an innate action by the body to balance the nervous system in a highly stressful scenario. His NHL boys were stressed going into battle on the ice and as they yawned, they were able to relax and focus better. Yawning is very similar to sighing. At its core, a yawn is an extended inhale combined with an exhale that is let go. The difference between the two is that the yawn is typically bigger than a sigh, it involves a massive stretch of the jaw muscles, and it often brings a whole-body stretch with it.

BREATHING UNDER HIGH PHYSICAL PRESSURE

I hear and I forget. I see and I remember. I do and I understand

CONFUCIUS

In becoming a breathing coach, I decided I needed to do more than just read the books and perform the breathing techniques. I needed to test breathing in action too. The first test I set myself was to fulfil a childhood desire and run a marathon. I'd always wanted to run a marathon but, given my education in strength and conditioning, I believed the traditional training for a recreational athlete was misguided at best and downright dangerous at worst. The amount of mileage people run in preparation for a marathon far exceeds their needs, and when you pile that amount of mileage on top of poor running mechanics and a poorly functioning breathing system, it's no wonder people develop so many injuries. In contrast to traditional running, I knew from my past experiences that breathing had a huge role to play in fitness. I still vividly remember the winter GAA training session when it all clicked in place for me.

With another twelve years of breath training, strength, and conditioning education, I knew I had a better way of training for a marathon. I thought that if people integrate breath training into their overall training schedule, then they could run a better race and recover faster without the need for so many miles in training and the very high risk of injury. I decided to isolate and test breath training against the norm. I chose to run the marathon using breath training alone, combined with some prehabilitation training for my body's joints, tissues and muscles. And this was on the back of no endurance training (running, cycling, rowing or swimming) for more than seven years. I hadn't run much farther than running for a bus in that time!

The first step in the training plan was to get tested as a baseline. I recorded breathing and heart rate scores daily and I performed two VO2 max tests in the lead-up to the race; one at the beginning of the 16-week training block and one towards the end. I'm delighted I chose the VO2 max test because it was one of the most fascinating and enlightening experiences for me through all my years of researching the breath. It gave me the data and insights to understand what is happening with the breath in exercise and how to train it properly. During the tests I discovered the relationship between my breathing level and energy systems. This was nowhere in research at the time and it provided a key insight for me in my race plans. We'll dive deeper into this discovery later in the book but just know that it was the catalyst for me successfully running the race with my mouth taped! Not only that but I also fully recovered within three days and used the breath training again to compete in the Irish Open Judo Masters a week later, where I achieved a bronze medal. Not bad for someone who only trained their breath and prehab in the previous 16 weeks!

Running that race and competing in the judo inspired me to learn more about the breath. I wanted to know if my results were a freak of nature or if they applied to other people trained in breathing. Luckily for me, I was able to recruit ten GAA sport players from a division 1 team I had been coaching for the previous two years. All were adapted nose breathers and all were willing to do the VO2 max test. Again, the results blew my mind; all the participants had similar results to me. My insights were not just relative to me; now I knew that any breath-trained sportsperson could achieve similar results, and I knew this training was imperative to the health and performance of every sportsperson. My experience of the breath, my gut feeling, and my research were further backed up by the experiences and research of friends and colleagues of mine in America, Brian MacKenzie and Rob Wilson.

Brian and Rob are the founders of *Art of Breath*, a breath training program originally aimed at athletes and the cross-fit community which has since expanded to the general population. They built this programme shortly after we had conversations on breathing in early 2017. In these conversations I shared my insights into nose breathing, breath-holding, CO_2 tolerance, and the Buteyko method, whilst they shared their insights on Wim Hof, free diving, and yoga breathing techniques. Over the following year, we all went away and did our own research into breathing and it became apparent that we had arrived at similar conclusions. Brian and Rob tested on their end, and I on mine. The results were starkly similar. Again, these were not random effects of breath training or freaks of nature. Now there was a pattern. Time and again, that pattern showed the relationship between breathing and energy systems.

Physical pressure is slightly different to mental pressure. When you are under physical stress, both your body and mind come under pressure; there are more signals to contend with. This means we need to

Direct Benefits of Better Breathing

- Better preparation of air for your respiratory system (filtration, moisture, heat)
- Better regulation of carbon dioxide
- Improved delivery of oxygen to your cells
- More efficient use of breathing muscles
- Larger breathing capacity
- More sensitive to stress and how it affects you
- Enhanced senses of smell, taste and hearing

With the ability to...

- Express emotion
- Meditate more deeply
- Problem solve
- Unleash creativity
- Provide strength to the body
- Energise the body and mind

Benefits to Overall Health and Performance

- Decreased symptoms of all lifestyle-related diseases with the potential to cure those diseases
- Decreased psychological disorders and diseases
- Decreased symptoms of allergic reactions
- Decreased response to pain, panic and anxiety
- Lower blood pressure and heart rate
- Improved sexual function and desire
- Improved balance to hormones
- Better blood sugar management
- Improved bone formation in children and young adults

- Process traumatic events and high stress
- Promote physical, mental and spiritual healing
- Regulate emotions better
- More relaxed
- More balanced nervous system
- More calm in the body and mind
- More regular and balanced menstrual cycle for women
- Improved mood
- Happier outlook in life
- More positive mindset
- Better cognition

- Better athletic performance
- Increased endurance
- Shorter warm-up periods
- Quicker start to sport
- Improved stress response
- Better regulated sweating
- More relaxed
- Better response to high levels of stress
- Think clearly
- Focus more sharply
- Concentrate for longer
- More energy
- Improved immune system
- Improved sleep

use the breath to regulate energy in the body to maintain focus and attention, and keep a clear mind. Typically, modern sports people have been taught to breathe in through the nose and out of the mouth for physical activity. More recently, people are being instructed to only nasal breathe. Which is right? Actually they both are. For sportspeople, breathing works progressively, like changing gears in a car. I call it the Breathing Level System.

Ideally, you should build a high aerobic base, using nose breathing only in training. The first step is to ingrain a naturally-centred breath pattern into your daily life. As pressure intensifies through a warmup and in sport, you progressively open your breathing system. You use more of your breathing capacity, and you turn that subtle naturally-centred breath pattern into a much bigger breath wave. Progressively opening your breathing system enables a better regulation of CO_2 and supply of air, to meet the body's demands. This is better than jumping to a nasal inhale and mouth exhale pattern. You can also learn to change your breathing patterns to suit your individual needs and that of your sport. If you need more strength, you can create that pressure by shaping a mouth-controlled exhale. You can focus your mind by releasing the exhale and calming your breath. You can dump CO_2 through a variety of approaches to reduce fatigue. When you've ingrained a quality breathing pattern in your system first, all these amazing and wondrous breathing techniques will help you breathe better under greater loads of physical pressure.

UNDERSTANDING BREATHING TECHNIQUES 10

The problem with breathing techniques and breath-work is not the limited supply of knowledge but knowing which ones to use for a particular purpose. For the past 16 years, I've looked at breathing and tried to decipher what is going on with it. In particular, over the last five years I have reviewed hundreds of research articles, read dozens of books, spoken with many experts in the field, and trained with some of the international pioneers of the breathing world. In all that time, I have only come across breathing techniques and methods, not principles and frameworks. Yoga, Wim Hof, Buteyko, Rebirthing, Zen, Coherent, Mindful, Shamanic Breathing are all examples of techniques and methods. Some of these techniques are good for rehabilitating the muscles of your breathing system; others for the chemistry, and more for the psyche. Some are good to get you riled up, and others calm you down. Each technique and method has pros and cons in its own right. However, it has always baffled me why a technique works for one person and not for another. It also confused me why some people hated a particular technique and someone else could love it. Take people immersed in the Wim Hof and Buteyko methods, for example. Ask a follower of the Buteyko method to supra-ventilate like Wim Hof and they'll think you are mad. Tell them it's beneficial to their health to mouth breathe or breathe big like Wim and they'll scorn you. Equally, you tell a 'Hoffer' they are harming their health by breathing big like Wim and they will laugh at you.

Unlike nutrition, sleep, and exercise, the development and understanding of breathing as a practice is still in its infancy. In the last year or two, modern breath practitioners have become more open to the different breathing methods. As they study the different methods, they understand that no method holds all the answers; rather, different people have different needs. That first-hand experiential knowledge is now filtering into research and academia. Research into breathing has only really been integrated and examined comprehensively over the last ten years. These are small timeframes considering it takes at least twenty years for that research to filter down to public application. This is partly the reason why doctors don't know about the power of breathing for mental and physical health, why therapists have great success with some clients and not with others, and why coaches often mistake their traditional knowledge of breathing as universal knowledge for all. In time, I think the breadth of experience and knowledge of breathing, the research, and the science will extend beyond techniques and methods into frameworks. It is already beginning.

Over the past five years I have peeled back the veneer of more than one hundred breathing techniques and dozens of methods in an effort to find the underlying principles of breathing and breathwork. I have broken through my own fears and opinions of seemingly opposing techniques, formed through the adoption of particular methods, to understand exactly what is happening in the body with a person's breathing pattern. I am not the only person doing this work. Particular aspects of breathing, such as the psychological, emotional and mechanical effects, have been detailed in books by Dr. Stan Grof, Judith Kravitz and Alison McConnell, for example. The mechanisms of these effects have been more deeply connected in books by Timmons and Ley, Chaitow and Morningstar. Finally, this knowledge is being simplified and communicated to lay people in great books like *Breath* by James Nestor, *The Breathing Cure* and *The Oxygen Advantage* by Patrick McKeown, and *Breath* and *Breathing for Warriors* by Dr. Belissa Vranich.

There are also people like Brian MacKenzie and Rob Wilson of Shift Adapt in the USA who are producing similar work to me. This work goes beyond methods, techniques and aspects of breathing into integrating all our knowledge of breathing. Laying all the cards on the table, I have been mapping out how anybody can gradually develop their breathing system and use breathing techniques for specific purposes in life and sport. In addition to building the framework for breath training, I also wanted to know how I can coach the weakest person in the room to restore their own breathing back to a natural centre, and use it to perform at their best in life. This whole process begins with understanding your state of being and the idea that we're strongest when we operate from a state of natural centre, rather than an adapted perceived centre of being. Then you need to know how stress affects your state of being. Stage three recognises the power of breathing in general to influence your state of centre. We have covered both these topics in some detail up to now. The next stage is understanding the power of individual breathing techniques on your state. Finally, you can begin to get much smarter about your approach by leaning on my experiences to train yourself to restoring your centre through the Innate-Strength framework of breath training.

STAGES OF UNDERSTANDING THE IMPACTS OF BREATHING ON YOUR STATE

1. Understanding your state of being and the concepts of natural and perceived centre
2. Understanding how stress acts on our state
3. Understanding the role of breathing in restoring you to your natural centre
4. Understanding the power of individual breathing techniques on your state
5. Restoring your breath using the *Innate-Strength* breath training framework

Now that you understand the first three stages to restoring your breath, we begin our journey into how you can use breathing to benefit you. The first step in any training programme is to become aware of what you're doing. Breath awareness is the fundamental aspect of training. Knowing how you breathe daily and respond to different stressors is incredibly valuable in learning how to restore your breathing. Sometimes, awareness alone is enough to change your state of being. Most times, however, it is very difficult to change that state of being when you're in the middle of a stressful scenario. This is where building strong baselines is important. You need to take time out of your day to practise, breathing to make it effective when you need it most. The most basic and effective form of breath training is to pick any technique and practise it. You can choose the same one every day or choose different ones on different days. Through awareness, consistent daily practise and a desire to improve, you are likely to restore your breathing in time. The next section dissects common breathing techniques to give you an understanding of their effects on you. If you are looking for more structure in your training, I provide a breath training framework for these techniques in part three.

THE POWER OF TECHNIQUES ON YOU

The power of a technique is determined by two main factors – the size of the breath and the time in the technique. Big or small, fast and long, slow and short, through the nose or through the mouth, with a long breath hold or none – these are the characteristics of a breath or the variables we can adjust to make the size of a technique more or less powerful. The impact of a technique depends on its innate variables combined with your alterations to those variables and your state of being at the time of performing the technique. Understanding this map helps you choose the right technique for you at the right time in your life. To lay out the map in full, I will show you the variables, their potential power, how you adapt them, and then how you choose the right ones for you. Here's the full list of breathing characteristics below:

BREATHING TECHNIQUE CHARACTERISTICS

(Variables to adjust size of the technique)

Breath-holding with movement

Static breath-holding

Extending the exhale

Extending the inhale

Humming or toning

Reducing the amount of air you breathe

Choosing the vent you use – nose only, nose/mouth, mouth only

Bigger breathing

Faster breathing

Full Breaths

Time in an exercise

The variables of breathing either pull you towards a lower state of arousal or rest, recovery and rejuvenation, or to a heightened state of arousal – they give you the feeling of energy, alertness, focus, and concentration. The power of a technique is determined by how much it challenges you, and how far it pulls you away from your centre. When you stack several variables on top of each other, the technique increases in power. Time is the other variable to consider, and it is the one variable which applies to both sides of the continuum. The longer you perform any technique, the more challenging it becomes and its effects have a greater impact on you.

PART 2 BREATH-ABILITY

Moving Breath Hold

Toning / Humming

Static Breath Hold

Extended Exhales

Mouth

Bigger

Faster

Naturally Centred Breath

5 – 10 Mins +

0 – 5 Mins

5 – 60 Mins +

Time

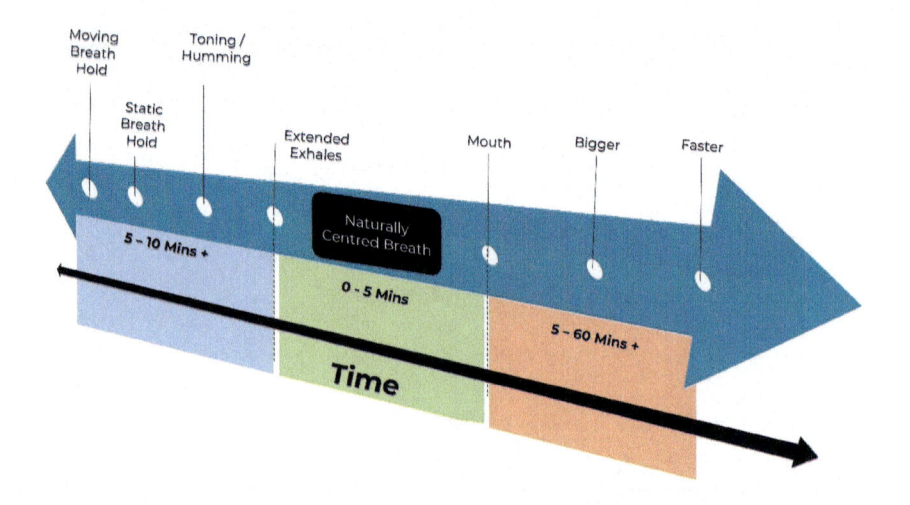

THE POWER OF TECHNIQUES

Variables	Lowering Arousal	Neutral	Heightening Arousal
	Reduced breathing Breath-holding Breath-holding with movement Extended exhales Toning and humming	Calm, subtle, nose breathing Techniques on either side of the continuum used for short periods (2-5 mins typically)	Mouth breathing Fast breathing Large breaths

By default, every common technique and method contains its own base power – either a lowering arousal technique or a heightening one. Some techniques are innately very powerful by the number of variables built into them, and others have less of an impact on your system. Finally, there are some techniques which I classify as neutral. These techniques are typically used as a short reset to your system to help you focus or relax in the moment but they do not necessarily have a long-term effect on your system. Opposite is my classification of some typical modern breathing techniques according to their impacts on your state:

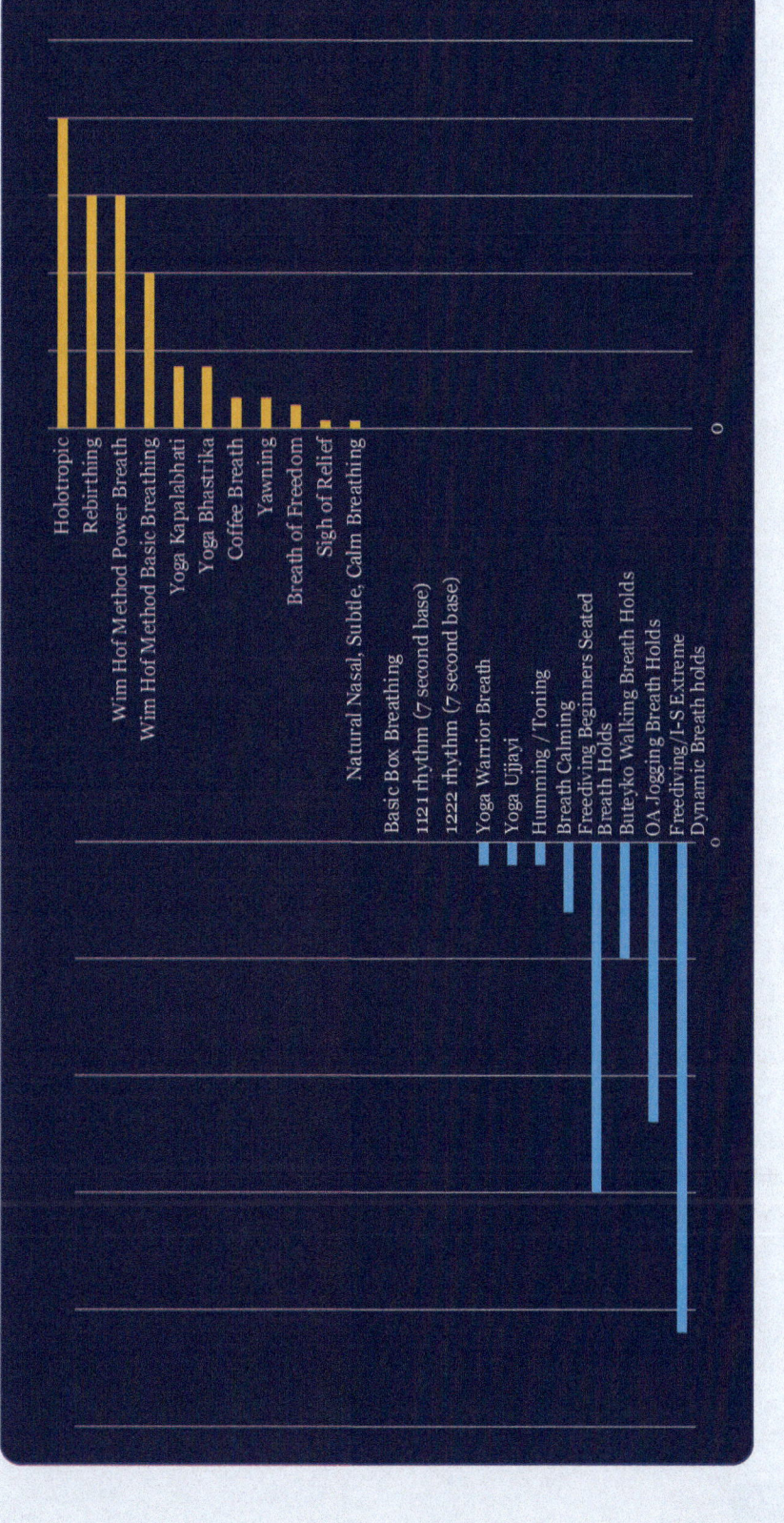

Holotropic
Rebirthing
Wim Hof Method Power Breath
Wim Hof Method Basic Breathing
Yoga Kapalabhati
Yoga Bhastrika
Coffee Breath
Yawning
Breath of Freedom
Sigh of Relief
Natural Nasal, Subtle, Calm Breathing

Basic Box Breathing
1121 rhythm (7 second base)
1222 rhythm (7 second base)
Yoga Warrior Breath
Yoga Ujjayi
Humming / Toning
Breath Calming
Freediving Beginners Seated Breath Holds
Buteyko Walking Breath Holds
OA Jogging Breath Holds
Freediving I-S Extreme
Dynamic Breath holds

This map is a representative illustration of breathing technique power based on the characteristics of each technique. There are four-time groups displayed on the map and five variables which impact the technique's power.

TECHNIQUE VARIABLES	
Time in Technique	Other Variables affecting the technique
5 mins 5-20min 20-60 mins 60 mins +	Vent Size Breathing rate Physiological breath-holding effects Interoceptive / Emotional Supraventilation effects

As you can see for yourself, most breathing techniques are only performed for a handful of minutes. Techniques longer than five minutes are generally used for breath training and breathwork. These are the ones which produce a strong response from the body and alter the biology of your body in the long run. The less powerful techniques are great for changing your state within minutes, feeling better, and finding some balance in your day (calm or energising depending on what you want). These are the ones closer to 0 on the map. These less potent exercises are also the techniques I'd recommend when starting a breath practice for the first time, without any coach to help you out. Techniques with neutral power don't build a stronger natural centre or explore the inside edge of your comfort zone from a physiological perspective. However, you can change this impact in two ways.

1. Change the power of the technique
2. Use a neutral technique in a highly stressful situation

The first way is to drastically change the technique variables and the original intent of the technique. A box breath is an example of a neutral technique. Box breathing is typically performed for up to two minutes. It uses an equal inhale – hold – exhale – hold pattern for a count of four seconds. It is best used to help you to calm and focus in moments of high tension; that is why it is often the technique of choice for service people in the Navy and armies worldwide. The box breath will not change your overall long-term state, it won't build your centre or explore your boundaries in its natural form but you could adjust its variables to produce a more powerful effect and use it for training. For example, extending the size of the box from four seconds to seven increases CO_2 levels in your system and challenges you to stay calm during a tough exercise. This alteration to the box will benefit your CO_2 tolerance, diaphragm contractility and states of mind under pressure. Altering the box further by changing the balance of ratio of inhale to exhale will also increase the box's potency. It then becomes a technique and an approach you can use to challenge yourself to improve your long-term health. In fact, altering any one of the breathing variables can change the effects of a technique rapidly. It comes back to principles again. Think of a squat exercise in a gym. Technically a basic bodyweight squat is not a powerful technique but can potentially become very powerful if you change the variables. Add a barbell with 60 kg weight, and it has a more powerful impact on changing your body than a bodyweight squat. Performing multiple sets of ten reps changes it again. Slow down the movement or speed it up, and the benefits of the technique differ. Breathing is no different to squatting or any other movement in the gym. Understanding the variables in the exercise and their power helps you to predict its effects, especially when it is mapped onto your arousal continuum.

The second way to make a neutral technique more powerful is to use it in highly stressful situations. Your ability to become aware of your breath and hold a neutral breathing technique in a highly stressful situation teaches your body, mind, and spirit to remain calm in the face of danger. Even breath awareness alone can be highly potent when you can maintain your attention on your breathing when highly stressed.

TECHNIQUES ARE GREAT BUT REMEMBER YOUR BASELINES

Now that you know the power of techniques, you can get to work on improving your own breathing. Start by finding a technique with the least power that delivers a state change for you. This is called the *Minimum Effective Dose*. Practise that technique daily until you feel inspired to try something else new. Then repeat the process. Like an artist experimenting with different colours, textures and techniques, you too select a breathing technique with an open inquisitive mind and a willingness to use your breath creatively. Some people are artists and love this way of experiencing the breath. I am a little different. My view is that your baselines, your natural centre, need to be restored in a focused and structured way. I have found this approach to be less frustrating for people like me who want to breathe free. It is also far more efficient and effective at delivering results for you.

In any practice, the biggest barrier to success is commitment daily over a long period of time. People enter half-committed to a program, they don't know their 'why', they don't understand how training works, they're not fully engaged with the technique, and they can't see the benefits of the training. In the end, I found the answers to my client's problems by structuring a breath practice into a framework of training; the focused intention of breathing free is the result of all that experience. This book is a culmination of all that work. I believe it forms the foundation for breath training in the future. The techniques I use in the framework may change over time as our collective experience and knowledge of breathing improves, but I feel the overall framework for breathing will remain intact. Now that you have read the background information to the breath, it is time for you to experience it for yourself and learn the skill of Breathe-Ability.

PART 3

THE INNATE-STRENGTH BREATH TRAINING PROGRAMME

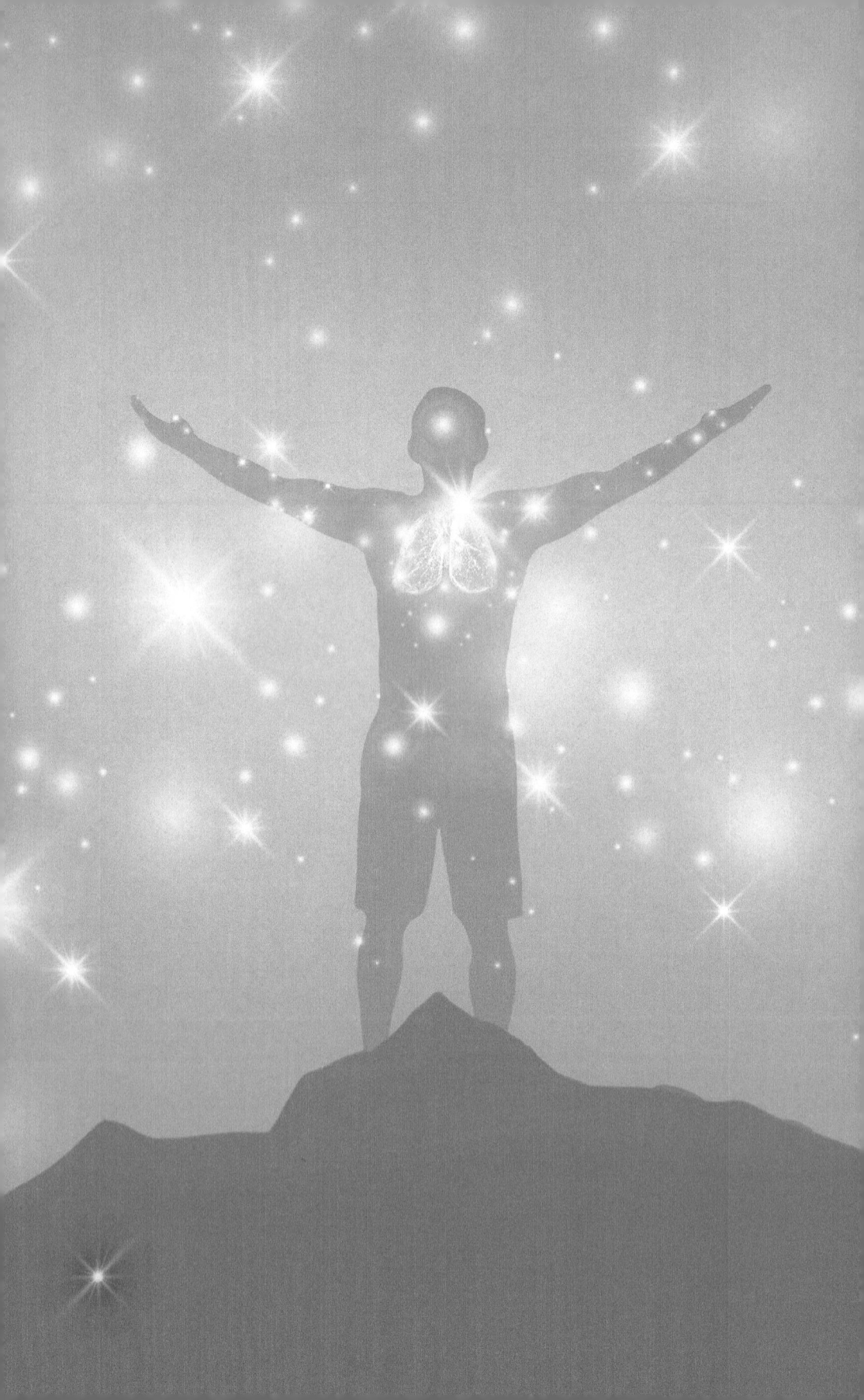

ROAD MAPPING YOUR SUCCESS 11

WHEN YOU SUCCESSFULLY PREPARE, PREPARE FOR SUCCESS

Many people consider breathing to be automatic, so it doesn't even occur to them that they should develop it as a skill. Rather than call it automatic, I think of it as subconscious. It is something that happens beneath our awareness during our everyday lives. By bringing awareness to our breath, we notice that it is responsive to our lives. Sleeping, exercising, eating, and moving all change patterns to match our needs. Some might ask, shouldn't I just leave it be and allow it to take its natural course? I would tend to agree with them if we lived a life aligned to our biological needs. However, our lives and our breathing have adapted to modern life to the extent that our breathing may no longer serve us efficiently and effectively. From this perspective, we can also consider breathing as a skill and training as the systematic approach to developing that skill. Breath training, then, is the process of gradually (re)learning the craft of breathing for health and performance purposes. I say (re)learning because most of us knew how to breathe well as a child; we've simply trained ourselves out of it because of our lack of attention and knowledge. It is rare for people to develop adapted breathing patterns overnight. Usually, it takes years and years to develop. Unravelling those patterns also takes time, focus, and effort. It took me eighteen months of daily practise to cure fifteen years of asthma. What I am trying to say here is: breathing free is ultimately down to you. You must do the training, perform the techniques, make the lifestyle changes, and integrate the practice into your life. You need to be determined to make a change and keep that determination throughout the process until you, too, feel like you have gained everything you want from the experience. In our modern age of 'insta-everything', many are looking for a quick fix. The only hack to developing your breathing system and your health is the experience of somebody further down the road than you.

Up until now I have suggested that you stay open to trying many forms of breathing to see what works for you. This approach does work, but it can take a very long time to achieve your ultimate goal. What I am presenting to you is a distillation of my own experience, and knowledge to deliver faster results for you. I stay true to the need to experience both sides of the breathing continuum, but I do it in a structured, safe and effective way. I also deliver the breathing programme in the broader context of life. Before I begin showing you the breathing techniques, I will share some insights from my experience of breath training in this chapter to help you on your journey. These are coaching and personal development strategies which I hope will enhance your experience, focus your mind, and help you achieve your goal of breathing more quickly. I start by sharing the importance of changing how you look at life. Next, I give you a template for creating a vision for your breath and your life. Then I define the steps you need to take to achieve that vision, and finally, I round off the chapter by sharing with you some ways to keep you on track and make the whole process enjoyable. Although you may want to jump straight into the programme at this stage, I encourage you to do these personal development exercises first and return to them throughout. They are the means to help keep you on track when times get hard and you're not overly motivated to continue your practice. They are not compulsory exercises, but they do come highly recommended.

CHANGING YOUR PERCEPTIONS

Your perceptions are your reality. Shortness of breath, low energy, dysfunction, pain, and disease are significant indicators that you are living out of synchronicity with your body, mind and spirit. You were created with the capacity for optimal health; that is your natural state, and this is the perception of health you need to hold in your mind. You need to clean your glasses and perhaps even replace the lens. You must look at health through a crystal-clear lens. With that clear lens, you can see the details of what it takes to have optimal health, like breathing freely, moving often, sleeping soundly, and nourishing your body, mind and spirit. As you change your perception of health, and put the practices of optimal health into action, you will realise you have an excellent opportunity to become even healthier, and live a more remarkable life – a life beyond shortness of breath, restless nights sleeping, afternoon energy slumps, disease symptoms, and medication. A life more resilient to viruses, bacteria, and infection. A life that you can then use to pursue your dreams, and live the way you want. This is what I call your great life. As you build these new healthy living practices into your life, your health slowly but surely begins to improve too.

Maybe it's time to let the old ways die

BRADLEY COOPER

This is a simple road but not an easy one. It takes courage to change your lifestyle. Finding optimal health takes pain, love, faith, hope, persistence, focus, and continual effort for years to find optimal health. There's no point in sugar-coating it. You need to decide you are changing once and for all, then you need to burn your boats, and give yourself no other option but to change. That doesn't mean you won't fall back into your old ways; you very likely will. It does mean when you get prompted to start anew, you forgive yourself for failing and find a way to pull yourself out of that hole and move forward with your health.

PART 3   THE INNATE-STRENGTH BREATH TRAINING PROGRAMME

LOOKING MORE CLOSELY AT YOURSELF

It's time we looked at what you are bringing to the party. This way you can prepare yourself better for training, execute it beyond the sticking points, and reap the rewards from your efforts. From the moment you were conceived, your history matters. Every major event in your life, every belief system passed onto you, and every habit you have created contributes to your current state of health and performance level. I call this process your growing pains.

In one way or another, you are in pain – the pain of low energy/disease/anguish/physical pain, or the pain of not being the sportsperson you know you could be. It's ok to be in pain. In fact, I think pain is the primary pathway for humans to progress in life. The only way to better this situation is to take responsibility for it and train it. Own your pain. Own your disease. Own your inability to execute a skill and your relatively poor performance. Take 100% responsibility for your life situation and do something about it. That 'something' is training.

The training itself is the easy part, once you know how to do it (that is what this book is all about), but sometimes executing that training requires more nuance than just a 'how to'. Life always throws you curve balls – a death in the family, financial pressure, an argument with a loved one or increased pressure in work are just some of the typical events that compromise people's training success. This is where coaching comes in. During my eighteen years as a coach, I have picked up more than a few tools to help my clients continue to train, even when they don't want to or when life forces them to take their eye off the prize. We all experience these times. Knowing what to do when they come is vital. Your preparation starts now. First, I want you to understand the pathway you are choosing; the training-life-cycle. These are phases or periods of training that almost everybody passes through when they progress from a training novice to becoming able to realise their goals and dreams. Next, I will show you how to set your vision and define your goals. This is the roadmap for you to succeed. I'll finish this chapter by giving you some great coaching insights to help you manage your motivation for breath training through the hard times and the good.

THE TRAINING LIFE CYCLE

There are four phases within the training life cycle. The first important period is *The Initiation*. The time when you decide you are going to get better. Motivation is high. The drive to train is easy. You execute the plan as prescribed. You are seeing small results, and everything appears fantastic. During this period, keeping a level head and riding the wave smartly is critical. There is no need to turn your world upside down. You simply need to be better than you were yesterday. Your body improves with small increments over time. Enjoy this phase of training. Settle into your new way of living and integrate it with your life as you know it.

I call the second important phase *The Drag*. It arrives when your motivation to train is low because you've taken your foot off the pedal, reduced your training frequency, and you're no longer seeing results. You're doing your training, and you still feel awful; you feel like giving up.

The third period arrives when you see some positive results; you're not in the pain you were in, yet you know your numbers are not that high. This is *The Witching Hour*. It's when your body is at ease, but you haven't built in resiliency yet. Then one or two stressful things happen in your life and all hell breaks loose. Your symptoms return, and you feel terrible. You're in a funk. The exercises you are about to complete become really important when you hit either of these two time periods in your training. When those times come, and they will, you can review this section to give you the hope, inspiration and motivation to continue on your journey.

The Homestretch is the phase of training where you have overcome all the major obstacles of change. You have integrated your training into your life, and it is now part of who you are. You are still training. You are seeing compounding results. You are not quite at the finish line, but that doesn't really matter; you know it is only a matter of time.

Training is easy when it's all going well and you are seeing results. Ask any trainer and they will tell you that these times don't last forever.

PART 3   THE INNATE-STRENGTH BREATH TRAINING PROGRAMME

Now that you are aware of the training life cycle we can empower you with tools and techniques to stay on track. The next chapter gives you these tools.

The information and exercises in these chapters are designed to help you through the most challenging times of your journey, The Drag and Witching Hour phases. When you take the time to execute these exercises before your training, you are giving yourself the best chance at realising your own potential for health and sports performance. The exercises all fall under the remit of creating a vision, an image of success you can tangibly feel with all five senses.

CREATING A VISION OF YOUR SUCCESS

A vision is simply a dream you feel you really, really want, and a dream you can see clearly. Once this image becomes clear in your mind, you move onto generating a plan for realising that vision. The final, and arguably most important, aspect is to act on the project and the image and enjoy the process along the way.

But first, before you create any vision, you need to change your state of being. As Einstein once said, 'We cannot solve our problems with the same thinking we used when we created them'. You need to raise your energy, and feel good before creating something new. There are many techniques to explore. I like to prime both the body and the mind to feel good. We must breathe, move, and think of something good. In the beginning, you can separate these steps. As you become better at it, you will merge the steps into one short and effective practice.

There are three components to designing a complete vision and attaining it. These are: wiring your brain, focusing your intent, and small wins to success. To wire your brain means connecting with your vision in body, mind, and soul. Your subconscious needs to feel like the vision is part of your core self. Goal setting is the most common path to focusing your intent. Breaking your vision down into specific and

PRIMING FOR A VISION

Breathe

- Inhale for 4 seconds and exhale for 6 seconds
- Inhale and exhale out of your nose only
- Fill your lungs with each inhale
- Repeat for two minutes or twelve breaths

Move

- Perform ten bunny hops on the spot
- Exhale every time you jump off the floor
- Stand tall in a victory posture, with hands outstretched overhead like you've just won a race
- Inhale and hold your breath
- Tense your whole body by squeezing all of your muscles
- Exhale and release everything
- Repeat the 'move' exercise three times

Think

- Think of something that makes you feel awesome. It could be a past physical challenge you completed, your favourite day, how you felt with a job promotion or the smile on a loved one's face
- Use one image or allow for a few images
- Hold the feel-good feeling the image brings you
- Magnify the feeling in your body by seeing the image vividly
- Hold the feel-good feeling for sixty-four seconds

measurable chunks is an essential part of the process of realising your vision. Last but not least, taking action on your vision is the primary way to achieve it. As you act on it, make sure to celebrate every mini-success along the way with your loved ones; there's nothing like the feeling of winning to make you want to continue winning some more. Let's dive into each of these areas a little deeper to help you structure the process a little more.

1. Wire your Brain

We begin the process by allowing our mind to imagine the extremes of what we want. Think beyond reality and imagine the impossible. Usually, these extremes contain the kernels of what we truly want in life. By thinking about the extremes, we bypass the negative voices

> **EXAMPLES**
>
> Become healthy, energised, and pain-free for the first time in ages and then be able to return to sport
>
> Enhance my training, mental resilience, and physical health through breathing
>
> Participate in a marathon, an ironman, or my own personal endurance event
>
> Set off on an adventure like climbing Mt. Everest, running Marathon Des Sables, or trek on an Arctic expedition
>
> Have more energy to be more productive in work and get to the position in my career I crave
>
> Have the energy and fitness to play with my kids after a long day's work and take them out on weekends to do cool activities like rock climbing

keeping us from what we actually want. Start by listing every outlandish thing you want to do in your life. In our case, hone in on things you want to achieve physically and with your breath.

Take some time out of your day, turn off your phone, and all distractions. Go to a quiet space or a place you feel good in (it could be in nature or a room in your house). Put on some light music if you like and dream. Play with each of these images and see which one feels best for you. From this point:

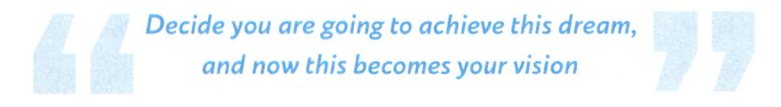

> Decide you are going to achieve this dream, and now this becomes your vision

You need to take time out daily to envision and feel this dream. Afterwards, you should journal all the positive and explicit aspects of your vision experience as if you are already experiencing them. Writing from your future-self consistently will wire your brain to live out your vision subconsciously.

Once your vision is ingrained in the subconscious brain, it is only a matter of time before it becomes a reality for you. It's an excellent tool for realising your dreams. As Big Séan once said, 'If you want a pair of shoes and they're at the store, they're at the store! It's not like they don't exist. You have to figure out how to get them'. And so it is when you envision your dream. The dream is at the store in your mind. It exists. You need to figure out how to make it a reality for you.

Wiring your brain to what is possible is an essential first step in creating your vision. If you are not passionate about your dream, and you cannot see it clearly, then there is no point in setting goals. The vision does not have to be crystal clear for you to get working on it, you do not have to see every aspect in advance, but knowing what you want and having the feeling and the passion behind what you want is critical to its success.

A LETTER FROM YOUR FUTURE SELF

Improve the vision creation process by writing a letter from your future self.

Date your letter and write it in the present tense. Write how wonderful you feel about living the experience. Describe with passion all the sensory details of life – how it looks, feels, smells, tastes, and sounds.

A vision is simply a dream you can see clearly. Once this image becomes clear in your mind, find pictures and headlines that represent that image (see below: the how-to vision board). Surround your life with images of this vision. Make it become a reality for you in your mind's eye.

2. Focusing Your Intent

To attain your vision you need to break it down into smaller chunks, specific goals, develop a plan to achieve these goals, and then adopt everyday activities to move you in the direction of your vision. Once you've defined your vision in Step 1, you need to focus your intent in Step 2 with goals and a plan as a guide to attain the vision. Start by listing every significant aspect of your vision you can think of right now; prioritise the three most essential parts and then detail a plan to achieve them.

> **EXAMPLE VISION**
>
> I have an abundance of energy for work, home, and play with some left over to grow!
>
> List of everything involved:
>
> - Eliminate brain fog and mid-afternoon slump
> - Sleep soundly
> - Become mentally more resilient
> - Develop my physical endurance
> - Become less anxious about things
> - Eliminate asthma medication and breathe free
> - Recover faster so I can live better
> - Have the sex drive (energy) to be with my partner
>
> Prioritise top 3 things that I want to achieve
>
> 1. Eliminate asthma medication and breathe free
> 2. Sleep and recover better for sport
> 3. Have the sex drive (energy) to be with my partner more often

THE GOAL SETTING PROCESS FOR HIGH ACHIEVERS

Once you have your priorities, you need to dig into them a little deeper. You can make them more specific and attach the feelings or create the 'why' for this priority. Being specific and attaching the feelings to the goals is what separates a typical goal-setting process from a process for high achievers.

PART 3   THE INNATE-STRENGTH BREATH TRAINING PROGRAMME

- You need to get specific about what it is you want, including dates for achieving it
- You need to attach a feeling to the event and remember why you want it
- Over time you will track your success and date when you achieve this goal

	GOAL EXAMPLES		
Goal #	What I want specifically	Why I want it	Date I achieved it
1	I finished a hard-slogging winter pre-season training tonight, and felt amazing. My lungs felt free, my body felt like it could run forever, my mind was clear and focused, and as I sit here, writing in my journal, I feel exhausted, yet accomplished. Ready for bed and a deep rest	I am sick several times per year with asthma, especially after pre-season training	Dated 3 months from now
2	I think clearly, I am resilient, I no longer need medication to live	I have suffered with anxiety, and lack of energy since my late twenties, and I'm sick of it	Dated 6 months from now
3	My partner and I are having sex every week now, and sometimes even more. It feels wonderful to connect with her so deeply. Amazingly it's also helped our relationship blossom in other areas too	We've drifted apart in the last year, and I want to bond more closely with them	Dated 12 months from now

REMEMBER GOALS SHOULD BE SMART

SMART goals are a structure for the most detailed level of goal-setting. SMART stands for Specific, Measurable, Achievable, Realistic and Time-bound. By using SMART goals, you are applying a time-tested method to analyse the progress you are making to attaining your goals and eventually realising your vision. This is the best way to know that you are pressing continuously, following the right path, and improving your process along the way. Let's take a closer look at the details of SMART goals:

Specific – What is it exactly that you want to achieve? Clarify your goal and break it down into several more achievable goals if necessary.

Measurable – There's a saying in business: 'What gets measured, gets managed.' By setting numbers to your goal, you know how close you are to achieving it. Then you can adapt your strategy to suit. The numbers are essential, particularly when starting this process – for motivation, for accountability, and progression.

Achievable – Success breeds success. Make 100% sure you can achieve your goals. As you succeed with every mini-goal, you'll prepare yourself to take on bigger goals.

Realistic – What time, resources and commitment are you putting towards achieving this goal? Have you the time in the day to do the work? Do you know how to cook, to eat better, or do you need to learn that first?

Time-bound – You must put a date on completion for the goal. The one thing common to all goal achievers is that they put a specific timeline on their goal; it challenges them and it is possible to achieve. Even if you fail the first time around, set another timeframe for completion. The brain is super smart and learns from the process when you set a new timeline.

SMART GOAL EXAMPLE	
\multicolumn{2}{|l|}{I finished a hard-slogging winter pre-season training tonight and felt amazing. My lungs felt free, my body felt like it could run forever, my mind was clear, and focused and as I sit here, writing in my journal, I feel exhausted, yet accomplished. Ready for bed and a deep rest.}
Specific	Breathe free
	No more asthma symptoms
	No more medication needed
Measurable	Yes, through the personalised breathing assessment
Achievable	Video analysis and questionnaire – all clear
	BOLT Score <40s
	MES <90s
Realistic	Yes – achieved by others before me
Time-bound	Six months – giving plenty of time to train everything I need, plus some extra room for error

LOOK UNDER THE HOOD OF THE GOAL

Finally, you need to account for everything you'll need to achieve your goals. Many people fail to achieve their goals because they're too afraid to face their weaknesses and see what's involved in making a dream a reality. By having the courage to look at everything you need to be successful, you free yourself from some of the fear of failure. You empower yourself to take on this big project and ace it, one step at a time. The questions you need to ask yourself are:

- What obstacles stand in my way?
- What skills and knowledge do I need to develop?
- Who will be my mentor/coach?
- What resources do I need?

As a note of encouragement, I know it can be overwhelming to dive into your vision with this much detail, but the deeper you go the better it will be for you in the long run. If you create your vision in advance, break it down to its tiniest parts and attach feelings to it, you'll easily be able to hold yourself accountable, and keep your focus when the going gets tough along the way.

SMALL WINS TO SUCCESS

As Tony Robbins says, the final aspect to realising your dream vision is to 'burn the bridges' and take 'massive action' on your vision. What Tony means is that you decide this is happening for you, and you cut yourself off from all other options. No matter how hard it gets and how long it takes, nothing will stop you achieving your vision of breathing free, improving your health, and performing at your best. No matter how many times you get side-tracked from your vision – it's happening for you.

Now I know that it's all well and good saying that, but it's another thing following through when the going gets tough. That is why you've taken the time to create the vision so clearly and feel really, really, really good about it. It's why you visualise your idea every day, and it's why you journal from your future self. There is one final step, and it is probably the most important one.

I have found that the only way to realise a vision is to create small wins for yourself and work on your vision every day.

CREATING HABITS

Every day you must do something to achieve your vision. I call these daily actions habits or rituals. 'Do not break the chain,' as Jerry Seinfeld once said. His idea was to become a famous comedian. He wrote scripts to become famous every day, and he'd put a big red X on his calendar to mark that day. He didn't want to see any blank spots on the calendar. He wanted his chain of success to remain unbroken. He wanted his habit to become ingrained in his life so he could attain his vision.

You need to do the same. You need to train your breath every single day, sometimes two to three times daily. Every time you practise, mark it off on your calendar and keep the chain unbroken. The longer the chain becomes, the more likely it will remain intact.

EVERY DAY GET BETTER AT GETTING BETTER

Success in any area of life depends on one thing only: a consistent, focused effort every day. Health is no different. Every day you should produce a slight advancement on the previous day, whether that is better technique, an extra rep, a little less rest or even gleaning an insight into an off-day. Let no day go to waste.

> *'When setting out to build a wall, you don't build a wall. You place one brick at a time, as perfectly as you can, day after day until one day you have a wall'*
>
> WILL SMITH

Breath training is not just a 12-week transformation, but a lifetime shift. Once you restore your breathing and health, you can use those skills to perform better in life and sport.

CELEBRATE AND HAVE FUN

When you think about it, the whole process of becoming healthy and performing at your best is about becoming happier. We are all human and all we really want is the feeling of contentment and happiness inside. One way to attain that feeling is to enjoy the process; the best way to do that is to treat everything as a celebration.

Did you train today? – Celebrate it

Did you get an extra rep today? – Celebrate it

Did you glean an insight from your session? – Celebrate it

Did you hit a goal you've been after for 3 months? – Celebrate it

Turn the whole process into a game. Create small wins relative to your goals and celebrate them every week. It feels good to regularly take the time to congratulate yourself, share your success with your loved ones and your coach and perhaps even treat yourself to something beautiful. The road to success is never straight, so it's essential to stop, breathe in the air and look at the scenery before moving onto your next step.

MAKING SENSE OF IT ALL

Throughout this journey you can easily get caught up in the small details of day-to-day training and life. It is essential, however, that you can step back and see the bigger picture. Breath training has a massive impact on all areas of your life. Some details are subtle at first and the only way to see them is when you have a timeline to look back on. Journalling is a good way to gain insights into your experiences, connect the dots of your training, and see the patterns of impact it has on your life.

The best way to gain insights into your breath training is to journal every night. It doesn't have to be a 'Dear Diary' scenario. You simply jot down anything that stood out for you that day. It could be an insight from your training; an emotional outburst, a recall of a long-forgotten memory, or a chance meeting with a friend – just jot it all down.

Here's a list of a few examples you could journal:

- Changes to your breath and health
- Different feelings within the breath training
- Synchronicities in life
- Vivid dreams
- Random emotional outbursts
- Insights into how you act and live
- Insights into your life

It's okay if you don't see any connections in the beginning; it can take up to six weeks to make sense of some of the things happening to you right now. Just journal and put it away. Give it 4-6 weeks then you'll be able to make sense of it all.

WHEN THE GOING GETS TOUGH, THE TOUGH GET GOING

Les Brown was giving a motivational speech to a large crowd one day. During the speech, he recounted the story of an experience he had as a door-to-door salesman. He approached the porch of a house and rang the doorbell. As Les waited for someone to answer the door, he noticed a dog whining on the porch. When a man answered the door, Les asked him, 'Why is the dog whining so much?' The man told Les not to mind the dog; he was just lying on a nail.

Les was incredulous. 'Why is the dog lying on the nail? Would he not get up?' To which the man replied, 'When the dog is in enough pain, he will get up off the nail'.

You may think the man was cruel. He could have easily helped the dog, and you're right, but is the dog not silly too? As the man saw it, the dog was responsible for taking care of itself. At any time, the dog could easily stand up off the nail and stop the cause of the pain.

And so it is for us right now. Through lifestyle, we are causing ourselves arguably more pain than the dog. All we have to do is to stop doing the things that harm us and start doing the things which will heal our bodies. 'Easier said than done,' you might say to me, and I agree with you. We generally know what is good for us, but, as we embark on a new lifestyle, we sometimes forget how much pain we were in. We do the hard work by getting off the nail, but after we're feeling a little better, we think, 'Maybe life over there lying on the nail was not so bad after all,' and we return to lying on the nail. This is perhaps the most dangerous phase of the whole programme for you. If you stop moving forward, or give yourself a little break because 'you deserve it', you may end up right back on that nail before you even realise it.

Trust me; it's happened to me on numerous occasions. I remember when I was 27, eight years after I cured my asthma symptoms, I relapsed. I gradually returned to a lifestyle my body didn't appreciate. I could see all the signs along the way. My BOLT was decreasing, I had less energy, my bodyweight decreased, and I began to develop the old cold again. I buried my head in the sand, and treated each of these signs as a misnomer. 'Sure, I can start again tomorrow,' was my attitude. It was not long before my scores dropped significantly, and my symptoms kicked back in again. I let myself slip so much I even returned to taking medication to offset my poor habits. It reached a point where enough was enough. Not only would I build myself back up to feeling healthy, but I would also maintain that healthy lifestyle with plenty of resilience. At the time, I swore to myself that this would be the end. I had tasted that deep pain again, I sat back on the nail, and it was too much for me. I decided there and then I would return to health and stay there. It took me another two years to gain complete health. It was a lesson hard-learned.

You don't have to go through the same process as me. You have an opportunity to be better than me by hearing my experiences, listening to the wisdom in them, and making them a part of your decision process. One of the skills I picked up through the relapse experience was the idea of remembering my pain. To remember your pain effectively takes five steps:

Step One: Feel the Pain

Right now, when you're at your worst, it's time to open up and feel your pain. Take ten minutes. Close your eyes and feel the pain in your body and mind. After your time is up, take out a journal and write down every aspect of the pain. Rate it out of ten. Describe it in detail, especially the feelings around it. Once you're finished, put the journal away and shake off the emotions by doing something physical. You can sprint on the spot, hit a punching bag, go training, get in cold water – anything vigorous.

Step two: Get Breath Training

Forget about the journal. Get breath training and get improving your life.

Step three: Remember Your Pain

If you find yourself relapsing, if you find pain creeping back in, remember the journal. Take it out. Read how much pain you were in. Take ten minutes out to meditate on the lifestyle you once had and what it meant for your body.

Step four: Reset Your Vision

Make the decision to move forward again with a plan. Affirm this decision by writing it down. Reinforce this decision by taking out your vision. Review who it is you want to become and the life you want to lead. Confirm all of this positive reinforcement by rewriting your vision in the present tense.

Return to your plan and your goals too. Analyse what went wrong by seeking the things in your control which you can improve. For example, if you found yourself in too much of a rush to train first thing in the morning, you could move the training session to your mid-morning break. Be ruthless. Find those weak links in your plan and strengthen them.

Step Five: Reaffirm with Action

Get breath training right now! Even if it's half of what you used to do. Get doing it straight away. Act before that monkey mind takes over and convinces you otherwise. 5, 4, 3, 2, 1 – GO!

Every time the wheels come off the wagon and you relapse, it is really important to return to steps three through five. A new lifestyle is not won on a single decision but in the many choices over time. There will be many setbacks on the way. Re-wire that thinking. The setbacks are simply part of the process. They are not nice but they are a reality when you want to achieve greatness in your life. Brian Peters, host of the podcast Chasing Edges, said it cleverly: 'A goal is a contract with yourself to be miserable until it is achieved'. That means, if this vision is something you really, really, really want, then don't give yourself the choice to ponder at this time – just get in and do it again. Your desire to train and 'motivation' will return. This is just a phase, and it too shall pass.

SUMMARY OF PREPARATION

Your success can be broken into three distinct parts: planning; the actions you take; and your review process. This is a never-ending cycle until you are breathing free. Creating the vision and planning your process is a fundamental way to keep your eyes on the prize. Times will get tough. Knowing why you chose this training and seeing the way-points along the path are vital in preventing you from getting stuck in moments of despair; having said that, the only thing that will actually move you forward is the training itself. Train. Train often and keep training. Breath training works every time you work. All the goals

PART 3 THE INNATE-STRENGTH BREATH TRAINING PROGRAMME

I lay out in the programme are attainable, provided you train often enough and long enough. Remember that you lived with adapted breathing patterns for years; the training only takes a relatively short period of time in comparison. Finally, as you take that journey, you always want to be improving your processes. Regularly review your vision to feel good about your future. Review your actions in comparison to your plan to see if you can improve how you're training.

By now, you should have created that vision and your goals. Your next steps are to find out your goal markers and your baselines. In the next chapter, I will provide you with the numbers and guide to breathing free. You'll then need to determine your starting point by assessing your breath as it breathes today.

12

BREATH TRAINING PROGRAMME CONSIDERATIONS

When it comes to breathing, it's all about training. Concepts get you nowhere, training gets you everywhere

MARK DIVINE, NAVY SEAL

It is said that the only way to know the taste of an apple is to take a bite; so it is with breath training. The only way to know the many benefits of breath training is to do the actual training. Give it time and you will savour the experience. There are so many techniques and methods on breathing nowadays, from yogic traditions to Western psychotherapy, physiotherapy approaches to breathing and performance breathing techniques. The question becomes not whether breathing is right for you, but which technique works for you and why. To date, no book has put together the techniques and methods into a comprehensive framework for breath training – one that any technique can fit into and where you can find the reason for using that technique. The aim of this book is to piece together a framework of breath training which restores your breathing system, enhances your health, and enables you to live your great life.

PART 3 THE INNATE-STRENGTH BREATH TRAINING PROGRAMME

Restoring your breath to its natural centre requires training in three specific areas; these form the daily habits associated with quality breathing and the supporting lifestyle practices to aid your breath practice and enhance your health. Once you've re-centred your breath, the breath can be used to enhance performance in life and sport. The three dimensions of breath training are:

1. Breathing mechanics
2. Breathing Resilience
3. Breathing rhythms

The first step to achieving these goals is to determine who exactly breath training can work for. Next, we determine how we manipulate the programme's variables to suit your needs. Then comes the breath training itself and the application of breathing in life and sport. Before we get ahead of ourselves, let's begin with who should train their breath and how we make it safe for you.

IS BREATH TRAINING SAFE?

The short answer is that breath training is safe for everybody; however, some people may need to take some extra precautionary steps. If you have any health condition, you should check with your medical provider before you start any training programme, including breath training. No matter how good you feel throughout the process, never stop taking medications without first talking to your doctor or medical advisor.

There are some guidelines for particular groups of people:

Pregnant women and people with epilepsy should not practice any of the more vigorous techniques – that is, the walking breath holds and the fast breathing, like Wim Hof breathing.

People with cardio-vascular and respiratory issues, diabetes, or people who've experienced trauma in their life may perform these techniques, but they should start gently and progress slowly.

WHERE SHOULD I PRACTICE BREATH TRAINING?

Safety always comes first; that is physical, psychological and spiritual safety. Always practise your training in a comfortable and safe space. Preferably at home or in a familiar environment. Never practise big or fast rhythmical techniques in water or when operating heavy machinery. In the beginning, I also recommend that you don't practise breath training in your workplace or in an environment where you may be socially uncomfortable.

HOW SHOULD I PRACTICE BREATH HOLDING TECHNIQUES?

When you are pushing a breath-holding-technique, always practise the hold when the breath is suspended after your exhale.

> *Example: breathe in, breathe out, then hold your breath. I prefer this method to holding your breath after your inhale.*

CLEANSING REACTIONS ASSOCIATED WITH BREATH TRAINING

Now that we're kicking into the breathing aspect of the programme, I want to give you a heads-up on some cleansing reactions you may experience and why. If you've ever started a weight training programme, you'll know that your body aches for the first few days after your initial training sessions. Similarly, if you ever had the pleasure of giving up your favourite cup of coffee, you would have experienced headaches, and fatigue for a few days. You might have been a bit grumpy, and your energy levels would likely swing. In both cases, this is your body getting used to the changes in your lifestyle. Breath training can be the same. When you begin a breath training programme you will probably experience a variety of physical, mental, and emotional reactions. These are called cleansing reactions.

PART 3   THE INNATE-STRENGTH BREATH TRAINING PROGRAMME

Everybody has a different experience of breath training and a different reaction to it. Some people's experience may be similar and some can be vastly different. Some experience deep cleansing reactions and others none at all. However, I have found a few common reactions with most people over the years. With this experience I have also figured out how to minimise the cleansing reactions. The most important thing for you to do when you do experience a cleansing reaction is to continue with the breath training. Reduce the power of the technique, practise fewer repetitions in every session; but make sure to keep training regularly. Ceasing the programme when you experience reactions may create a block in your body; this means the reaction may be more severe the next time you try to overcome it. Similar to Albert Einstein's advice for life, breathing is like riding a bicycle; to keep your balance you must stay in motion. So please, persevere with the programme and utilise the strategies below to minimise the experience too.

The common cleansing reactions to breath training are a flare-up of your own typical disease symptoms. Emotional outbursts are common if you usually keep emotions locked inside. Headaches, fatigue and inflammatory symptoms are all typical reactions to the training during the first few days.

COMMON CLEANSING REACTIONS

Mucus build-up in nose or lungs

Cold and flu-like symptoms

Joint pains

Headaches

Fatigue and tiredness

Emotional reactions

In addition to continuing with your programme, there are a few ways to reduce the severity and length of the reactions. Water, movement, time in nature, and sleep are the best tools to mitigate any cleansing reactions.

Hydration is a powerful way to help you deal with the changes your body's chemistry with breath training. As the saying goes, 'The solution to pollution is dilution'. Drinking plenty of water is the simplest way to hydrate your body and help it work optimally. If you want to level up your hydration practise, you could add some vitamin C and reduce your intake of tea and coffee. Vitamin C can be included in the form of a supplement or naturally by adding some lemon or lime to your water.

'Movement is the song of the body' (Vanda Scaravelli), and it's the next powerful way to help you with cleansing reactions. Moving helps your lymph system to clear toxins and detoxify your body. Without movement, you become stale and suffer with your symptoms for much longer. It doesn't really matter what form the movement takes; just move your body. Start gently with practices like yoga, dance or walking. If you feel up to it, you can move more vigorously.

Getting out into nature is another powerful way to help reset your body, calm it down, and deal with cleansing reactions. We weren't built to sit around all day in offices, commute in cars and watch TV in the evenings. Biologically, we are built to live in nature. It isn't a place to visit, as Gary Snyder says, it is home. Walking barefoot on grass, going for a swim in the sea, or taking a hike at the weekend are all brilliant ways to use nature to help you with your breath training.

Last but not least, sleeping better will help ease the cleansing reactions to breath training. Without good quality sleep, there is no chance you will achieve your goals with breath training because your body only truly restores itself when it is sleeping. Develop sound sleeping habits, such as going to bed early and at a similar time. Sleep in a cool room and tape your mouth at night if necessary.

Remember, if you perform additional exercises to the programme or push yourself excessively within the exercises, the BOLT score may progress more quickly. You may happen upon more severe cleansing reactions too. So be careful not to push yourself too hard, or you will just have to bear the brunt of your body's natural reactions to your intense training.

Finally, these cleansing reactions are not the same as exacerbated symptoms of your [possible] disease. If you have anxiety or asthma, rhinitis or allergies, or any one of a number of other respiratory diseases, then those symptoms may emerge at various stages throughout the programme. This is normal until your breathing scores improve, as per the next chapter's programme guidelines. Just in case you need it, please, always have your medication at hand.

The simple rule to remember is this, if you have symptoms during this programme then:

- Gently begin your exercises immediately
- Perform the exercises for 5 minutes
- If your symptoms ease, then continue the exercises until they completely subside

However, if the symptoms persist beyond 10 minutes or you are uncomfortable, then take your medication immediately and follow all medical advice as normal.

BREATH TRAINING PROGRAMME LAYOUT

The structure of the programme is simple and takes one of two shapes. The first approach proceeds in the order I have laid it out; you train Phase 1-2-3 in that order. The second option for the framework reverses Phases 2 and 3. In this case you train Phase 1-3-2.

Regardless of the approach you want to take to your training, you can see that you always train Phase 1 first. This is the breathing mechanics phase. Why? you may ask. I train breathing mechanics first for two reasons. Firstly, I've found that when you begin with the mechanical techniques, they can hugely influence and speed up the effectiveness of the more potent techniques. And I've found them to be safe, every time I've used them. In other words, everybody gets something from them, everybody likes them, and whilst there is often an emotional/psychological response from the techniques, it is never too powerful.

Phase 2 of the training acts on the physiology of your body. This is the resilience building phase. Its purpose is to decrease your sensitivity to CO_2, increase your CO_2 tolerance, and begin to calm the rhythm of your subconscious breath.

Rhythmical breathing patterns follow the breath-holding phase of the programme. Rhythmical breathing acts more on the psychological and emotional aspects of breathing, and it can also help improve the subconscious rhythm of your breath.

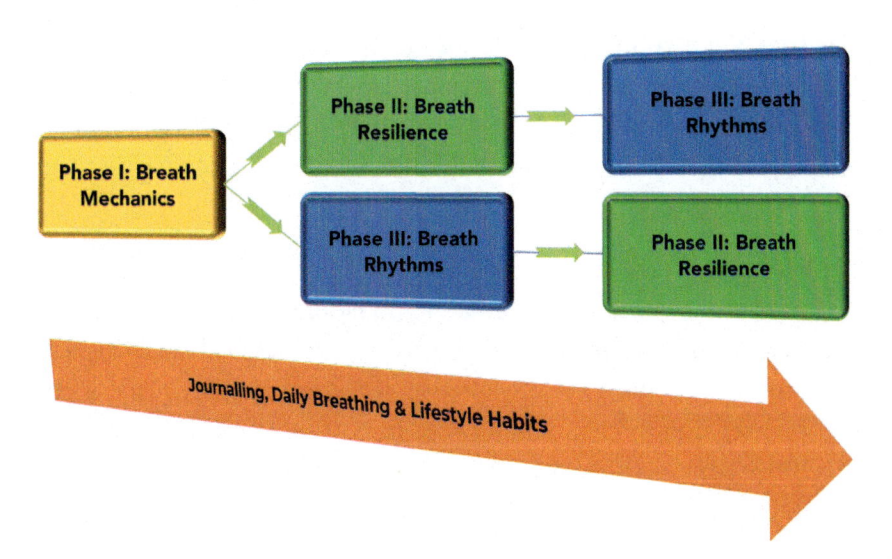

The Two Approaches to Innate-Strength Breath Training

PART 3 THE INNATE-STRENGTH BREATH TRAINING PROGRAMME

Throughout the course of the programme you'll need to instil daily habits that complement the breath training in your life; I'm talking about exercise, connection and sleep lifestyle here. Furthermore, journaling your experiences throughout all three phases will be essential to the programme's success for you. Through the journaling, you'll find synchronicities of life regularly; there will be weird co-incidences, strong feelings, and unusual reactions occurring in your life as you improve your breath. You want to document them at the time to help you make sense of them throughout the programme.

Rather than train the programme in the initial order I laid out, you can also train it as Phase 1-3-2. The order now becomes physical – psychological – physiological. The reason you can switch Phases 2 and 3 around is because, throughout my years of coaching, I have found some people really disliked the Phase 2 techniques (Buteyko). They found the suppression of the breath too intense, they got bored with the techniques and they dropped out of the programme before they felt the benefits. Meanwhile, other clients became emotionally overwhelmed with the rhythmical breathing techniques (Wim Hof Breathing). You may think this is a bit far-fetched, but you will know it is true when you experience, in time, the full power of these techniques. Remember, one of the original modern masters of the breath is Stan Grof. He is a medical doctor and psychiatrist who uses breathing techniques to explore the human psyche, cure psychological disease, and heal people.

At this point in time, the original layout of the programme is my preferred choice because it is subtler and gentler on you emotionally, it covers all bases and people tend to have a better overall experience. However, there are always two sides to the story. That's ok, just be prepared to clear some space in your life, and go on a deep dive into your psyche from the word go, if you choose the latter approach.

And so, the question is not do breathing techniques work for me, but which ones are best for me now? Where do I start?

I suggest you begin with these questions:

- Do I feel like now is the right time for me to:

    a) Create emotional upheaval?

or

    b) Do I need to take my time and create that space mentally and physically for myself?

If the answer is B, then please proceed with the programme as I have originally laid it out: Phases 1-2-3.

If the answer is A, then proceed to the next question.

- Can I dedicate one to two full days to processing this emotional upheaval? (Low demands on life, from work, sport, family, etc.)

If the answer is no, then please proceed with the programme as I originally laid it out.

If the answer is yes, then choose the alternative order to the structure, and practise the training as Phase 1-3-2.

Whichever approach you choose to restore your full breathing system and ensure the benefits stick, you still need to finish the path. You need to build resilience in your system so that when life does hit and it takes a huge gulp of your health, you still have ample reserves in your glass of water to take the hit and continue on your journey, pain and symptom-free.

TRAINING TIMELINES

The length of time it will take you to restore your breathing patterns and breathe free varies from person to person. It will depend a lot on your current health status, the length of time you've had the underlying disease conditions, and their severity. I took longer than anyone else I know to achieve my goals. I had asthma for roughly seventeen out of twenty years of my life. It took me eighteen months to fully restore my breathing, remove all medications and remain stable. Most of my clients that commit to their training are successful within three to six months. This is because I was a particularly tough case and I have since found better ways to help people achieve their goals faster.

Regardless of your health condition, you may start to feel the difference in your breathing almost immediately after your first session; freeing your breathing mechanics feels like somebody has just loosened a corset around your body. The freedom of movement in your diaphragm and ribs feels great.

After that initial freedom, it takes a little time to restore your CO_2 tolerance with the resilience training in Phase 2, balance your nervous system with the breathing rhythms in Phase 3, and free your whole breathing system. This phase may take as little as four weeks for the athletes among you. Athletes tend to achieve their breathing goals in a faster time because their fitness levels are generally high, and they tend to be very diligent with their training. For us mere mortals, it can take some extra time to become familiar with training so frequently and for the effects to take place. Generally, I allow up to six months for this process to be completed.

Complete health is the final expectation for you, I am sure. In some cases, restoring the breath alone is sufficient to re-establishing your health. Afterall, the breath is the foundation stone for health and performance. There are some diseases, however, where we can only improve the symptoms because there is structural damage in your body that is perhaps irreparable. The poorer your health is and the longer you have been unhealthy, the longer it will take you to restore that health and feel great again. Makes sense, right?

Having said that, everyone has the opportunity to improve their health and breath training will drastically improve everybody's health. If you developed a disease as an adult, your body has probably been in a state of incomplete health for many years, perhaps even decades, before the symptoms began to show. Please give the training the commitment and time it needs to work. This is not supposed to be an overnight transformation. This is a block of committed practice to restoring your breathing system. After your breath training, you will need to continuously improve other specific aspects of your life to gain complete health. These include exercise, nutrition, financial health, relationships, etc. With this perspective, I want you to know that it is usually possible to achieve your health goals. I've seen it too many times to know otherwise. It can take many years and a lot of effort, but it's possible. Below is a summary of all of these timelines for you:

	Some Underlying Health Conditions	Relatively Healthy With No Underlying Health Conditions
TRAINING TIMELINE EXPECTATIONS		
Feeling the Difference	1 Session - 1 Month	1 Session – 1 Week
Breathing Freely	8 Weeks – 6 Months	4 – 16 Weeks
Complete Health	It's Possible	3 – 10 Years

TRAINING FREQUENCY EXPECTATIONS

Now we come to the nitty gritty stage of preparation. 'How often do you need to train to achieve your goals?' is perhaps the most important question when undertaking this programme. The answer is: often! The more frequently you train your breath, the better. From a practical and sustainable point of view, I have found three training sessions per day to be optimal. This training frequency delivers great results in a timely fashion. The sessions are only fifteen minutes long, which is a total of one to one and a half hours of training per day. Some people are happy with doing a little less and taking their time. In this case, I recommend a minimum of two training sessions per day, and a total of approximately thirty to forty minutes of training. Any less than this figure and you will be unsuccessful with the programme.

PART 3   THE INNATE-STRENGTH BREATH TRAINING PROGRAMME

Considering we breathe more than 20,000 times per day on average and yet you are only training for approximately one hour per day, you'll understand why you have to train so frequently. If you break the numbers down, you affect approximately nine hundred breaths during your training, and this leaves another 19,100 breaths to be influenced. These figures make frequency of breath training the most important aspect of the programme. If you train often enough, the benefits will come. The more frequently you train your breathing, the quicker your body will adapt and the sooner you'll be breathing free and feeling great again.

Time commitment:	10 mins-30 mins
Frequency per day:	x 2-3 times
How long:	Every day until you are breathing freely, feeling great, and scores are high

My final words in your training schedule are these: treat this block of breath training as an athlete would prepare for the Olympics, and commit to it wholly with everything you've got. Once your training period is over, use the skills you have developed here to maintain your breathing, aid other aspects of health, and live your greatest life as you see fit.

TRAINING STRUCTURE

The training programme is built in phases, with linear periodisation, similar to skill development in a strength training program. Each training phase and block within a phase serves a specific purpose. The goal of that phase/block is to enhance those physical qualities of the breath, integrate them with the previous block (if necessary) and then move onto the next phase. There are three training phases and seven blocks to the program:

BREATH TRAINING PROGRAMME CONSIDERATIONS

Preparation: Road mapping Your Success

Phase 1: Breathing Mechanics (2 blocks)

Phase 2: Breath Resilience Training (1 block)

Phase 3: Rhythm Training (3 blocks)

SPECIFIC TRAINING CONSIDERATIONS

Women's Menstrual Cycles

A woman's menstrual cycle affects breathing, and breath training will also impact the cycle. The fluctuations of progesterone levels during different phases of her cycle may make her more or less prone to CO_2 sensitivity. This will appear in a woman's BOLT and Maximal Exhale scores. Therefore, it is important that a woman tracks her scores over a longer period of time so she can have a better grasp on a truer baseline for her and remain positive about her training outcomes.

On the other hand, both strong breath-holding and supra-ventilation breathing techniques may have an immediate and powerful impact on a woman's cycle. Many of my female clients have reported changes to their cycles throughout breath training. Whilst there is no data in research to support this yet, the anecdotal evidence from my own clients and that of other breathing teachers I've spoken with suggests that a woman's cycle goes through a period of change (sometimes heavier, sometimes lighter, sometimes more painful, sometimes less so) and then it normalises. The new normal for the cycle is usually a natural 28-day rhythm with decreased pain and more regularity.

I think this is happening not because breathing has some magical effect on a woman's cycle, but because the woman has calmed her body, for the first time in a long time, with breathing practise. Her nervous system tone has been rebalanced by the breathing techniques, and her hormone system has subsequently come into alignment with the natural rhythms of her body. So through breathing techniques, the woman has realigned her internal chemistry to its natural state. This results in a more regular and less painful menstrual cycle.

Pregnancy

Women go through many changes while pregnant, and these changes impact a woman's breathing through the three phases of pregnancy. The most apparent changes to a woman's breathing during pregnancy arise due to the following:

Physiological changes:

- Progesterone gradually increases throughout the course of pregnancy. It acts as trigger for the primary respiratory centre by increasing the sensitivity of the respiratory centre to carbon dioxide.
- The smooth muscle tone of the lungs dilates, resulting in a bronchodilator effect
- It causes nasal congestion
- The woman will increase her breathing volume up to 48%, and yet her breathing rate will remain the same
- Up to 70% of women report the feeling of breathlessness during pregnancy, starting from the very first trimester. Such an early onset suggests that there is a physiological reason for the sensation or an awareness of the changes in her body

Mechanical changes:

- Due to the growing baby, progressive uterine distension is the major cause of lung volume and chest wall expansion. This distension compromises the elevation of the diaphragm and alters thoracic configuration.
- The diaphragm can be displaced up to 5 cm upwards as a result of the growing baby

- The woman's chest height becomes shorter, and consequently, she changes to a more lateral breathing pattern
- There is higher inspiratory intercostal recruitment, and there is more work from the accessory muscles
- There are also a myriad of psychological and spiritual changes a woman experiences during pregnancy

The physiological and mechanical alterations in breathing patterns during pregnancy suggest that women need to move slowly with breath training. It is recommended that pregnant women stay away from any exercise that drastically changes CO_2 levels as it could influence progesterone levels and place the pregnancy in jeopardy. This includes both strong breath-holding techniques in Phase 2 and supra-ventilation techniques in Phase 3.

Children

In general children are free to try out most of the techniques in this book. There are a few exceptions which I strongly suggest a child does not try until their lungs have developed fully and they have matured. In my opinion, children should not perform the supra-ventilation techniques for a sustained period of time; fast and big breathing patterns. This is because the impact of these techniques on a child's development is unknown. I have heard some horror stories from fellow breath teachers and parents online, which I would never like to see in person. For that reason, I coach children on the exercises in Phase 1 and 2 only, and I refrain from using any technique from Phase 3. 16-18 years old is generally the accepted age to allow children to begin some of the deeper work, but always be aware of the child's medical and psychological history.

Epilepsy

There is a long history and body of research connecting breathing rates, carbon dioxide, and the onset of epileptic seizures. CO_2 in particular, appears to have a connection with seizures, but the research is thin and inconclusive. It is the opinion of most breath teachers that we should avoid using techniques with strong breath holds or supra-ventilation techniques with people who have epilepsy to avoid the risk of bringing on a seizure. Some breathing methods, however, do allow for these methods to be used under competent support and guidance.

As a breath coach, I recommended that people with epilepsy start with the foundation techniques in Phase 1 and very slowly progress through the programme. I am happy for people with epilepsy to perform the techniques in Phase 2 with caution, but I ask that they only push to 80% of a maximum breath hold. Take it easy, progress slowly and listen to your body. I ask people with epilepsy to seek professional advice if they choose to perform the techniques in Phase 3.

Remember, this is not a race, and no, there is no end-point, just a journey into self-discovery and the health of your own body.

Traumatic Events and Mental Illness

People with traumatic events in their past or mental health problems, are free to use the programme as they wish. However, you need to know that breathing is very closely linked with emotions.

Both strong breath holds and supra-ventilation techniques may bring up a lot of emotions you haven't experienced since your trauma. Breathing will help you to process those emotions and allow you to move forward in your life.

You will most likely find that you get turned off by Phase 2 training if you are pushing too hard or if the emotions are overwhelming for you. If this happens, it's ok. Make sure to continue journalling every day. Reduce the intensity of your technique (push to 80% instead of

90%) and reduce your training volume. This means you should still step up to train daily, but perhaps you will do only one or two reps of the exercise instead of six.

When you're ready to train Phase 3, it's recommended you do so with a qualified and experienced practitioner; a lot of emotion can surface, and you need to know how to deal with it effectively. If you choose to perform these techniques on your own, you should train them very slowly – reduce both intensity and volume – or you may end up in a much worse psycho-emotional condition than if you never did them in the first place.

If you have ever had a traumatic event or a mental illness please, please, please listen to these recommendations. I've come across far too many people who dived into a breathing technique without knowing this information, and it caused them a lot of needless pain and suffering as a result. On the other hand, those that follow the recommendations tend to benefit enormously from breath training.

Cardiovascular Disease

People with cardiovascular disease are fine to breath train. You should heed the usual medical advice and take a sensible approach to training.

Like lung diseases, the severity of your cardiovascular disease will influence the intensity of your training. You are free to choose the training route of your choice. It's better to train more often with less intensity than to train hard for a short time.

Diabetes

Dr. Buteyko did a lot of work with people who had diabetes, and he felt that the breathing techniques could help regulate the blood sugars of those with type 1 diabetes in particular. While this area of research is thin, we have found some interesting studies in recent times to support his ideas. The benefits of breathing for people with diabetes in particular are:

- Chronic hyperventilation and supra-ventilation techniques increase sugar usage and decrease blood sugar levels
- Most people with diabetes have a low parasympathetic tone. Low, slow, calm and relaxed breathing improves blood sugar management
- In the long run, breath-holding techniques improve blood sugar management for people with type 1 and type 2 diabetes. However, this needs to be medically supervised as strong breath-holding techniques can strongly influence blood sugars in the short-term

It is recommended that people with diabetes can do all training phases; however, care must be taken. It is recommended that the blocks be trained in the order 1-2-3 and that blood sugars be carefully managed during the training periods. In particular, people with diabetes need to be careful using the supra-ventilation techniques in Phase 3. Careful management of blood sugars is recommended around these techniques, just as it is for general exercise. Breathing will exacerbate the same symptoms of your diabetes as a long cardio training session but in a much shorter time period (possibly minutes). Therefore, you should carefully manage your blood sugars in breath training, and in the same way as you would for general exercise.

Respiratory Diseases

Obviously, the respiratory system will be the most sensitive system in the body to change as we begin breath training. You are free to train the blocks in any order you like, but simply be aware that the training will directly impact any underlying disease you have. No matter what respiratory disease you suffer from, training your breathing will improve your symptoms, and may even cure them.

There are no major contraindications to breath training when you have a respiratory disease; just take your time, consult your doctor, and manage your symptoms sensibly. Don't even consider removing medication from your life until you speak with your GP and gain medical advice.

PERSONALISED BREATHING ASSESSMENT 13

Like with most systems in the body, there is no one universal measure of breath quality. Rather there are indicators for the overall system function. There is no universal definition of a quality breath. The closest definition scientists and practitioners have come to an agreement on, is that when you are resting, the breath should be:

Nose – inhale and exhale using the nose

Gentle – the breath is quiet

Low – breathe into the stomach using the diaphragm

Slow – both the breathing rate and volume is calm

Let go – the exhale should be passive

A second way of describing this optimal resting breath is to illustrate it by using the analogy of a wave. A quality breath at rest is a light breath, and the air is gently pulled in by the nose. The air fills the body like a wave; belly rises first followed by the chest. The breath transitions smoothly from an inhale to an exhale, like a wave cresting, and falling back into the ocean. The exhale is relaxed, long, and extended. It's almost as if the air falls out of the body the same way a wave washes out on a shore line. There are no pauses in the breath and no sharp phases; all is smooth, calm and gentle, as seen in the illustration below.

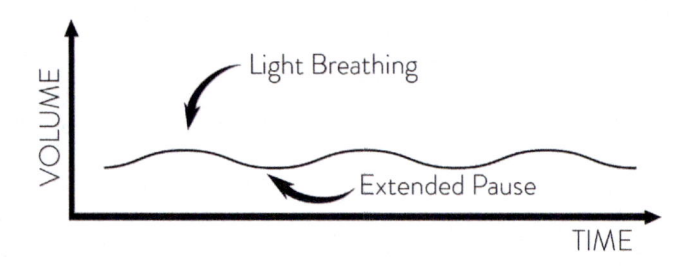

[Figure: A graph with VOLUME on the y-axis and TIME on the x-axis, showing a gentle wavy line labeled "Light Breathing" with an "Extended Pause" indicated.]

The lack of definition in the literature makes it very difficult for us to put numbers on a quality breath. Even more so, this definition doesn't encompass our ability to use our whole breathing system for performance.

When we investigate sports performance, for example, there are no standards of measure for the breath, like for fitness or strength. There are, of course, lab-based medical tests for measuring the breath. Unfortunately, their application does not transfer to the practical world of using the breath, and the equipment used to take these measures is not accessible to everyone. The purpose of these tools is usually to measure a single breath or a forced exhale. I found some clients made huge progress with a particular technique and that progress wasn't reflected in the individual tests; this led to frustration, decreased motivation and in some cases, the people stopped training altogether. In my opinion, this was unacceptable; I needed a better way to coach them.

That is why I use a triangulation approach for measuring the breath. Taking a few different data points gives me a bird's eye view of the health of your breathing system. I brought them together into a framework and renamed them. The integration of the tests and their new names more accurately describe what they are measuring and how they fit together in the overall framework of training. Like 99% of the exercises in this book, you will find these tests elsewhere in a specific breathing method. Each of the tests does a good job of measuring the specific aspect of breathing that it is supposed to measure.

The four measures I take to assess the quality of your breath are:

1. Breathing rate
2. Video analysis of the breathing pattern with a questionnaire
3. BOLT score or maximal exhale score
4. Maximum breath-hold paces

BREATHING RATE

Perhaps the easiest and most common test, assessing the number of breaths you take, will give you a very quick and approximate assessment of your breath efficiency. Your breathing rate only accounts for one-half of efficiency; your breathing volume is the second.

According to clinical guidelines, a normal breathing rate is 12-15 breaths per minute. People with different lifestyle diseases are known to breathe up to 25+ breaths per minute. Optimal breathing, however, has a lot lower breathing rate. Someone with a high-quality breath rate would breathe 8-12 breaths per minute at rest. According to some research, if you wanted to drop into a meditative state, you're looking at 3.5 – 6 breaths per minute. Many people are reporting on research nowadays to indicate that a breathing rate of approximately six breaths per minute is ideal. However, when I investigated this research, I found that this breathing rate is a conscious breathing pattern the participant used to elicit particular benefits. It is not the natural subconscious breathing rate of the person. The research into breathing needs to be expanded before we assume that everybody should be breathing at a rate of six breaths per minute for ideal health. However, it is becoming widely acknowledged that slow breathing is extremely important for your health and wellbeing.

*The normal 24-hour breathing rate averages
12-15 breaths per minute*

VIDEO ANALYSIS & QUESTIONNAIRE

Origins of the tests

Many breathing teachers speak about breath awareness as the first step to a breathing practice, but you don't know what you don't know. What if you think you are breathing one way, but in reality, you are breathing quite differently? The video analysis and breath pattern recognition questionnaire (BPQR) arose from my education and experience coaching people over the years.

Purpose

Create awareness of your current breathing patterns. 'Do you breathe efficiently or do you compensate in some manner to make the breath work for you?' is the central theme of the analysis.

The video is a phenomenal tool, and the feedback gives you a visual of your breathing at rest when played back to you. Many people think they are breathing one way, but when they see it, they soon find out they are breathing in a completely different manner.

The BPRQ investigates your breath pattern during the video, at rest, and during your daily living tasks. People may breathe ok while at complete rest, but can change their pattern to an adapted one pretty quickly once they get on with their day.

Reasons

Through the years, I have found that people who come to train their breath for the first time are usually aware something is wrong, but they have no idea how their breath looks from a mechanical perspective (it is the same when you analyse someone's walking gait or running pattern for the first time).

Measurement

The benefits of having efficient breathing mechanics are numerous:

- ✓ Speeds up results you obtain from the other breath training
- ✓ Gives you a sense of freedom in your breath
- ✓ Releases many pent-up emotions gently
- ✓ Enables better use of breathing for postural strength and core stability
- ✓ Improves pelvic floor stability

Ideally, your breathing should look like this at rest:

- Inhale through nose only to begin with for 5 breaths
- The inhale is active
- There is no breath-holding at the top
- The exhale is passive, and you let it go
- As you inhale the belly rises first, then the chest
- As you exhale, the belly falls first, then the chest
- There should be a noticeable rise and fall of both belly and chest

Technique for video analysis

1. Record the technique on video for analysis later
2. Perform this technique lying down on your back, with knees bent and feet flat on the floor
3. Breathe in through your nose and out of your mouth
4. Inhale fully – filling all of your body with air
5. Just let go of the exhale through the mouth

PART 3   THE INNATE-STRENGTH BREATH TRAINING PROGRAMME

BREATH PATTERN RECOGNITION QUESTIONNAIRE
Place a Number in the Corresponding Box

Part 1	0	1
Breath Patterns at Rest	Never / Rarely	Sometimes / Regularly
Do you use your mouth to breathe at all?		
Do you feel short of breath often?		
Do you sigh or yawn often?		
Do you gasp or heave for breath at rest?		
Has your breathing worsened or do you cough after laughing?		
Sub-Total Score		

Part 2	0	1
Video Analysis	No	Yes
Is your chest still as you breathe?		
If it moves, does your chest rise first (before your belly)?		
Do your collarbones and shoulders lift up, even a little?		
Do you hold your breath?		
Take a few deep breaths. Do you get a headache or feel dizzy?		
Sub-Total Score		

PERSONALISED BREATHING ASSESSMENT

Part 3	0	1
Take a few big, deep breaths and notice what you feel...	No	Yes
Is your breathing restricted, stuck, or jumpy anywhere?		
Is there tension, soreness, or pressure anywhere in your upper body (jaw, neck, shoulder, or chest)?		
Do you have breathlessness, air hunger, or shortness of breath?		
Time yourself humming with your mouth closed on a single breath. Is your score less than 10 seconds?		
Sub-Total Score		

Part 4	0	3
Hook your fingers under your bottom ribs and press in when you exhale. What do you feel?	No	Yes
Is the tissue quality tough, like a well-done steak?		
When hooking your fingers, is there pain anywhere?		
Sub-Total Score		

PART 3   THE INNATE-STRENGTH BREATH TRAINING PROGRAMME

Part 5	0	1
Breath Patterns & Exercise	No	Yes
Do you use your mouth to inhale or exhale during long-distance exercise?		
Do you gasp, heave, or get shortness of breath when walking?		
Do you find it difficult to catch your breath during more vigorous exercise (i.e. jogging, running, or intense exercise)?		
Does it take you a while to get your second wind?		
Do you find it more difficult to breathe when exercising in cold weather?		
Perform a side plank with nose breathing. Is your score less than 70 seconds?		
Sub-Total Score		

Part 6	0	1
Breath Patterns & Lifestyle	Never / Rarely	Sometimes / Regularly
Do you get respiratory disease symptoms (i.e. asthma, bronchitis, sinusitis, rhinitis, etc.)?		
Do you have allergies (airborne, food-related or animal etc.)?		
Does your nose get stuffed/runny often, or do you find it difficult to nose breathe during hay fever season?		
Do you wake in the morning with a dry mouth?		
Do you mouth breathe after eating a meal?		
Does you nose get stuffy / blocked after you eat dairy / eggs / wheat?		

PERSONALISED BREATHING ASSESSMENT

Part 6	0	1
Breath Patterns & Lifestyle	Never / Rarely	Sometimes / Regularly
Does you nose get stuffy / blocked after you eat dairy / eggs / wheat?		
Is your voice thin, weak or raspy?		
Sub-Total Score		

BREATH PATTERN RECOGNITION QUESTIONNAIRE	
Indicators of Quality Breathing	Your Score
Part 1 – At Rest	
Part 2 – Video Analysis	
Part 3 – Video Analysis	
Part 4 – Feeling the Tissue	
Part 5 - Exercise	
Part 6 - Lifestyle	
Total	

Ideal	High Quality	Low Quality
0	1 - 10	11 - 30

You want to score a 0 in this test. A 0 is your baseline for a quality breath, and it is very achievable with breath training. Every point where you have more than a zero reflects how adapted your breathing mechanics are at rest and during your life.

THE BOLT SCORE

Origins of the test

The Blood Oxygen Level Threshold, or BOLT score, originated as the Control Pause by Dr. Buteyko and was popularised as the BOLT score in *The Oxygen Advantage* by Patrick McKeown. It was designed by Dr. Buteyko himself after years of laboratory-based research.

Purpose of the test

BOLT measures your breath efficiency at rest, and it measures your first urges to breathe or the chemo-sensitivity of your brain to CO_2. Remember, CO_2 is the only substance that crosses the blood-brain barrier and the body has many ways of measuring CO_2 at critical junctures. This makes the brain super sensitive to any changes in CO_2 levels. The slightest shifts of CO_2 in the body lead the brain to adjust your breathing as needed. This makes the measurement of your first urges critical to your overall breathing health.

Reasons for the test

Most people tend to have an unnaturally high sensitivity to CO_2 or a low tolerance of the gas. These terms are similar. CO_2 sensitivity relates to the brain's response to a rise in CO_2, whereas CO_2 tolerance refers to the amount of CO_2 gas you can withstand; it involves willpower in addition to brain signals. When the brain notices a rise in CO_2 levels for a while, it resets its gauge to a higher sensitivity. According to Dr. Buteyko, re-setting your brain's gauge has drastic knock-on effects for your whole health. This vicious cycle of detecting CO_2 early and over-breathing to get rid of it alters your daily breathing pattern habit and can lead to over 150 diseases of hyperventilation syndrome.

The measurement

As shown below, BOLT measures the length in time of a relaxed breath hold. It measures the breath hold in seconds ranging from 0-60 seconds. The longer the relaxed breath hold is, the more normal the breath and the healthier you are.

RELATING BOLT TO BREATH-HOLD TIME TO DISEASE

BOLT (s)	Symptoms of Health
60+	Optimal health - No disease of civilisation
40 – 60	Great health - very resilient
30 – 40	Good health with some resiliency
20 – 30	Vulnerable System
15 – 20	Highly symptomatic of disease
11 – 15	Severe symptoms and daily medication usually required to manage health
<10	Severe symptoms and strong medication usually required

The technique

Measuring CO_2 Sensitivity with the BOLT Score

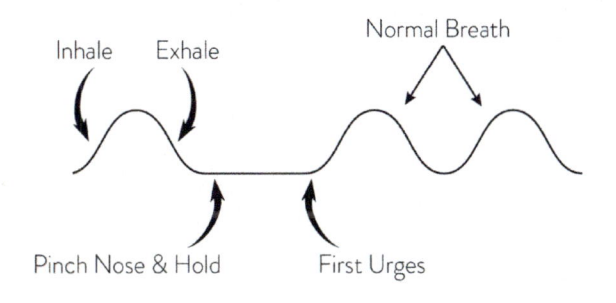

PART 3   THE INNATE-STRENGTH BREATH TRAINING PROGRAMME

1. Relax for 2-5 minutes before taking the BOLT test
2. Adopt a tall seated posture
3. Close the mouth and breathe in through the nose
4. Take a small breath out of the nose, and pinch the nose at the bottom of the breath when the lungs are almost empty. Hold the pinched nose
5. Using a stopwatch, time the number of seconds you hold the breath
6. Release the nose when you experience the first signs of air hunger (needing to breathe). This may be an involuntary contraction of the stomach, neck, or just a feeling of need to inhale
7. Record your BOLT score in the success diary

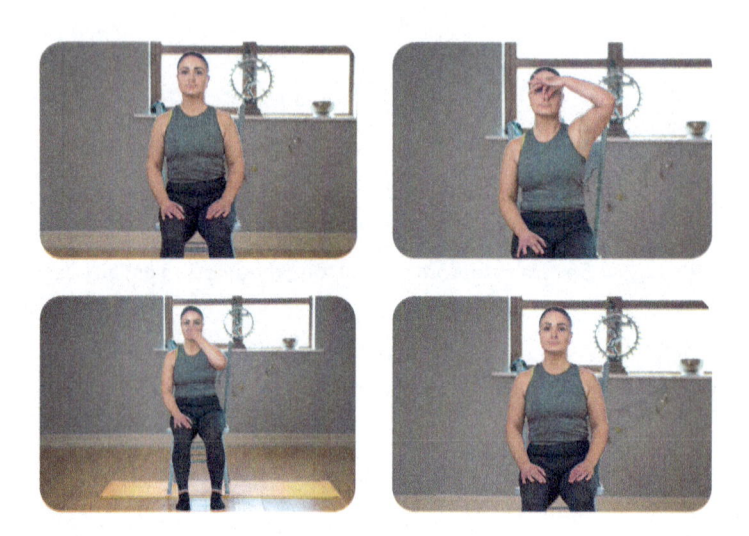

THE MAXIMUM EXHALE SCORE

Origins

To the best of my knowledge, this test originates from the freediving community. It was adapted to the general population by Brian Mac Kenzie and Rob Wilson at Shift Adapt. They have started to develop correlations between scores in this test and anxiety levels.

In Brian Mac Kenzie's words:

> *Freedivers used it to set breathing rhythms and O_2 / CO_2 tables ... Not everybody uses it but what we found was that it was an under-utilised tool that they were using. It really exposes some holes in people. I don't know if it is that important to high level freedivers because they are so in tune with things and they know how to set things so well that they have their own ideas and methods to set things.*

Purpose

People may have a low sensitivity to CO_2 and a good CO_2 tolerance level, but they can still have a reduced ability to use the capacity of their lungs when required. This test measures your ability to fill all of your lung space with air, CO_2 tolerance, and fine motor control of exhalation muscles. The results of this test give us the first quantitative measurement of the fine muscular control of the breathing system and your ability to use it. The test has several components to it:

Maximum Capacity – your ability to access maximum lung capacity improves your score in this test; anything less will result in a weaker score.

Fine Muscular Control – This test includes a strong element of complete muscular control combined with CO_2 tolerance. All expiratory and inspiratory muscles are challenged including the throat, rib cage, diaphragm and abdominal cavity.

CO_2 Tolerance – CO_2 levels rise in your body as you perform this test. Your brain will receive these signals from your body to try to override your conscious control of your exhale by forcing you to take its next inhale. A better test result indicates a high ability to tolerate CO_2 and the brain's signals to breathe.

In my interview with Brian MacKenzie, he told me they have a research paper under review at the moment (2021) but from their work at Shift Adapt, they have seen that 'Anybody under 30 seconds are anxious-prone people. What we found in our work (I can't reveal the research work until the paper comes out) is that state of anxiety is predictable through this test. If you're under 30 seconds you are likely to be high anxiety'.

Reasons

Breathing is not just a subconscious act; it is supposed to be actively used to enhance our lives. After respiration, its major functions are an expression of emotion (communication) and postural strength. For your breathing system to be working optimally, all three functions must be intact. The MES measurement is a wonderful tool to assess your ability to use your full breath for expression. It also guides the person as to what type of training they should begin with.

According to Brian MacKenzie, people can have perfect breathing mechanics but their CO_2 tolerance is weak and this results in anxiety traits and an inability to perform, even at elite-level sport. 'A lot of elite athletes have fairly decent breathing mechanics but their CO_2 tolerance is shit and yet why I am meeting these people is because they are having panic attacks and they are anxious . . . [People] with a higher MES (over 60 seconds) work on that advanced [CO_2 tolerance] concept stuff.'

Measurement

On their site, Shift Adapt discusses the correlations between the test results, breathing ability and health (particularly anxiety). The most noticeable steps are above 40 seconds and above 80 seconds. Those with a breathing skill score below 40 seconds probably have an issue with breathing mechanics, and very likely have a low CO_2 tolerance. It is also predictive of emotional reactivity and may have some health issues. A score above 80 indicates you have decent control of your breathing mechanics, a quality CO_2 tolerance level, your breathing is good, and its impact on health and performance is pretty good overall.

MES	% of Users	Rating
80+	2%	Excellent
60 - 80	5%	Very Good
40 – 60	10%	Good
20 – 40	35%	Fair
< 20	47%	Poor

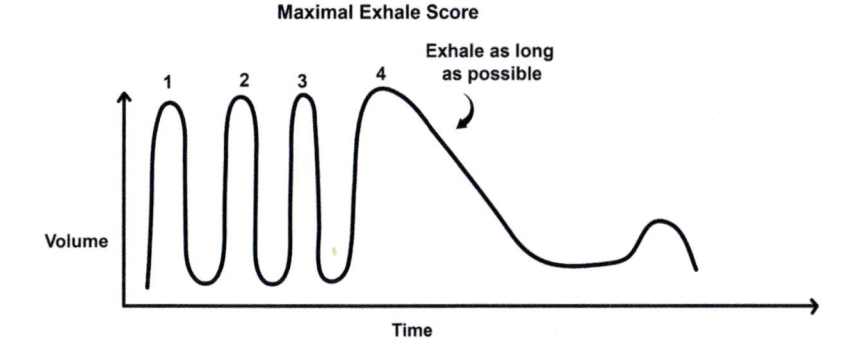

Maximal Exhale Score

SCAN ME

Technique

1. Use a stopwatch and nose breathing only
2. In a seated posture, take 3 large breaths in through your nose, trying to fill every corner of your lungs
3. On your 4th breath, inhale fully
4. Start your stopwatch and begin to exhale slowly. Time the length of your exhale
5. If you need to swallow, hold your breath or inhale some air, then stop the watch and finish your test
6. Be aware: your body may over-ride you and sneak in some air; if this happens, that is the end of the test
7. Recover afterwards and record your score
8. Ideally perform this technique first thing in the morning on an empty stomach

THE WALKING BREATH HOLD TEST

Origins

This is the second of Dr. Buteyko's original measurements, previously known as the maximal breath hold test. Similar tests, known as the CO_2 tables, are found in the free diving community. Their purpose is to enable you to hold your breath under water for longer periods. The background of this test is to measure the health of your system.

Purpose

The Walking Breath Hold test (WBH) is a great measurement of your ability to handle metabolic stress and the resulting fear from a rise in CO_2. Technically, it measures the maximum number of paces you can walk whilst holding your breath.

As you attempt to walk further and further during a breath hold there are strong elements of rising CO_2 and wilful control. The breath hold itself retains CO_2 in your system, and the walking generates CO_2. To do well in this test, you need to train yourself to be relaxed in a very stressful environment (holding your breath) and you need to have a high tolerance of CO_2 (due to the retention and walking).

Reasons

Breath retention only occurs for three reasons. The first is if you are being suffocated/drowned, the second is an embedded response to a long-term stress/deep trauma, and the last is a wilful retention of the breath. Training yourself to retain your breath in a safe environment is key for several reasons:

- Unwinding the habit of chronic subconscious breath-holding
- Helping you to deal with past trauma and long-term stress
- Restoring calm and peace to your body
- Improving fitness
- Decreasing CO_2 sensitivity
- Improving the efficiency of your aerobic energy system
- Enhancing the parasympathetic tone of the nervous system

Measurement

The goal for this test is to walk more than 100 paces whilst holding your breath after an exhale. To achieve this goal and make the results stick, you will end up walking up to 120 or even 140 paces in one effort, but you will need all of your results over the course of a week to be above 100. This wasn't always the case, but as I have coached more and more people over the years, I found the original goal of 100 paces insufficient. Typically, people would reach the goal, stop the training and they wouldn't be able to retain a sufficient score. So I changed it over time to an average of 100 paces and then a goal of more than 100 paces over the course of a week. Once that happened, I found clients obtaining better health benefits and longer-lasting results.

PART 3   THE INNATE-STRENGTH BREATH TRAINING PROGRAMME

Paces	Interpretation
Above 100 for the week	Excellent score – move onto different training depending on your goal
Average 100	Almost there – you need to keep going to make the training stick long-term
One-off 100	Big shifts in fitness, calmness of body and mind, and sleep quality
80+	Noticeable differences in fitness and states of mind
	Bring in higher degrees of CO_2 tolerance training and lactate-based training to continually improve your score - Train twice per day minimum
60+	Another noticeable point on the scale. May notice shifts in both fitness and calmness – keep up the training frequency
40+	You'll notice the difference in a calmer system by now
Below 40	Train three times per day

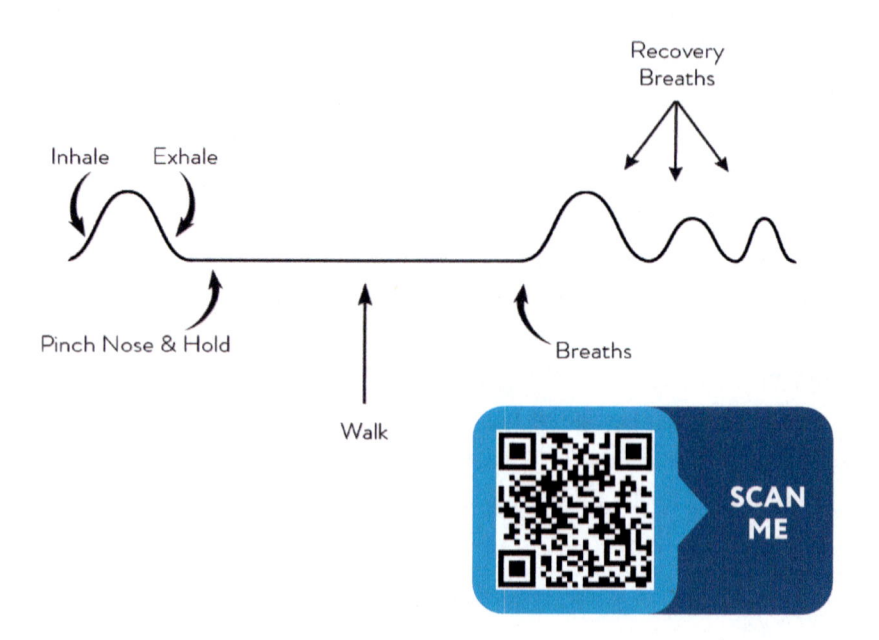

Technique

1. Take a normal-sized inhale through the nose and a normal exhale out of the nose
2. Pinch and hold the nose
3. Walk as many paces as possible, counting your paces
4. When you've reached 95% of your maximum ability, release the nose
5. Inhale through the nose fully, exhale out of the nose
6. Recover and calm your system quickly and gently with nose-only breathing

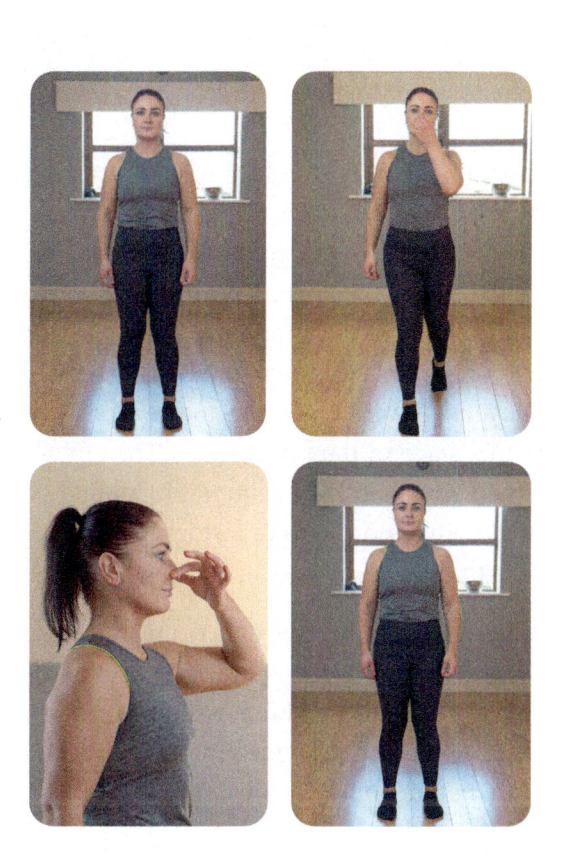

PHASE 1 TRAINING DESIGN – BREATH MECHANICS

14

The Innate-Strength Breath Training programme opens with restoring movement quality to your breathing. Every exercise I've chosen for this phase focuses on either improving the exhale's relaxation or the inhale's freedom. You want to train yourself to let go of the exhale and to be able to inhale fully into zones one and two of your breathing. I also want to make sure that other tissues aren't impacting the breath's movement, and so I've included flexibility and somatic movements in this stage of the programme. The end goal of Phase 1 is to improve both your naturally centred breath and your deliberate breath. However, it may not be fully restored until you complete the full Innate-Strength Breath Training programme.

By the end of Phase 1 you should be able to create a wave of breathing from belly to chest, then let go with the exhale. In particular, parts 1, 2, 3, and 4 of the personal breathing assessment questionnaire will improve, so make sure to take a video of your breathing and answer the questionnaire before and after this training phase.

I recommend you work out at least once per day. In Block 1 there are additional stretches to practise. Highly dedicated people will practise these stretches daily, which brings your total training sessions to two per day. If you're struggling to commit so much time to the programme, then practise the stretches at least three times per week.

Typically, Phase 2 will be completed within two to four weeks, and this time allows one to two weeks per block. Some people may need less or more time depending on their specific needs. You will only know this by checking the state of your breathing mechanics against the video analysis and personal breath assessment questionnaire. When your breathing mechanics are moving nicely, it's time to move on to Phase 3 of the programme.

PHASE I TRAINING DESIGN	
Purpose	Restore Natural Breathing Mechanics
Goals	1. Relaxed exhale 2. Ability to use diaphragm and rib cage naturally
Result Tracking	Personal Breathing Assessment – Video & Questionnaire
Recommended Workouts/Day	1 - 2
No. of Training Blocks	2
Time to Completion	2 – 4 weeks

BLOCK DESIGN

You'll notice that the workouts are laid out similarly. Each exercise has a specific order, a required number of breaths, and some additional notes. The specific arrangement of the programme is a principle of fitness and a key aspect of all good physical training programmes. Like all good science, you need to keep this order to the training so that you can evaluate its effectiveness when it's over. Only at that point should you consider changing some of its parameters.

The order of the exercises is important. They are laid out as A, B, C. Practise all of exercise A first before progressing to exercise B. If you are stuck for time, prioritise the first exercise in the block. It has the highest potency and will deliver the best benefits, especially in the beginning. Sometimes, an exercise will be repeated in the workout, so I've written it in again to save confusion. The length of time in each exercise is guided by the number of breaths you take in most cases.

Exercise Order	Exercise	# of Breaths	Comments
A.	SAMPLE 1	5 - 10	
B.	SAMPLE 2	5 - 10	
C.	SAMPLE 3	5 - 10	

BLOCK 1 LAYOUT

There are two distinct parts to Block 1. The first is the breathing techniques, and the second is the stretching. Both are important; however, the breathing always takes priority if time is tight. The purpose of the breathing techniques in this block is to let go of the exhale and to use your diaphragm effectively. The way you achieve those goals is to uncouple the stress response from your jaws to your diaphragm. First, bring awareness to your breathing pattern by practising the breath of freedom a few times. Next, use an intentional yawn to teach the muscles of the jaw, mouth, face, and throat to let go. Then rewire your brain to innervate your diaphragm better by self-massaging it with the diaphragm release technique.

BLOCK I WORKOUT I – BREATHING (PRACTISED DAILY)			
Exercise Order	Exercise	# of Breaths	Comments
A.	Breath of freedom	5 - 10	
B.	Intentional yawning	5 - 10	
C.	Diaphragm release technique	5 - 10	4/10 pain – no pain when fingers press in
D.	Breath of freedom	5 - 10	

Finally, you teach the rest of the body to let go of tension by stretching it out. The stretching exercises and their sequencing were specifically designed to aid your breathing mechanics. The stretches themselves work from the diaphragm out to the hips and the shoulders – these are key areas of tightness that frequently play havoc with your breathing. The sequencing of the stretches is designed to unravel the tissues rapidly. Pay attention to the details in the techniques, and they'll fast-track your breathing progress.

\multicolumn{4}{c}{BLOCK I}
\multicolumn{4}{c}{WORKOUT 2 – STRETCHING (PRACTISED 3-7 TIMES / WEEK)}
Exercise Order	Exercise	# of Breaths	Comments
A.	Diaphragm stretch (back)	5 - 10	Find your tightest spot – train that one first and more frequently than the other positions
B.	Diaphragm stretch (side)	5 - 10	4/10 – no pain
C.	Diaphragm stretch (front)	5 - 10	
D.	Hip flexor series	5 - 10	
E.	Modified child's pose	5 - 10	

BLOCK 2 LAYOUT

The layout for Block 2 is slightly different to Block 1. In Block 2, you practise alternating workouts each day. Workout 1 continues to focus on freeing the mechanics on the breath. The workout again begins and finishes with bringing awareness to your breath by practising the breath of freedom. This is an important stage for you to familiarise yourself with your own breath and how it feels compared to how it should feel. Next, I look to connect whole-body movement with breathing using somatic exercises. Somatic exercises reduce the stretches from Block 1 as they enhance the connection between brain and body movement. These movements can quickly reduce body-wide pain and promote ease of movement. The final exercise in Workout 3 is the breathing bands. The emphasis here shifts from innervating the diaphragm (as in Block 1) to expanding the ribcage. This is not something many breathing coaches focus on, but it is vitally important to breathing free and having the ability to use your breath as your life demands it.

	BLOCK 2		
	WORKOUT 3 (PRACTISED EVERY 1ST DAY)		
Exercise Order	Exercise	# of Breaths	Comments
A.	Breath of freedom	3 - 5	
B.	Flower	3 - 5	
C.	Dishrag	3 - 5	
D.	Breathing bands	10 - 20	
E.	Breath of freedom	3 - 5	

Meanwhile, the second workout focuses on calming the breath's rhythm and instilling relaxation into the body and mind. The workout begins with the same somatic movements as in Workout 3. These movements are still included because breathing mechanics can frequently become stuck due to the brain holding tension in other tissues and preventing you from breathing freely.

Ultimately, Exercise E is where the money is at with this workout. Breath calming is the king of breathing techniques, in my opinion. If I had only one technique to choose, this would be it. I've included Exercises B and C because some people need to be guided toward the breath-calming technique. From this perspective, humming is a great way to extend your exhale, stimulate the vagus nerve and relax the body. 4:6 breathing is equally as effective at relaxing the body but in a different way. It has been shown time and again in research to synchronise breath, heart, and brain rhythms to create a calm rhythm throughout your whole being.

BLOCK 2
WORKOUT 4 (PRACTISED EVERY OTHER DAY)

Exercise Order	Exercise	# of Breaths	Comments
A.	Flower	3 - 5	
B.	Dishrag	3 - 5	
C.	Humming breath	3 - 5	
D.	4:6 Breathing	10	
E.	Breath calming	3 – 5 mins	
F.	Meditation	As desired	

PHASE 1 TECHNIQUES

You've come across some of these techniques earlier in the book. The difference is now you are putting together a structured programme of progressive training with the aim of restoring your breathing. This is the critical difference between breath training and breathwork. The steps to practising each of the techniques in Block 1 are laid out in this chapter, along with some coaching notes. Each technique has a specific goal in this program, with the ultimate aim of training you to breathe free. Goals, benefits, progressions, when to use the techniques, and when not to use them are included. Finally, I'll include a skill development aspect to a technique where appropriate.

Once you have restored your breathing mechanics at the end of Phase 1, it will be time for you to move on to either Phase 2 or 3. As I said in the last chapter, you are free to choose either path next. Just remember that you need to train both Phases 2 and 3 to fully restore your breathing system, breathe free, and be healthy. For now, let's get going with the exercises of Phase 1.

PART 3   THE INNATE-STRENGTH BREATH TRAINING PROGRAMME

THE BREATH OF FREEDOM

The breath of freedom is a mirror for the quality of your breathing mechanics, and it reflects the quality of your deliberate breath and your readiness for the next training phase. Use it as an overall assessment of your breathing mechanics at the start and end of the programme, during all stretching movements and I also ask you to use it as a daily assessment before and after your training throughout Phase 1: Breath Mechanics.

Purpose

Asses the quality of your breathing mechanics

Ideally you can exhale with complete relaxation and inhale fully into the body during the breath of freedom. As you exhale you can feel your body let go of the tension in your breath. The muscles of the jaw, face, mouth, tongue and throat all release and let go on the exhale. It's only when you can let go of your exhale that your whole body and mind begin to let go of tension. Muscles relax, the body moves with ease, stress dissipates, and the mind calms. Next, you inhale through your nose and fill your body with air. A nasal inhale not only cleans and filters the air but it also engages the diaphragm up to 50% better than a mouth inhalation. With a slow, full nasal inhale, you will clearly see and feel the belly rise followed by the chest expanding. This movement indicates that you can use all of your breathing muscles, when required by the demands of life, such as in sport, when singing, or expressing emotion. Life becomes fuller and more vibrant, and at the same time it flows easier with a quality, trained breath of freedom.

Breath of Freedom Goals:

1. Have a relaxed exhale through the mouth
2. Inhale through the nose fully into the body – belly rises first, then chest expands

PHASE 1 TRAINING DESIGN – BREATH MECHANICS

Outside of a breath assessment, I use the breath of freedom as the foundation for all tension-releasing techniques of both the body and mind in breath training. Here I am referring to physical rehab techniques like the diaphragm release technique and the breathing bands (both found in Phase 1), all stretching and movement techniques (again found in Phase 1), as well as mental/emotional releasing techniques like circular breathing and the Wim Hof Breathing (found in Phase 3).

Breath of Freedom Functions:

1. Assessment of quality breathing mechanics
2. Improve stretching
3. Vital for somatic movements
4. Foundation technique in all breathwork

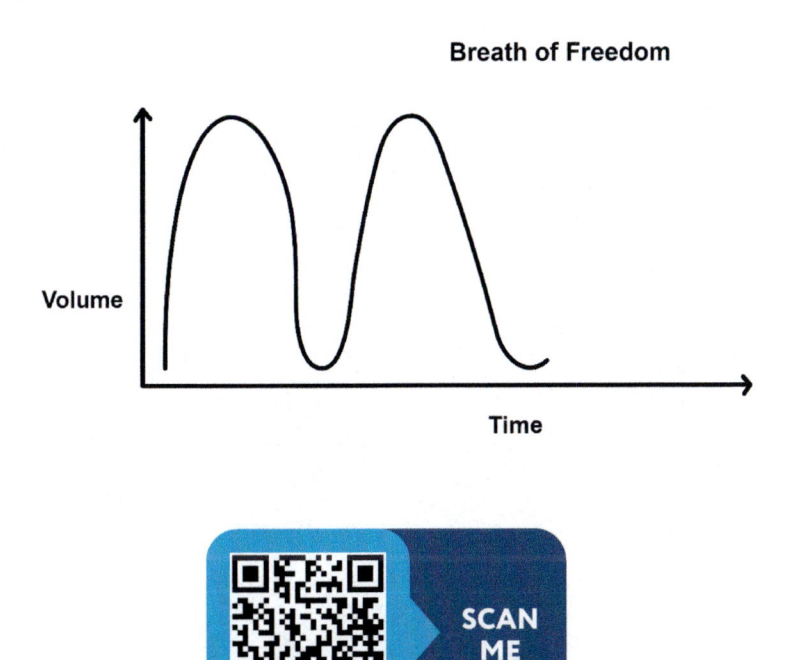

Breath of Freedom

Technique

1. Lie on your back in a relaxed position with knees bent and feet flat on the floor.
2. Breathe in through your nose and out of your mouth for three to five breaths.
3. The breath is continuous, there are no pauses at the top or bottom of the breath. The air is just pulled in naturally and flows out of the body at ease.
4. As you inhale, the belly should rise naturally. There is no need to push the belly out or force anything. If it does not rise, it simply means that the diaphragm is stiff and needs some training. This will be achieved with the diaphragm release technique.
5. The chest should expand on the inhale too, following the rise of the belly. Think of your breath like a wave flowing through your body from belly to chest. Again, if the chest does not move significantly, that's ok. We will train it to expand more with the breathing bands exercise.
6. An exhale that is relaxed makes a 'haaah' sound in your throat. It is the same noise you'd make when sinking into a nice hot bath. This is a sighing action and a sign that all of the tension is being released from the mouth, jaw, tongue, and throat. Don't worry if you can't get it the first time, as the intentional yawning technique in Workout 1 is designed to improve it.

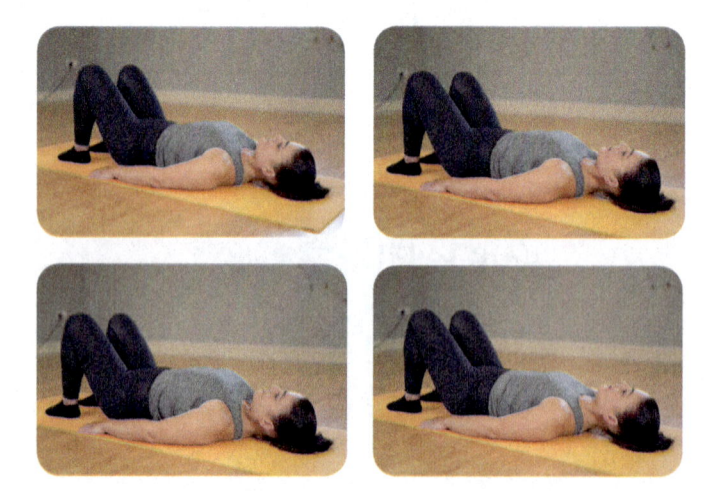

Skill Development

- Remember to breathe the breath of freedom when practising all stretching and movement techniques. Combining the breath of freedom with movement helps to release tension from the breath out into the whole body, it improves suppleness in the body, eases pain, and paves the way for a strong body.

INTENTIONAL YAWNING

Yawning is an innate process God created in your biology to rebalance your nervous system after a stressful period or when you're tired. It helps you to breathe more easily. That is why everybody loves a good yawn, right?

Purpose of a yawn

Rebalance your nervous system and maintain a supple breathing pattern

Why is it that you stifle a yawn when you need it most? In an office meeting, during sport or even when watching TV with your friends and family – you often suppress your yawn even though your body is crying out for it to help you rebalance.

When you continuously stifle a yawn, you are hardwiring an imbalance into your nervous system more deeply. The brain listens to your conscious demand to over-ride it and it drives more power to suppressing the yawn. Because of the neuro-anatomical wiring of your nervous system, your brain takes power from your diaphragm and redirects it to the jaw area. This rewiring of your nervous system compounds the effect of a suppressed yawn by adapting your everyday breathing pattern and stress response even further. Now you have ingrained an adapted breathing pattern with every breath of the day. That adapted breathing pattern is a retracted diaphragm, a controlled exhale and frequent breath-holding. It also leads to TMJ pain, frequent headaches, migraines, and teeth grinding. The pattern is ingrained even deeper with each suppressed yawn and stress reaction.

Effects of a suppressed yawn:

1. Suppressed yawn = clenching the jaw
2. Gradually drives power to the jaw area consciously
3. Gradually reduces power to the diaphragm creating a retracted diaphragm
4. Creates an adapted breathing pattern
5. Produces pain, earaches, headaches, migraines, teeth grinding, controlled exhale, and breath-holding

Yawning on purpose, then, has the opposite effect of suppressing it. An intentional yawn uncouples the adapted stress response. It stretches the muscles of the jaw, mouth, tongue and throat, and it teaches you to let go of stress and breathe easier.

Purpose of the intentional yawn

Decouple stress from the jaw, mouth and throat area and rewire your brain to breathe naturally with your diaphragm and let go of an exhale.

In particular, an intentional yawn releases the exhale. It helps you to let go of the exhale and trains you to stop holding your breath during every moment of your life. Sometimes, intentional yawning can automatically rebalance your breathing mechanics on its own. More often than not, though, you will need to train the other techniques in this phase to restore your breathing mechanics fully.

Benefits of an intentional yawn

1. Relaxes the exhale
2. Releases the muscles of the face, jaw, mouth, and throat
3. Rewires the brain to strengthen the diaphragm
4. Reduces subconscious breath-holding, pain, and tension in the head
5. Reduces TMJ pain, teeth grinding, migraines, and headaches
6. Improves shoulder mobility

Technique

1. Slowly inhale through your mouth and fully stretch open your jaw. Repeat this for three to five breaths
2. After repeating a few intentional yawns, the body may automatically yawn. This is a good sign; let it happen
3. Once you get a handle on the gradual inhale and stretch, then focus your attention on the exhale
4. Allow the exhale to recoil. Let it go. Let it relax and fall out of your body. The exhale is completely passive
5. You may notice a 'haaah' sound with the passive exhale

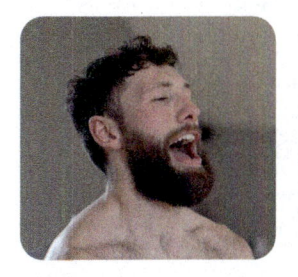

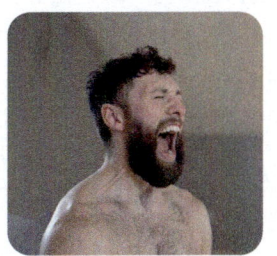

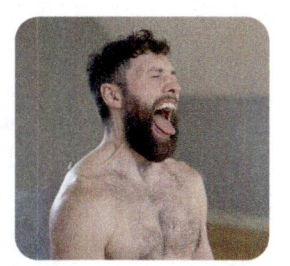

SCAN ME

PRO COACHING TIP

- Remember to always keep the focus on the inhale and stretching the jaw – make the inhale as long as you can and the stretch as big as you can. The passive exhale will come.
- If you find it hard to make the 'haaah' sound as you sigh out through your mouth, then I suggest you strengthen the muscle tone of the throat by gargling water for 30 seconds as loud as you can every time you brush your teeth (twice per day hopefully!).

Skill Development

As you become proficient with the yawn, begin to release more of the tension in the body by making the movement bigger. As you inhale, wiggle your tongue, jaw and move your head gently (in any direction). Stretch your arms out and arch your back. Bring a full upper body stretch into the yawn. This is the start of your somatic exercises and the progression to the intentional yawn.

THE DIAPHRAGM RELEASE TECHNIQUE

Background

I learned this technique from Pasquale Silvestre and Alex Mauri. These two men came to Ireland to teach an introduction to Dr. Danielle Raggi's *Posturology* course. Since learning this technique, it has become a staple in my breath training programme. It is undoubtedly one of the best self-myofascial-release techniques I've found to restore pliability to the diaphragm – it's an absolute gem. Think of it as giving yourself a massage. By restoring the diaphragm, the technique almost immediately resets your breathing mechanics; it brings the body to a more rested state, reduces pain and improves performance. I've personally seen this technique benefit people with breathing problems, heart arrhythmia, high blood pressure, gut issues and back pain.

Purpose of the Diaphragm

The diaphragm is your key breathing muscle. Restoring the pliability and power to the diaphragm is the foundation to breathing free

Purpose of the Diaphragm Release Technique

Restores innervation and pliability to the diaphragm

Functions

The diaphragm is located in the middle of your body and has very few sensory nerve endings, meaning it's a difficult muscle to feel, compared, say, to a leg muscle. The breath, combined with the focused touch of your fingers, is responsible for the success of this technique. The aim is to inhale into your fingers and relax your body as you hook your fingers deeper under your lower ribs. As you breathe and hook your fingers under your ribs, you bring kinaesthetic awareness to your diaphragm. The brain naturally does the rest of the work under relaxation to wire power and suppleness to the diaphragm.

Functions of the Diaphragm Release Technique:

1. Restores movement to the diaphragm and induces Zone 1 breathing naturally
2. Eliminates pain and restriction when nasal breathing

Benefits

By re-wiring your brain to breathe with the diaphragm, you restore natural Zone 1 diaphragmatic breathing. Diaphragmatic breathing is a part of your natural resting breath, and it is crucial for managing the efficiency of your breath when life demands it. Not only does it improve breathing but it is also critical for all other body systems to work well.

A quality moving diaphragm beats the heart gently with every breath. As you inhale, your heart rate and blood pressure increase, and as you exhale, they decrease. There is no separation between breath and heart. With a slow diaphragmatic breath you improve mental health by synchronising breath, heart, and brain rhythms. A diaphragmatic breath improves gut health by bringing blood flow, oxygen, and nutrients to the abdominal organs. It is key to removing toxins and waste by enhancing the flow of lymph through the body. Finally it is great for sexual function and pelvic and core health because the diaphragm works together with these muscles to contract and release as needed.

Benefits of the Diaphragm Release Technique:

↑ Diaphragmatic breathing

↑ Ability to breathe full breaths

↑ Gut motility

↑ Blood pressure and heart rate

↑ Lymphatic drainage

↑ Sexual function

↑ Core strength and health

Technique

1. Lie on your back in a relaxed position with knees bent and feet on the floor
2. Use the breath of freedom breathing pattern during this technique – exhale passively and inhale fully through the nose
3. Trace the middle of your breast bone with your fingers. Find the bottom of the breastbone. Place the finger-tips of both hands under your ribs (1 inch or more from your mid line)
4. As you exhale, sink your fingers deep into your abdomen, just under the ribs
5. As you inhale, hold your hands there
6. Breathe out; sink the fingers deeper
7. Continue this process in a relaxed state. There may be a lot of pressure but there should not be any pain. The pain level should be 4/10 max. If it's any higher, then you're pushing too hard
8. Eventually, you'll be able to hook your finger under your ribs
9. When you finish that section, move your hands laterally across the ribs (away from the middle) and repeat the process the next section

PHASE 1 TRAINING DESIGN – BREATH MECHANICS

10. Continue until you have reached the bottom portion of your ribs (usually 3 sections)
11. Relax the hands. Breathe the breath of freedom a few times. Can you feel your lower rib cage and belly move more with your breath?

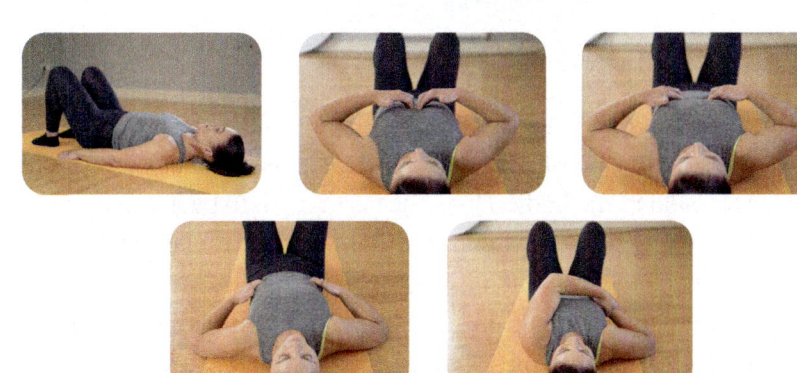

SCAN ME

PRO COACHING TIP

- The diaphragm has roles to play in both posture and breathing. If you are seated or standing during this exercise, the diaphragm is recruited more for posture, making it more difficult to release the diaphragm. Similarly, if you are lying down with your legs straight, it can pull your body out of alignment. For these reasons I recommend you practice this technique lying down with knees bent.
- After you hook your fingers under your ribs for a few breaths, deliberately cough hard through your nose. The diaphragm powerfully contracts during a nasal cough. The odd deliberate nasal cough during this exercise will help to restore the diaphragm even more quickly.

PART 3   THE INNATE-STRENGTH BREATH TRAINING PROGRAMME

Contra-indications

Your heart sits above the diaphragm on the centre-left side of your body. Your liver is below it on the centre-right and your stomach is right in the middle of your bottom two ribs. For these anatomical reasons, practise this technique gently if you have any cardiovascular issues or gut. It is still a perfectly safe technique for you to practice. More to the point, a quality moving diaphragm is excellent for people with all of these conditions. So just be gentle, breathe calmly, and have no pain during the exercise.

BREATH PATTERN FOR STRETCHES

The somatic nervous system innervates the muscles and tissues of the body to move. Some physical therapy modalities teach that all emotional traumas are held in the body. This space is thought to be in the somatic nervous system and fascial tissue. Moving the body in particular ways can free the body of these traumas through the somatic nervous system; realign posture; relieve pain in the body, and improve performance. Stretching is the most simple and powerful way to teach your somatic nervous system to release tension and increase the length in a tissue. In the Innate-Strength Breath Training Programme, we begin with stretches during Block 1 and advance to whole-body somatic movements in Block 2. All stretches, practised effectively should align with the same principles of the whole-body somatic movement patterns.

Principles

- The chosen breathing pattern is essential to connect the mind to the movement, enhance blood flow and nutrients to the area, relax the body, and release the hold of the nervous system. Your breath either works with the movement or competes against it. To simplify, an inhale works with any expanding and opening movement. An exhale combines with a closing movement or relaxation in a movement

- Relaxation is integral to stretching and somatic release
- The essence of quality movement is a conscious connection between the movement and the brain – in other words, you have to feel exactly what you are doing

Process

If you want to increase the tissue length, you must release it first, and then stabilise it.

Releasing means getting the nervous system to let go, and allowing the myo-fascial network to unbind.

Stabilising it secures the joint at the new tissue length. Without stabilisation, the tissue would just return to its normal length.

The breath is integral to this relationship.

BREATH OF FREEDOM WITH SOMATIC MOVEMENTS

As described earlier in the chapter, the breath of freedom, is the key breathing technique for effective somatic movement. All somatic movements flow with the breath. The body naturally folds over with the exhale, and conversely it opens with an inhale.

Once you are familiar with the breath of freedom, you can then exaggerate both the breath and the movement to feel your body more. Exhaling hard and squeezing the body closed sends a powerful signal to the brain which will help you to feel it more. As you release out of the exhale and into an inhale, the brain unravels the body and lets go of any unnecessary tension. The same happens when you inhale fully and contract the muscles of the body, albeit in the opposite pattern.

DIAPHRAGM STRETCHES 1-2-3

As you know by now, the diaphragm is located horizontally across the lower ribs. It's also a three-dimensional muscle in the sense that it wraps around the front, side and back of the body. For these reasons we need to choose stretches for each aspect of the diaphragm to give us the best chance of restoring it. These stretches come from a specialised form of therapy, called ELDOA. They were created by Guy Voyer D.O., a world-renowned osteopath and rehab specialist, and they were taught to me by world-renowned strength and conditioning coach, Paul Gagne.

These stretches are great for restoring movement to the diaphragm, rib cage, and mid- and low- back. Positioning the body in these stretches and breathing into them helps with the ventilation-perfusion ratio of the lungs. In other words, it helps transport oxygen/carbon dioxide into and out of the lungs. With these stretches, you begin to access parts of the lungs you may not have used in a long time. The rolled-up yoga mat is my own little addition to the technique. Using the mat in the stretches positions you better, creates an even more effective stretch, and helps the body and lungs to open further.

Technique

Rear of Diaphragm Stretch

1. Lie on your left side with your head supported by your left hand. Have your knees bent and place your top knee (right knee) in front of your lower knee. Place a rolled-up yoga mat under your ribs to exaggerate the stretch. Place your top hand (right hand) at your temple
2. Combine the breath of freedom with your stretch by inhaling through your nose and exhale with relaxation through the mouth
3. As you inhale, expand your ribs from the inside out. Drive your right elbow diagonally away from you, keeping your right hand in contact with your temple

4. At the same time, pull your coccyx (base of your spine) away from you
5. Exhale through the mouth, making sure to let go of your exhale. As you exhale, hold the position
6. Repeat the stretch with the flow of your breath
7. Inhale – try to stretch the elbow and the hips further. Exhale, hold the position, and relax into it
8. You should feel this stretch across the side and back of your ribs on the right-hand side

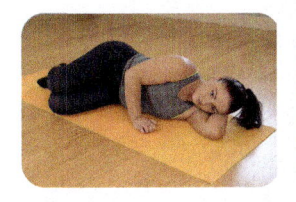

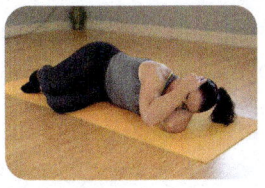

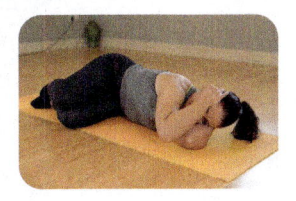

Side of Diaphragm Stretch

1. Start in a similar position as above, but straighten your torso a little this time. Keep the rolled-up yoga mat under your lower ribs
2. Your right arm straightens above the head
3. Cock your wrist backwards, like spiderman casting out a web
4. Use the breath of freedom with the same stretching pattern as above
5. Inhale – extend the wrist of your right hand away from you. At the same time, pull your coccyx in the opposite direction
6. Exhale – hold position and relax the breath, then repeat
7. You'll feel this stretch more along the right-hand side of the torso and ribs, through the arm-pit and into the arm

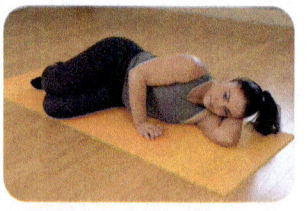

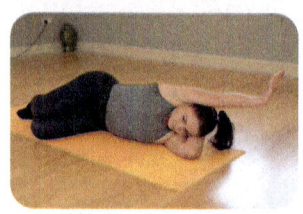

PART 3   THE INNATE-STRENGTH BREATH TRAINING PROGRAMME

Front of Diaphragm Stretch

1. Lying in the same position as the Side of Diaphragm Stretch, return your right hand to your temple
2. Open your elbow and chest so that your body rotates open
3. Practise the same breathing and stretch as before
4. Drive the elbow away from you and open your body up more with the inhale. Exhale, relax, and hold the position

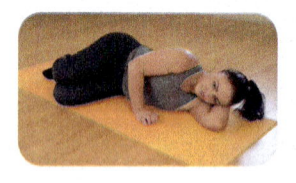

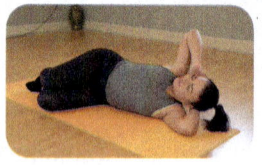

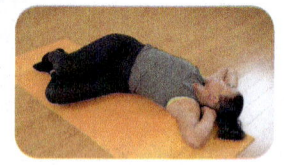

Once you've finished all stretches on the right-hand side, turn over and practice them all on the left.

After the technique, relax for a moment, and then breathe the breath of freedom a few times. Can you feel your rib cage move more?

> **PRO COACHING TIP**
> - If the left happens to be tighter than the right, then begin on the left-hand side in future.

THE COUCH STRETCH

The hip flexor group comprises three major muscles: the psoas, iliacus and quadriceps. Their primary function is to flex the hip and the spine. These primary hip flexors are supported by many other muscles to the front of the body, which run along both the deep and superficial fascial lines of the body. The deep and superficial fascial lines connect the head, through the rib-cage, into the abdominal region, over the hip and down the front of the legs to the toes.

Perhaps one of the most important muscles of the body, the hip flexor group is conventionally regarded as a problem muscle by many therapists and trainers. Generally, it is thought that over-working hip flexors are primarily responsible for low-back pain and recurring hamstring tears, while weak hip flexors contribute to abdominal tears and tight quadriceps in the legs. This may well be partially true; however, you also have to remember the hip flexors' location in the body. The hip flexors are attached directly to the diaphragm on the lumbar spine, and because breathing has a higher priority than posture, this means that they are subservient to the needs of breathing. If your diaphragm is retracted or your breathing is adapted, the brain can pull power from the hip flexors to help with breathing. This adaption for better breathing unfortunately changes your posture. The resulting posture can lead to all of the downstream pain and problems over time. Your first job in restoring your breath, then, is to improve the diaphragm; the next is to restore the length of your hip flexors.

The second way the hip flexors can affect your breathing is through movement. The hip flexors are shortened when you sit, squat and run.

PART 3   THE INNATE-STRENGTH BREATH TRAINING PROGRAMME

Considering that we are now more sedentary than ever between home, office, and commute, it is no wonder the hip flexors often become shortened. A shortened hip flexor group pulls on your diaphragm, contributing to poor breathing mechanics. When you view the hip flexors from both of these perspectives, you can begin to appreciate the need to restore length to them in order to benefit your breathing. A long and strong hip flexor group provides for efficient posture and breathing mechanics. It relieves pressure on the lower back and helps the pelvic floor to work efficiently. It allows the diaphragm to move freely and your breathing mechanics to work effectively.

Technique

1. Assume a ½ kneeling posture, by kneeling on one knee
2. Enhance the stretch by pushing your front knee as far forward as possible
3. Breathe the breath of freedom – nice, calm, and full breaths in, followed by a relaxed exhale

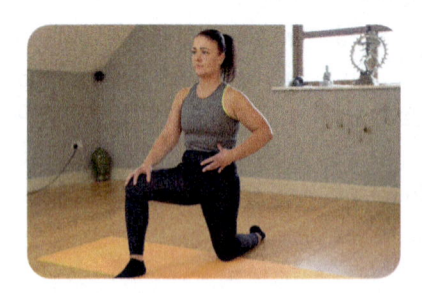

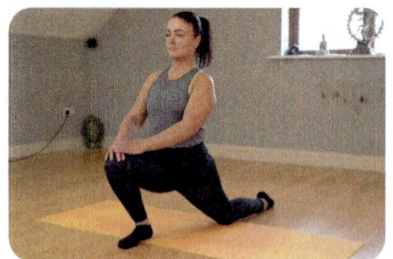

Advancing the Stretch 1

1. This is a serious progression from the previous stretch
2. Place your rear leg on a wall so your shin runs along the wall. You are kneeling on the rear knee, and your front foot is on the floor
3. Place your hands on the floor to support your body and open up the hips
4. If it's too tight in this position, kneel further out from the wall to release some of the stretch
5. You should be able to breathe calmly and stay relaxed throughout the stretch

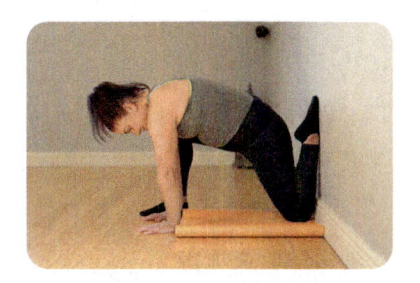

Advancing the Stretch 2

1. Kneel taller by placing your elbows on your front knee
2. Then progress to kneeling taller by placing your hands on your front knee
3. The ideal position is to have your shin, shoulders, and head touching the wall behind you
4. Remain relaxed and able to breathe the breath of freedom at all times

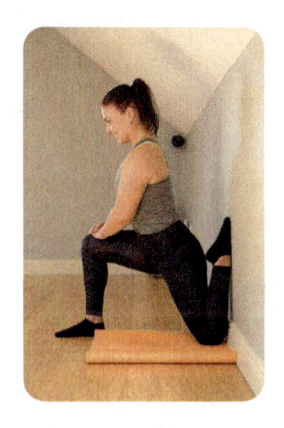

Advancing the Stretch 3

1. Reach your arm above your head, so you have one 'long side' from knee – hip – arm
2. Breathe as above
3. Feel free to play with the position by tilting and twisting. Find the tightest area and breathe into it

After the technique, relax for a moment, and then breathe the breath of freedom a few times. Can you feel your rib cage move more?

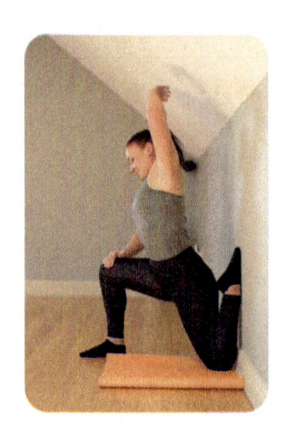

(MODIFIED) CHILD'S POSE

The Child's Pose is quite a famous resting posture in yoga. Here I change it a little to give more of a stretch on each side of the back. The emphasis is on the latissimus dorsi muscle, or the lats. The lats are big superficial muscles that run from the inside of your bicep to form the back of your arm pit. They stretch out over the back of the rib cage, through the thoraco-lumbar fascia and connect into the hip. They're among the largest muscles of the upper body, and they're a powerhouse of a mover. They contribute hugely to sprinting and all pulling techniques. Although the lats don't directly influence your breathing, they do contribute greatly to posture, and to an overall tightness in the ribcage if they become tight themselves. Lengthening the lats in this stretch helps you to breathe more freely into the back and sides of the ribcage.

Technique

1. Kneel on your shins and shift your bum back onto your heels. Reach your hands in front of you on the floor
2. Walk your hands out as far as you can whilst keeping your bum back on your heels

3. Breathe the breath of freedom and breathe into your back. Feel your ribcage expand, and contract in your back as you inhale, and exhale
4. Shift both arms to one side, say the left first. Feel the stretch across your right armpit and ribcage. Breathe into this area, focusing on expanding, and lengthening the rib cage on the right. Repeat a few breaths here
5. Move both arms to the opposite side and repeat

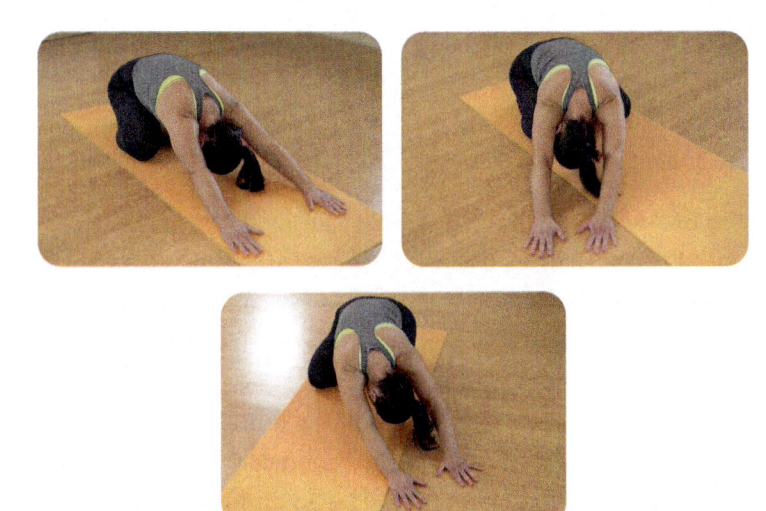

After the technique, relax for a moment, and then breathe the breath of freedom a few times. Can you feel your rib cage move more?

WORKOUT 3 EXERCISE TECHNIQUES

The purpose of Workout 3 is to help the ribcage move more freely. Freedom of movement in the rib cage is vitally important to breathing free. It allows for natural breathing patterns to occur subconsciously and gives you the flexibility to breathe fully when life demands it.

The first two exercises in Workout 3 are somatic movements. Each of these exercises capitalises on the innate innervations of the somatic nervous system to move the breath, body, and mind as one. The breathing bands exercise is at the core of this workout. Its purpose is to bring you a very powerful sense of rib cage movement through breathing and some very simple tools. The remaining three exercises aim to reduce your breathing rate, slow your breath rhythm, and calm your breathing. The humming breath and 4:6 breathing are stepping stones to the final technique, breath calming. Breath calming is the king of breathing techniques, in my opinion. It is the one that directly slows and calms your daily breathing patterns.

SOMATIC EXERCISES

Moshe Feldenkrais was an Israeli engineer and creator of The Feldenkrais Method. The Feldenkrais Method was developed in the early to mid-twentieth century. It is one of the first movement practices to arrange a set of exercises to purposely connect mind and body. In the 1960s, Thomas Hanna built on this work by Feldenkrais, calling his work Somatic Therapy. Somatic Therapy refined the connection between body and mind. Somatic Therapy aims is to restore ease to the body by helping you experience the connection between body and mind even deeper than Feldenkrais. The Somatic Flower and Dishrag exercises in Workout 3 come directly from Thomas Hanna's work. They are two of the primary exercises in his work, and I have found they work fantastically well to:

- Improve breathing mechanics, particularly your whole rib cage movement
- Improve ventilation-perfusion ratio and gas exchange in the lungs
- Connect your breathing and movement patterns together
- Reduce pain and movement restrictions
- Restore ease and freedom to the body

Technique for all Somatic Exercises

1. Find a comfortable space in a room, with no or few distractions and noises going on. This helps you focus internally on the technique
2. All somatic exercises are practised lying on the floor. Feeling the floor under your whole body gives your brain the most sensory feedback – it can feel where it is in space. By using the floor, the brain orients itself in space quickly, it feels the movement better and it rebalances itself efficiently
3. All somatic therapy exercises begin with small movements. The smallest movement the body can make is simply breathing. Gradually increase the size of your breath and add the movement of the exercise. Exaggerate the movement by squeezing and feeling the body part you want to move. Each movement starts in your core, and then grows bigger until your whole body moves in unison with the breath
4. Begin with inhaling and moving the selected body part. As you exhale, relax the body and allow it to fall back to the floor. Feeling both the inhale-squeeze and exhale-relax are essential to the overall success of the technique. Don't worry if you're not *feeling* the exercise initially – it may take some time

> **PRO COACHING TIPS TO ALL SOMATIC EXERCISES**
>
> - Believe it or not, it's not actually about the inhale and the squeeze in these techniques, it is more about the exhale and the relaxation. The inhale and squeeze give you the feeling of a moving body, and the exhale and relaxation signify that your body is re-centring itself. It's only when the body is re-centred that breathing improves, and the body moves more easily.

PART 3   THE INNATE-STRENGTH BREATH TRAINING PROGRAMME

Skill Development for Each Exercise

Over time you'll be able to role-reverse these two patterns. Once you've tried the exercise with emphasising the inhale and squeeze, turn your attention to an exhale and squeeze.

At the highest level of this technique, you alternate between inhale-squeeze-exhale-relax and exhale-squeeze-inhale-relax. When you can practise either pattern alternatively, you know you've mastered the connection between your brain, breath and body in this movement pattern. Your brain's flexibility to move swiftly between movements provides the freedom in your body and breath that you've been seeking.

SOMATIC FLOWER

Purpose

The Somatic Flower intentionally connects your breath to one of your natural whole-body movements.

Technique

1. Find a comfortable space in your room, without too many distractions, or outside noises
2. Lie on your back, with knees bent and arms by your side
3. Take 5 breaths during each layer of the exercise, then progressively add the next layer of the technique until you practice the full movement
4. Using the breath of freedom, inhale fully into your body. Feel your belly rise and then your chest
5. Arch your lower back and squeeze it tight as your belly rises. Exhale and allow your lower back to return to the floor
6. Build the squeeze of the back arch with your inhale into your mid-back once you've mastered the low-back arch squeeze

7. Next, open your legs as you inhale and back arch. The knees fall to either side, opening the hips up like butterfly wings. When you exhale, the back flattens once more, and the legs close
8. Once you've got the hang of the back arch and open legs, then turn to the arms. Twist open your arms with every inhale-back arch-open legs. Unravel the arms and allow them to relax with every exhale
9. Finally, add in the head. As you inhale, back arch, open legs, and open arms, then tuck your chin into your chest. This will lengthen the neck at the back and stretch your spine even further. Exhale and allow the body to return to a resting state
10. The next part of the technique is the exact opposite movement as above. This time you exhale as much as you can and follow with the body
11. The back flattens, knees come together. The arms rotate inward, and the chin lifts

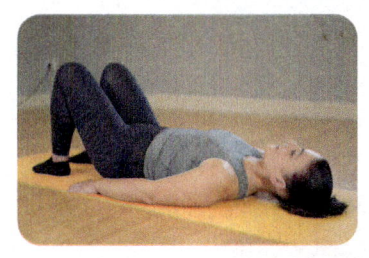

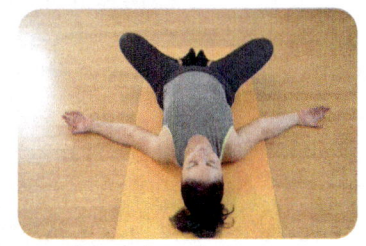

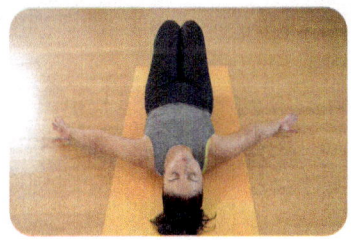

After the technique, relax for a moment, and then breathe the breath of freedom a few times. Can you feel your rib cage move more?

SOMATIC DISHRAG

Purpose

The Somatic Dishrag intentionally connects your breath to a second of your natural whole-body movements.

Technique

1. Find a comfortable space in your room without too many distractions or outside noises
2. Lie on your back, with knees bent and arms by your side
3. Take 5 breaths during each layer of the exercise, then progressively add the next layer of the technique until you practice the full movement
4. Using the breath of freedom, inhale fully into your body. Feel your belly rise and then your chest
5. Arch your lower back and squeeze it tight as your belly rises. Exhale and allow the lower back to return to the floor
6. Build the squeeze of the back arch with your inhale into your mid-back once you've mastered the lower back arch squeeze
7. Next, drop both of your legs to one side of your body as you inhale and back arch. Make sure to squeeze the movement at the end range by pushing the knees to the floor, arching the back further and inhaling fully into the body
8. When you exhale, the back flattens once more and pulls the back to the starting position
9. On your next inhale, drop your legs to the other side of your body, then return on the exhale. This alternation between left and right sides continues with each breath through the remainder of the exercise

10. Once you've got the hang of the back arch and dropped knees, turn to the arms. As you drop your legs to the left, twist open your right arm and twist closed your left arm. When I say open, I mean turn your right hand towards your head and continue the movement until you can't go any further. The opposite twist occurs with the left hand – it turns down towards the feet
11. Unravel the arms with your exhale, draw the knees back to the start, and allow the back to relax with every exhale
12. Finally, add in the head. As you inhale, back arch, drop the legs, and twist the arms, twist your head in the direction of the open arm. In this case, it is the right arm
13. Exhale and allow the body to return to a resting state, then alternate sides

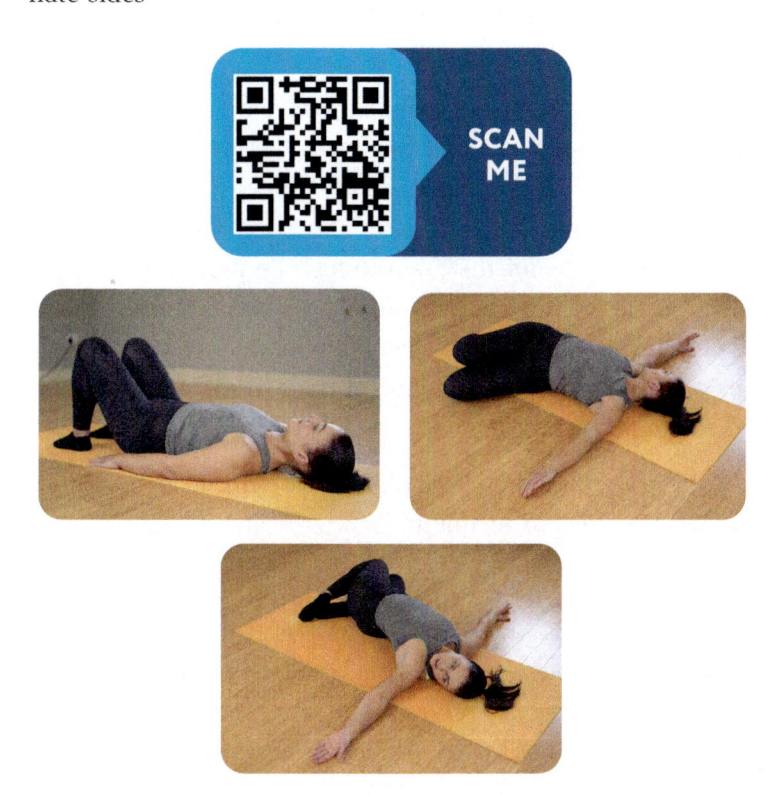

After the technique, relax for a moment, and then breathe the breath of freedom a few times. Can you feel your rib cage move more?

BREATHING BANDS

After I began using the diaphragm release technique to free up the diaphragm and get people breathing into Zone 1 better, I began to notice that some people don't breathe very well into Zone 2, or their chest. Their rib cage is inflexible and doesn't move very well with breathing or with body movement. And so I began to seek out ways to move the rib cage better. The typical way to encourage someone to breathe into their ribs is to either place a yoga block or kettlebell on their chest and have them move the item with their breathing. The only problem with that idea is that the ribs are 360° around the torso; I found the techniques to be a very long and ineffective approach to retraining the breath. With all my research, I couldn't find one exercise which restored rib movement swiftly and effectively. In the end, I created one, which I named 'Breathing Bands'.

The concept for the breathing bands exercise originated from a variety of backgrounds. Pilates, occupational therapy, personal training, emotional anatomy, and being a parent, believe it or not, all contributed to the formation of the exercise. The essence of the technique is to provide a stimulus for the brain to feel the movement of the ribs. I achieve this by pulling some bands tight around the entire rib cage. When you inhale, you imagine yourself bursting out of the bands laterally. Sometimes, just one to three of these breaths are sufficient to bring awareness and movement back to the rib cage.

You can use normal strength bands that you'd find in a gym or any martial arts belt for this technique.

Technique

1. Exhale fully through the mouth – breathe out as much air as you possibly can
2. Wrap the breathing bands around your rib cage. If you're male then wrap one below your nipple line and one above. If you're female, wrap one just above your breast (where the logo of t-shirt would typically sit) and one on the lower ribs, under your breast

PHASE 1 TRAINING DESIGN – BREATH MECHANICS

SCAN ME

3. Wrap the bands as tight as possible (with the fully exhaled breath from Step 1)

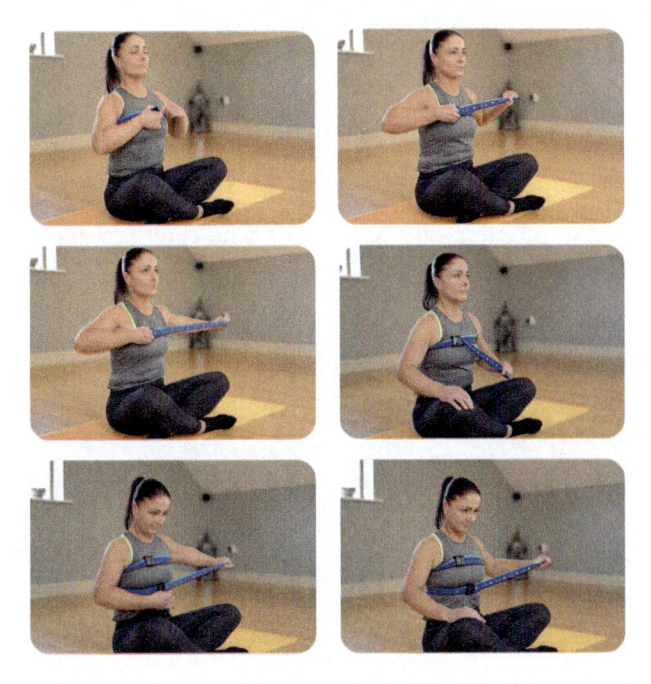

4. Lie down with your back on the floor, knees bent and feet on the floor
5. Inhale fully through your nose and then see if you can suck some more air in through your mouth. Think of the breath like a tornado – starting small at the bottom and then opening up as you suck more air in
6. Do your very best to 'break out of the bands' or burst the bands open by breathing fully into your ribcage
7. Repeat ten to twenty of these breaths, where you try to burst out of the bands
8. Stay lying down. Open the bands

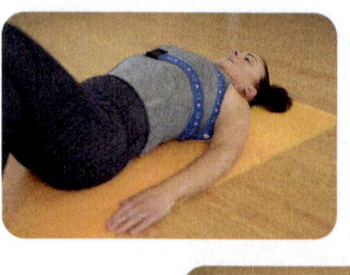

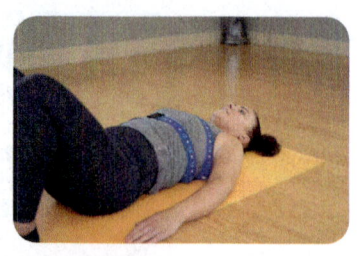

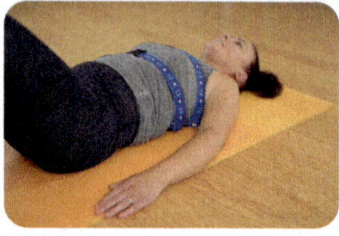

PART 3   THE INNATE-STRENGTH BREATH TRAINING PROGRAMME

After the technique, relax for a moment, and then breathe the breath of freedom a few times. Can you feel your rib cage move more?

> **PRO COACHING TIP**
>
> - Most times, the rib cage will move better after just one session. Sometimes, you need to give it more time. If you're in doubt about how much it is moving, then record your breath after the exercise and compare it to your original video of your breath at the beginning of the programme.

4:6 BREATHING

The 4:6 breathing technique is one of the most recognised and scientifically researched breathing patterns. The technique produces a six-breaths-per-minute breathing rhythm. This has been linked with improving heart rate variability, balancing the nervous system and synchronising the brain, heart and breath rhythms. It has positive effects on cardiovascular health, mental health, and overall well-being. You should be aware, however, that many breathing experts recommend you should be breathing at a rate of six breaths per minute throughout the day. This opinion is not supported by any research I can find, nor have I seen it proven in people I coach.

The reason I have brought this technique into the programme is to gradually decrease your breathing rhythm using numbers. By training your brain to comfortably breathe less, we end up breathing more efficiently. And because Westernised people aren't so familiar with feeling, but they love numbers, I have included it here. The ultimate aim is to reduce your breathing without the need for numbers; this is the breath-calming technique you'll see soon.

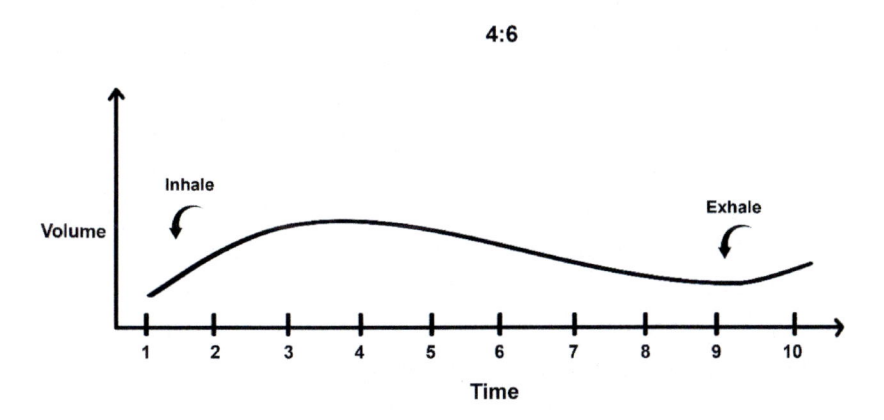

4:6

Technique

1. You can practise this technique any place you like to calm your breathing down. Within your training programme, please practise it seated.
2. Breathing with the nose only, inhale for four seconds
3. Exhale for 6 seconds
4. Repeat for a total of two minutes, or ten repetitions

After the technique, relax for a moment, and then breathe the breath of freedom a few times. Can you feel your rib cage move more?

PART 3   THE INNATE-STRENGTH BREATH TRAINING PROGRAMME

> **PRO COACHING TIPS**
> - Don't worry about breathing into your belly or chest with this one; just breathe.
> - 4:6 breathing for two minutes is great when you're stressed and need to think clearly or if your mind is racing and you're trying to sleep.

HUMMING BREATH

This is another great technique for slowing the breath down and calming the rhythm of your breathing, leading you to a gentle resting breath. The humming breath works a little differently from 4:6 breathing. By humming as you exhale, you naturally extend your exhale, stimulate the vagus nerve, and secrete up to fifteen times your natural nitric oxide level. The net gain of humming is a stimulation of your parasympathetic nervous system. Your body downregulates, gut function improves, lymph drainage flows better, blood circulates through the body more easily, and oxygen is delivered to your cells more effectively. For all these reasons, this is another great technique to employ throughout your day in addition to your training. For training purposes, I use it to prepare you for the breath-calming technique, similar to 4:6 breathing.

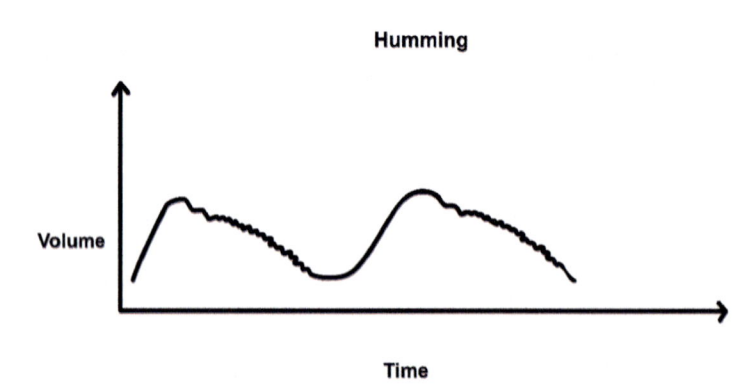

Humming

Volume vs. Time graph

Technique

1. Sit upright in a chair with feet placed firmly on the floor
2. Inhale fully through the nose
3. Keep the mouth closed, exhale and hum. Humming louder better stimulates the vagus nerve and delivers results quicker
4. Hum until your exhale is finished. There's no need to force out the exhale
5. Inhale and repeat for two minutes

After the technique, relax for a moment, and then breathe the breath of freedom a few times. Can you feel your rib cage move more?

> **PRO COACHING TIPS**
> - Although it works perfectly well, don't feel like you have to be sitting cross-legged and chanting 'om' like a yogi for this technique. Feel free to hum your favourite tune!
> - This is a great technique to use if you're constipated. Hum strongly for a few minutes and you'll soon get the urge to go.

BREATH CALMING

Breath calming originates from the Buteyko method. Dr. Buteyko found that breath counting techniques, like 4:6 breathing, were less effective at ingraining a natural calm and slow breath, so he created this technique. The technique was initially known as reduced breathing by relaxation and it is commonly known today as 'breathe light to breathe right' from *the Oxygen Advantage*. I renamed it because I felt the name breath calming was understood more easily by clients.

Breath calming is the king of all breathing techniques in my opinion. It is great for relaxation, recovery from sport, staying calm and attentive and for dealing with stress and fear. The goal of the technique is to minimise your breathing to create the feeling of air hunger whilst maintaining relaxation at the same time. Air hunger and relaxation are counter-intuitive sensations to your body. Air hunger on the one hand is your brain sensing a rise in carbon dioxide and communicating with you that it is more used to taking bigger breaths. Being able to relax into this feeling is an art which comes with practise.

By leaving breathing by numbers techniques (like 4:6) and using feeling alone to reduce your breathing, you are able to sense the rising signals of your brain and body more accurately and respond with relaxation more effectively. As you breathe less and relax into that feeling, your brain tends to listen to this technique better than 'breathing-by-numbers' or extended-exhale techniques. The result is that a slow, calm, and gentle breathing pattern is ingrained as a natural breathing pattern for the rest of your day.

Breath Calming

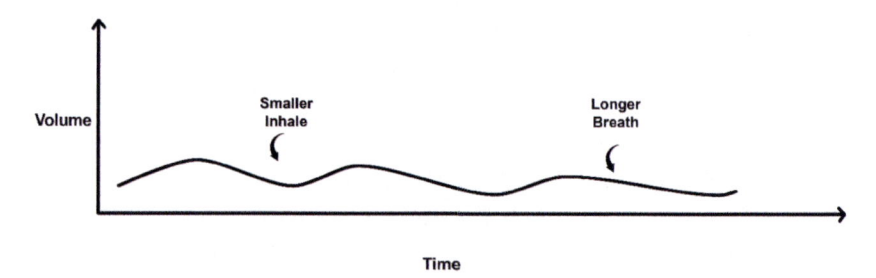

Technique

1. Find a comfortable environment with little distractions to practice this technique
2. Sit tall on a chair and adopt an upright posture
3. Tense your abdominal muscles and then relax them

PHASE 1 TRAINING DESIGN – BREATH MECHANICS

4. Focus your attention on the air flowing into the nose. Breathe in a little less air than normal by taking a smaller inhale
5. The primary goal is to feel air hunger while staying relaxed by slowly reducing the amount of air you take in. Once you have achieved an air shortage, move your attention to your hands
6. Relax your chest and stomach by placing one hand on your chest and one hand on your stomach. This provides great neural feedback to your system, calming it down even quicker
7. Let air flow naturally in and out of the stomach, like a balloon. You do not fill your body with air; rather you are trying to reduce your movement to as little as possible with relaxation
8. There is no need to mechanically exhale or force your exhale

PRO COACHING TIPS

Use different cues, mantras and images to slow your breath down. For example:

- Imagine yourself breathing just an inch deep (in other words take less air in than you would normally inhale).
- I breathe quietly. I breathe calmly. I breathe gently.
- Remember, it is said that the perfect breath breathes as if it does not breathe at all. You are so quiet your neighbour can't hear you breathe. You're so calm you can't hear yourself breathe, and your breath is so gentle that the fine hairs in your nostrils hardly even move as you breathe.
- Imagine your breath like a wave in the ocean. See your normal breath as a big forty-foot wave out in the middle of the Atlantic Ocean. It rises high into the sky, rolls over at the top, falls back into the ocean and then immediately swells again. Slowly reduce the size of your breath-wave until you can imagine your breath as a gentle wave, lapping upon the shore of the beach on a fine

summer's day. There's a gentle rise to wave. It crests over at the top and folds back in to the sea. Then it washes out on the shoreline. So too, does your breath rise gently in your tummy as you inhale through your nose. It flows into your exhale. Your exhale then gently falls out of your body and continues to fall long before the need for a new inhale arrives.

- Use your hands as visceral feedback. Place them on your tummy and chest to feel the body move with the breath, or place a finger under your nose to feel the air move in and out of your body.

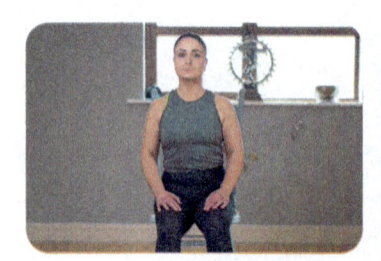

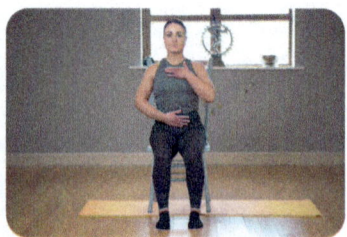

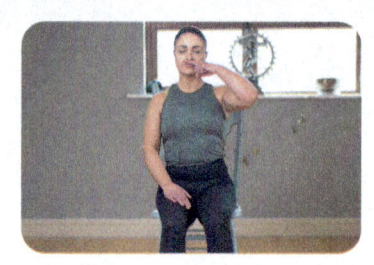

PHASE 2 TRAINING DESIGN – BREATH RESILIENCE

15

You have now moved into the core of the Innate-Strength Breath Training Programme. Remember, you can choose to train Phase 2 or 3 first, whichever you prefer. To help you decide which may be more appropriate for you right now, refer to Chapter 12: *Breath Training Considerations*.

Phase 2 is vitally important to restoring your naturally centred breath. This phase helps to ingrain a nice, smooth, relaxed subconscious breathing pattern as you go about your day and sleep through the night. Typically, this breathing pattern is fully restored by the end of this phase, once you've hit your goals, leaving only the deliberate breath to be trained in Phase 3.

PHASE II: BREATH RESILIENCE	
Purpose	Restore your naturally centred breath by improving CO_2 tolerance and your breathing rhythm

The goals of this phase are to:

1. Increase your tolerance level to CO_2
2. Ingrain a naturally centred breath

PART 3   THE INNATE-STRENGTH BREATH TRAINING PROGRAMME

The main assessment tools for Phase 2 are the BOLT score or the MES combined with your initial walking breath hold score. Here's a quick reminder of the scores and their meaning for your reference. If you want to review these scores more in-depth, review Chapter 13: *Personal Breathing Assessment*.

The BOLT score is a more traditional measure of your breathing rhythms and CO_2 sensitivity; however, due to the nature of the technique, it has some issues with reliability. The MES is a more recent way of measuring your breathing. It is very similar to the BOLT but it is a more objective measure of your breath. Trying both scores for the first week and then choosing the one you prefer. Your goal is to raise the BOLT Score beyond a forty-second breath hold with comfort or to raise the MES over ninety seconds.

The second measurement in this phase, then, is your initial walking breath hold score. Your goal is to score above an average of one hundred paces in this exercise for a full week. It's vitally important you don't just touch the one hundred mark but you continue training until your seven-days average is above one hundred paces.

SPECIFIC GOALS FOR PHASE II TRAINING	
BOLT Score	<40s
MES	<80s
Walking Breath Hold	Average of 100 paces for one week

Achievement of these goals is only attainable by consistent training, with a high frequency, over a period of time. Remember, the typical person has been breathing in an adapted state, heightened or lowered, for many years and even decades. Therefore, it's going to take some focus, time and patience to restore your breathing back to a naturally centred breath but, trust me, the benefits will be worth it. Each training session takes approximately ten to twenty minutes practise, and two pieces of trainings per day is an absolute minimum. Ideally, you need to train three sessions per day. You need to continue this training frequency until you've hit your goals.

PHASE II TRAINING DETAILS	
Time Allocated Per Session	10 – 20 mins
Frequency of Training Per Day	2 – 3 sessions
Length of Training Phase	Until scores are achieved (typically 12 weeks to 6 months)

There is only one training block in this phase, with two workouts and three exercises. The exercises in Phase 2 are synthesised from the Buteyko and Oxygen Advantage methods. Throughout the last ten years teaching these two methods, I have concluded that many other techniques found in the original methods distract people from their core goals: restoring your functional breathing patterns. The three exercises I've selected for this phase produce massively positive results for you every time and typically restore your breathing completely. This is a bold statement to make but it is true; however, it comes with some caveats. They are:

- You should free your breathing mechanics by training Phase 1 first
- You must stick to the plan for Phase 2 as it is laid out
- Your need to continually train with high frequency until your goals are reached in this phase

PHASE 2, BLOCK 3 LAYOUT

There are various choices to how you piece your own personal programme together in Phase 2 to make the training work for you in your life. The critical factor is that you train three times per day, and two of those sessions are Workout 5. Your final session can be a repeat of Workout 5, or it can be Workout 6.

PART 3   THE INNATE-STRENGTH BREATH TRAINING PROGRAMME

Workout Number	Number of Sessions / Day
Workout 5	2 - 3
Workout 6	0 - 1

Workout 5 is most important to me as a coach because you can control more of its variables and see continual progress every single week. If you hit a plateau or you're not achieving your goals, it is much easier to troubleshoot these exercises in this workout than any other techniques.

WORKOUT 5

Exercise Order	Exercise	Sets	Reps / Time	Recovery	Comments
A.	Breath Hold 1 - Walking	1	4 - 6	60s	Count your paces in every rep and record them
B.	Breath Calming	2	3 – 5 mins	60s	

Workout 6 is easier to fit into your lifestyle than Workout 5, so I included it in the programme. You're now stacking a breathing technique while you go for a walk, so you're getting the benefits of being outside, going for a walk and breath training all in one. If you choose to practice this exercise while you're out walking with a friend be careful not to speak with them in between your breath holds. Unfortunately, talking whilst practicing the technique will ruin your results; instead, save the chat until after your training. For more coaching tips on both techniques, be sure to read the exercise description for each technique.

PHASE 2 TRAINING DESIGN – BREATH RESILIENCE

WORKOUT 6

Exercise Order	Exercise	Sets	Reps / Time	Recovery	Comments
A.	Walking		10 mins	60s	Warm up
B.	Breath Hold 2 – On a walk, active recovery	1	12+	30 - 60s	
C.	Breath Calming	1 - 2	3 – 5 mins	60s	Practise this technique when you finish your walk

Remember to add the breath calming technique from Workout 4 at the end, no matter which workout you choose to practise. It's easy to practise at the end of Workout 5. If you are practising Workout 6, do the breath-calming technique when you get home from your walk if it makes it easier for you.

ADDITIONAL BREATHING HABITS AND ACTIVITIES FOR PHASE TWO

Breath training alone is not enough to ingrain a naturally centred breath. You also have to change your daily breathing habits and improve your lifestyle to make the training stick. During Phase 2, it is vitally important that you gradually improve both your daily breathing habits and your lifestyle to ensure success on the program and breathe free for life.

Breathing through your nose all day and all night is perhaps the greatest change you can make to your breath to benefit your health. It is more powerful than any one technique you'll practise. Why? Because it directly and positively affects each of the ~ 24,000 breaths you take each day.

PART 3   THE INNATE-STRENGTH BREATH TRAINING PROGRAMME

You should naturally own a quality breath pattern and use it effectively, without training. Unfortunately, your inputs, which are your daily activities done wrong, influence your breathing into an adapted state. Changing your activities of daily living and the way you breathe in them is the last piece of the jigsaw to restoring your breath in Phase 2. Learning what stress is and how to use it to benefit you is critical to your breathing and your health. Exercise, heat exposure, cold exposure, sleep, and nutrition are all core activities we need to improve to breathe free and live a happy, healthy life. The details of daily breathing habits are covered later (in Chapter 18) and your activities of daily living are explained in Chapter 19. A synopsis is displayed below.

Daily Breathing Habits	Complimentary Lifestyle Activities
Nose breathe all day	Stress Management
Nose breathe all night	Heat Training
Expressing the breath	Cold Exposure
Nose breathing during exercise	Sleep
	Nutrition

PHASE 2 – TECHNIQUES

There are only three exercises in Phase 2. Two of them are breath-hold exercises. The final one is the breath-calming exercise from Phase 1. Many people mix up the goals of the two breath-hold exercises. Let me be clear; although they have the same over-riding purpose – to improve carbon dioxide tolerance – the goals within these exercises are completely different. Please, watch out for the difference between them.

If you like the 4:6 breathing and/or the humming breath from Phase 1, feel free to incorporate those exercises into Phase 2 in addition to your programme. These are best completed between the walking breath-hold and the breath calming exercises, but they are not essential exercises.

PHASE 2 TRAINING DESIGN – BREATH RESILIENCE

BREATH HOLD 1 – WALKING WITH RECOVERY

Along with training your breathing mechanics to be supple and instilling a calm breathing rhythm, breath resilience is one of the key aspects to breathing free. Breath Hold 1 specifically improves CO_2 tolerance. The exercise is the exact same as the walking breath hold test you performed in your assessment. The difference is now you are turning it into an exercise that is repeated instead of a one-off test. This means you practise your maximum walking breath hold, then rest for sixty seconds and repeat.

The whole point of this exercise is that it is highly structured. The structure makes it easy for me as a coach and you as a trainee to review your improvements. It also gives us an opportunity to rapidly find the weaknesses in your practise. This analysis leads to a progression in the quality of your training and greater results delivered faster. Before you dive into the nuances of the technique, feel free to remind yourself of the benefits and reasons for training walking breath-holds by referring to the WBH test in Chapter 13.

SCAN ME

Walking Breath Hold

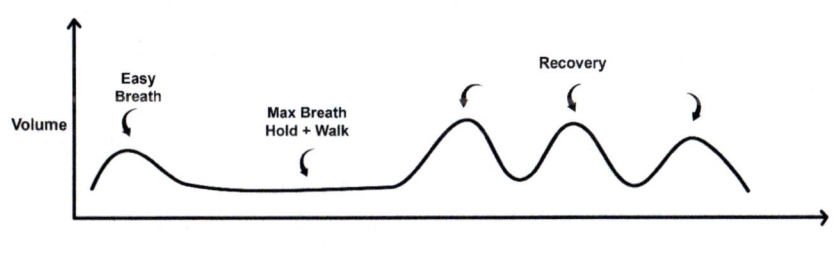

Volume — Easy Breath — Max Breath Hold + Walk — Recovery

Time

337

PART 3 THE INNATE-STRENGTH BREATH TRAINING PROGRAMME

Technique

1. Practise the Walking Breath Hold 1 in a safe environment, without any trip hazards. Particularly when you first start training the exercise, make sure there are minimal distractions in your environment so that you are able to concentrate on the exercise exclusively. This includes phones, laptops, and conversations, as well as social distractions in your immediate area
2. You will need a journal to record your scores daily and weekly
3. You will need a watch or phone, preferably with a timer. Set your timer for fifty seconds. This will be your rest period between sets
4. Standing upright and relaxed, take a small breath in through your nose and let it out of your nose gently
5. Pinch your nose after the exhale to prevent airflow. Keep your mouth closed
6. Walk as many steps as possible while pinching your nose and holding your breath
7. Count the number of paces as you walk

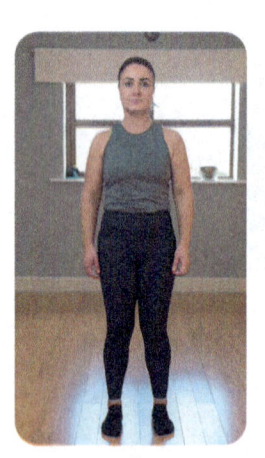

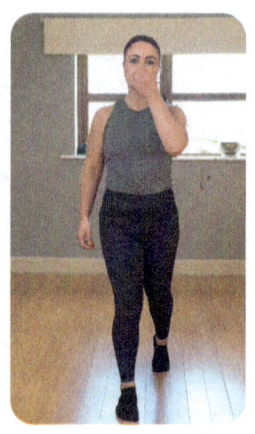

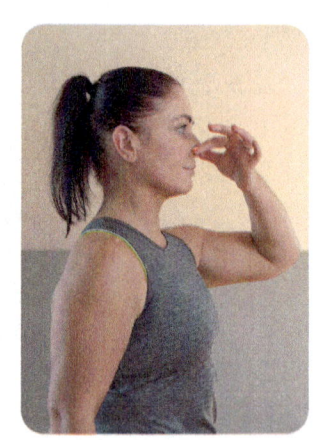

8. When you've walked your maximum distance, stop walking, let go of your nose, and inhale through your nose
9. The first three breaths after your breath hold will usually be quite large. Calm your breathing as quickly and gently as possible

PHASE 2 TRAINING DESIGN – BREATH RESILIENCE

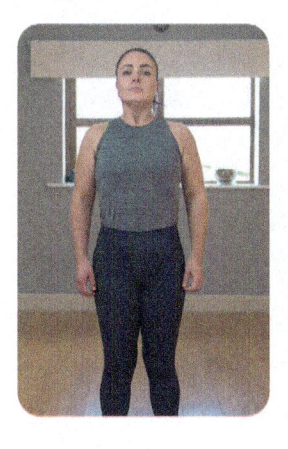

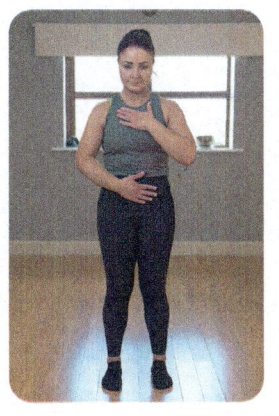

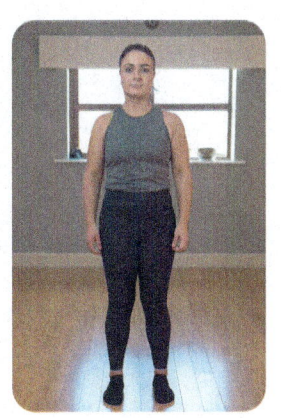

10. As soon as you release your nose, start the timer on your watch
11. Record the number of paces taken in your training journal
12. Once your timer expires, calmly take a breath or two and compose yourself for your next set
13. Compare your weekly average paces for progress. Your aim is an improvement of ten paces per week

PRO COACHING TIPS

- Relax during the exercise. The more relaxed you become, the further you can walk with your breath held, and your results will improve more quickly.
- The same advice goes for after the breath hold – relax. The more relaxed you are after you release the nose, the quicker normal breathing is recovered.
- Make sure you time your rest periods between your rounds of breath-holding. This has to be accurate. A difference of a ten second rest (more or less) will change the outcome of your next set.
- Preferably use a timer. A timer enables you to focus on relaxation during your rest period instead of worrying about starting the next set on time.

> - Only push yourself to 95% of your maximum ability. This is not an exact measure; give it a good shot but keep a little energy in reserve. If you continuously push yourself to your limit day after day, your brain will eventually override your ambitions and you will become demotivated. This is a hard tip to take for the athletes reading this book, but it is one of my best pieces of advice.

BREATH HOLD 2 – WALKING WITH ACTIVE RECOVERY

This exercise feels very different to Breath Hold 1 but it produces the same net effects when practiced correctly. In Breath Hold 1, you rested between sets, allowing CO_2 levels to decrease significantly; during Breath Hold 2 you continue walking – this generates some CO_2 in your body while still recovering. For this reason, you start with a sub-maximal breath-hold, and gradually build the length of your breath hold as your body gets used to the substantial rise in CO_2. The difference between breath hold 1 and 2 is a similar to high-intensity interval training with low-intensity intervals in strength and conditioning circles. The principles of fitness remain the same; the only real difference is that here we are exclusively working with the breath in this situation.

One of the benefits of this exercise over Exercise 1 is that the continuous walking in Breath Hold 2 enables you to practically integrate your breath training into your day more easily. For example, you can practise it during your commute to work to save time in your day, or you could do it during a walk and get the added benefits of walking with your breath training. However, keeping your concentration on this exercise is more difficult than Exercise 1 because you may be distracted by elements in your environment. This is why I only prescribe it in one of your breath training sessions out of three per day.

PHASE 2 TRAINING DESIGN – BREATH RESILIENCE

Walking Breath Hold with active recovery

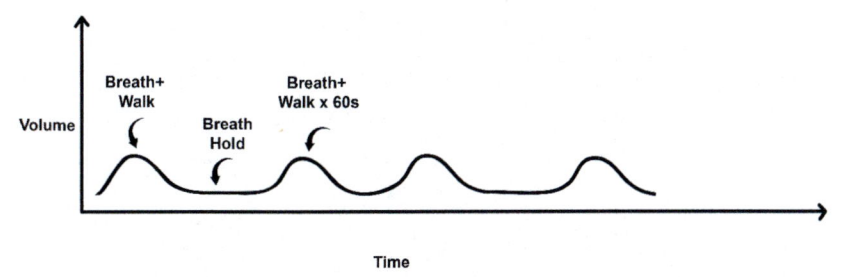

Technique

1. Walk for ten minutes with nasal-only breathing to generate a little CO_2 and warm up for the exercise
2. After the warm-up is finished, continue your walk
3. As you walk, practice twelve sub-maximal breath holds with the same technique as Breath Hold 1 (pinch the nose after the exhale and close your mouth)
4. Recover for sixty seconds between each breath hold. Continue walking in your recovery period
5. Practice three repetitions at the same level, then advance the number of paces by five steps
6. Practice maximum breath holds in your final three repetitions
7. When you're finished, continue your walk

Example: 15-15-15-20-20-20-25-25-25-max-max-max

PART 3 THE INNATE-STRENGTH BREATH TRAINING PROGRAMME

PRO COACHING TIPS

- There is no right or wrong number of paces to begin. It may take a few sessions to get a feel for your level. As a guide, start with fifteen paces if Breath Hold 1 was below thirty paces in your test. Start this exercise at twenty paces if Breath Hold 1 is between 30-50 paces. If Breath Hold 1 is more than fifty paces, begin here at thirty paces.

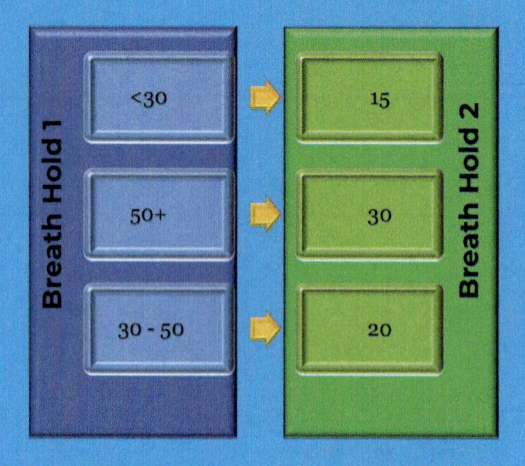

Breath Hold 1	Breath Hold 2
<30	15
50+	30
30 - 50	20

- Instead of using a timer for sixty seconds, you could use landmarks to indicate your rest period. I'll often use lamp-posts, trees, or blocks of houses to mark my rest periods
- Don't start with too many breath-hold-paces. The idea is to progress to maximum-breath-hold-paces so the first set of three breath holds will be relatively easy

Skill Development

There is no end to the layers you can add to this exercise. However, advancing this exercise comes at a cost in some cases. Breath-holding can produce many unwanted cleansing reactions. If you progress too fast, you will suffer unnecessarily along the way. The more advanced techniques add in traditional elements of fitness work. There are progressions to jogging, running, sprinting, adding weight, and/or reducing rest periods. These are the variables I use as a trainer when writing strength and conditioning programs. Now I customise all elements of training, including breathing, to produce the exact result I want for you. Honestly, there's no need to practice these techniques from a health perspective. They become most valuable if you're looking to optimise certain aspects of sporting performance. I hope to cover these techniques and their programming in a future sports performance breathing book. In the meantime, this programme is about building strong foundations for your breathing. The next phase is all about rhythmical breathing patterns.

PHASE 3 TRAINING DESIGN – BREATH RHYTHMS

16

Welcome to Phase 3 of the Innate-Strength Breath Training Programme. By this stage, you have optimised your breathing mechanics in Phase 1 and restored your naturally centred breath in Phase 2. It is possible that you skipped Phase 2 will return to it after this phase. That's ok; some people prefer the style of breathing techniques in Phase 3 over the techniques in Phase 2. Just remember, you need to train both phases to optimise your breath. See the questionnaire panel in Chapter 12: *Breath Training Programme Considerations* to help you decide which phase is better for you to do first.

The purpose of this phase is to experience the full expression of your breath through by varying its rhythms, combining it with your mind, and vocalising it. You may notice sensations arise in your body as you breathe the rhythms of your breath. The breathing and the sensations can lead to the emergence of emotions from your subconscious. Most people have a truly joyous experience in these breathing sessions. However, the true benefits of this phase are not the highs you can experience in the sessions themselves (although they are pretty cool) but the integration work of your breath, body, mind and spirit in the hours, days and weeks during this training phase. This phase leaves you feeling notably more energised and happier when the breathing sessions are integrated through journaling. To find out more about the integration, please re-visit the 'making sense of it all' section in Chapter 11, *Road Mapping Your Success*.

PHASE III: BREATHING RHYTHMS / BREATHWORK	
Purpose	Experience your breath alone and all of its rhythms
	Feel your body
	Allow emotions to emerge
	Integrate your breath and life

There are no set goals to achieve in Phase 3. Think of this phase as more like having a dance with your breath. The goal of dancing is not to get to the end of the dance but to enjoy it for what it is. Enjoy the music, the steps of the dance, and the movement of your body. In the same way, you want to enjoy the rhythms of your breath and the experience of your breathing sessions during Phase 3.

There is no need for an assessment in this phase of training as we don't have a specific goal for it. However, I would recommend that you retake the whole personal breathing assessment every week during this phase and especially at the end of it. I recommend you retake the assessments is because this training phase can dramatically change your BOLT, MES, and maximum walking breath hold scores. Your breathing mechanics may improve and your answers to your personalised breathing questionnaire will change.

I have seen a BOLT score jump more than ten seconds after just one training session in Phase 3. I have seen breathing mechanics completely restored and I have witnessed people have surreal experiences all during one of these sessions, let alone a whole phase of training. Equally, the negative impacts of this phase can be felt just as much by people. That is why you should read the preparation guide for this phase in the appendix; perform Phase 1 of the training first and only undertake this phase if you are ready to change your life. Have no doubt, this phase of training is very powerful, especially as you notice the shifts in your mind and begin to connect all of your life together with your breath.

> **PHASE III PRE-REQUISITES**
>
> Read the guide in the appendix to prepare you
>
> Perform breath training Phase 1 to ease you
>
> Clear your schedule to ready yourself mentally, spiritually, and emotionally for the journey

The training schedule is much less hectic in this phase; however, I do suggest you give more time per training session. I recommend that you perform any of the workouts one to seven times per week, depending on how you are feeling and how busy you are. Think of these sessions like a shot of vodka – some people just need one or two shots to get them drunk whilst others need a lot more. In the same vein, some people only need a breath session or two per week and others prefer to do it every day. Remember, the sessions themselves usually feel great (and there are scientific reasons for that) but it is the integration of the session where you will bring the most meaning to your life and peace to your body, mind, and spirit.

Set aside at least one hour for your breathing session. Clear the decks, set up a nice environment, get comfortable and give yourself time. Most techniques will only take about twenty minutes but it's important to leave time afterwards for meditation, journalling, and time to unwind. You will thank yourself for allowing the added time after just the first session!

PHASE III TRAINING DETAILS	
Time Allocated Per Session	60 mins
Frequency of Training / Week	1 – 7 Sessions
Length of Training Phase	One month

PHASE 3 LAYOUT

Phase 3 is structured a little differently to the other two phases. There are two primary techniques maintained throughout the month. However, the depth of the technique (how long you do it for and how fast) is expanded week on week. I also add more experiential parts to the session as the month goes on. I do this to gradually deepen your experience throughout the month. The same way as the climax of a movie is made all the more enjoyable when the build-up is tense, a breathing session is made better as you gradually explore and integrate your breath.

In week one I keep the number of rounds of breathing low: three to four rounds. Three to four rounds are the standard number for a beginner in the Wim Hof method, both in research and amongst its instructors. It's a powerful technique and I want you to enjoy every step of the experience. I also encourage you to build into the Wim Hof breathing by gradually opening the breathing levels. In round one, I encourage you to use only your nose to breathe. Inhale with the nose and exhale with the mouth in rounds two and three. Then in the final round, you could open up your breathing fully and use only the mouth to breathe. This progression from small to bigger breathing helps you to have a positive experience all round.

Phase III	Exercise	Progression
Workout 7	Progressive Wim Hof Breathing	3 – 4 Rounds + Meditation

Once you have some experience in the first week of Phase 3, I'm happy for you to take the training wheels off and open up your breathing yourself in week two. Feel free to breathe with your nose or mouth and extend your rounds to five or six, depending on how you're feeling. If the sensations become overwhelming for you, then pull back and start small again. Remember to check the guidelines for breathwork in the appendix for any further advice.

Phase III	Exercise	Progression
Workout 8	Wim Hof Breathing	5 – 6 Rounds + Meditation

During week three, I recommend you continually dive deeper into your breath by adding more rounds to the breathing. There is no set amount you should do; rather, do a minimum of six and then go by feel.

Phase III	Exercise	Progression
Workout 9	Wim Hof Breathing + Experience Enhancers	3 – 4 Rounds + Meditation

Adding additional components to your session can be a real game-changer in week three. The music, environment and people all have a key role to play in any breathing session. At this stage, I recommend you using some breathwork music in your sessions. You could also attend a breathwork session with a guide. There are a few breathwork sessions online, but I don't really recommend those ones because I feel you are missing out on being in a room of people. There really is no substitute for a live breathwork experience. It's similar to watching a football match on television compared to being in the stadium itself. Live breathwork sessions are so popular nowadays that you should be able to find one close to you. Check out my website www.innate-strength.com, to find any of the sessions I run. Read the next chapter (*Breathwork Magic*) to learn all about the experience enhancers for your own sessions.

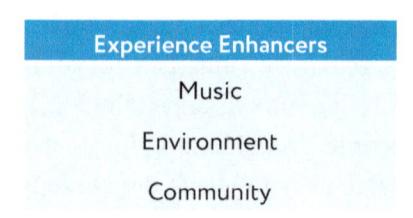

Experience Enhancers
Music
Environment
Community

The final week in Phase 3 involves the Ultimate Visualisation Process (UVP). This is a technique I have developed myself over years of practice and reading. It has four components to it. The process begins with Wim Hof breathing. As you breathe, you begin to think of things that make you feel great. Once you're feeling great, you then visualise an aspect of your future vividly. Finally, you relax and let go by meditating and enjoying the remainder of the session. Remember a key aspect of breath training is aligning your life – breath, body, mind and spirit. Only when you can accept your past, be happy in the present, and be excited for the future, is your breath truly at ease and health flows through you. I highly recommend trying it for yourself to see how powerful it can be.

Phase III	Exercise	Progression
Workout 10	The Ultimate Visualisation Process	> 6 Rounds + Visualisation + Meditation

BLOCK 3 TECHNIQUES

The foundation techniques in Phase 3 are Wim Hof breathing and meditation. Over the years, I've included a variety of other techniques in the programme, but gradually, I realised that Wim Hof breathing is the most well-rounded of all these techniques.

Wim Hof breathing has active circular breathing combined with breath-holding in each round. Some breathwork methods dislike the breath-holds but I think they bring a beautiful balance to the experience. The breathing activates your breath, body and brain while the breath-holding allows time for you to relax into the sensations that arise during the experience. In this sense, active breathing and holding your breath are the yin and yang of any breathwork technique. There is also great fun and variety in other breathwork techniques too. Double inhales, yawning and vocalising your breath can all be brought into your session. Some of these techniques happen naturally during your session – allow them to happen and flow with them if they occur naturally. Otherwise you can also learn specific techniques and bring them into your experience. Like the ocean, the breathwork world is vast and deep; if you want to dive deeper into it, try out the additional breathing techniques at the end of this chapter and visit Chapter 17: *The Magic of Breathwork* for some experience enhancers. Even better, attend a breathwork session with other people and a professional instructor.

The meditation aspect of the breathing session is quite simple. Lie down, focus your attention on your breath, relax, and enjoy the experience. Allow the mind to wander wherever it wants to go. Often people fall asleep during this meditation, and that's perfectly fine. The famous Buddhist monk Thich Nhat Hanh once famously said that sleep 'is the deepest form of meditation'. If you do manage to stay awake and your mind wanders, simply focus your attention on your breath as soon as you remember. When you feel like waking back up again or getting on with your day, slowly and gradually wake up. Progressively squeezing your muscles and slowly opening your eyes is a great way to come out of a breathing session.

Visualisation

Visualisation has been around in sports and business psychology for decades. The UVP is my process that I've tried and tested over the years to get the most out of my mind. I have also seen variations of it from various sources. The *Celestine Prophecy* book series has a similar process; Joe Dispenza, Tony Robbins, Abraham-Hicks and many sports psychologists all employ similar processes. The principle behind the UVP is to use your body (or breath in this case) to change the state of your mind. When you're in that altered state you evoke positive feelings through mental imagery. Finally, you create a vivid image of how you want your future to be. It's a fantastic technique for bringing creativity to problem-solving and for realising what you want to do with your life. The mind knows no difference between past, future, and present. It knows only now. From this perspective I hope you can see how powerful the UVP can be for you. In reality, the only way to find out is to try it out for yourself.

Coming out of your session

After you get up from any of your Phase 3 breathing sessions, take time to get back to life (that's why I recommended taking an hour per session). Go for a walk barefoot in nature, splash some cold water over your face, do some light movement, some journalling, or simply relax into your day. All of these activities are important throughout your week but some may be more important for you to do directly after your session.

PROGRESSIVE WIM HOF BREATHING

There are two types of basic breathing in the Wim Hof culture. There is the structured approach, which the instructors are taught and the Academy promotes; and there is Wim's completely unstructured approach. While I often use Wim's approach in a guided class, I highly recommend a structured approach when self-learning. This is the approach I'll be explaining here.

The official technique of Wim Hof breathing follows a very structured approach because this is the way of science. Scientific research demands structure, and that way, the researchers can tease out the mechanisms of the technique and its effects. The structures also enable official instructors to create safety for beginners and gradually increase the technique's potency. All in all, the structure is a good thing. Over time and with experience you can feel free to break from the structure and breathe as your body desires. I recommend beginners to practise the technique daily for a month before experimenting.

Beyond the official Wim Hof breathing technique, I place an additional regression into the exercise during the first week. The regression allows for three things to happen:

- Everybody tends to have a more enjoyable experience
- The regressions fit in line with the rest of your breath training
- It teaches you that more is not necessarily better, even with Wim Hof breathing
- From this perspective, I recommend breathing through your nose only during the first round. Use your nose to inhale and mouth to exhale for the second round. Finally, feel free to breathe only with your mouth during the last round or two.
- This regression is a gentler stimulus to the nervous system and your brain. By starting more gently, you change your brain gradually and you are more likely to enjoy the experience, rather than worrying about some unwanted emotional or physical reactions.

Technique

- Find a safe environment to practice the technique. Your bedroom is ideal. Minimise distractions from your environment; NB: never perform the technique before swimming under water or when driving heavy machinery like a car
- Practice the technique lying down or sitting tall and comfortably

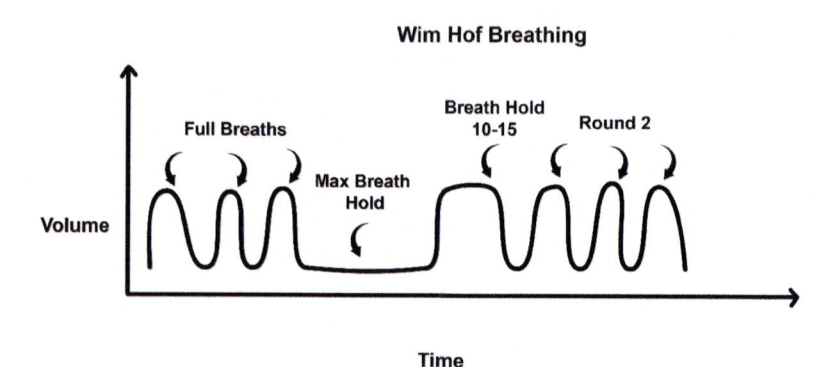

Wim Hof Breathing

Round one

1. Take 30-40 breaths in and out of the nose
2. Inhale deep and full breaths. Exhale and let go of the tension in your breath
3. At the end of your breathing, take one final breath
4. Exhale comfortably and hold your breath but don't pinch your nose
5. Relax into the breath hold. Hold for as long as you feel good
6. Take one breath in and hold your breath at the top of the inhale for 10-15 seconds
7. Exhale and start Round Two

Round two

1. Take 30-40 breaths in through the nose and out of the mouth
2. At the end of your breathing, take one final breath
3. Exhale comfortably and hold your breath by closing your throat
4. Relax into the breath hold. Hold for as long as you feel good
5. Take one breath in and hold your breath at the top of the inhale for 10-15 seconds
6. Exhale and start Round Three

Rounds three and four

1. Take 30-40 breaths in and out of the mouth
2. At the end of your breathing, take one final breath
3. Exhale comfortably and hold your breath by closing your throat
4. Relax into the breath hold. Hold for as long as you feel good
5. Take one breath in and hold your breath at the top of the inhale for 10-15 seconds
6. Exhale and start Round Four
7. Repeat the same for Round Four
8. After your breathing rounds, meditate

> **PRO COACHING TIP**
> - Remember, as long as it feels good, you're all good to continue. If you become overwhelmed by bodily sensations, reduce your breathing, calm down, and meditate.

MEDITATION

People generally think meditation is about getting rid of thoughts, but I have found that it is not quite that. Three years after I restored my breath, I asked a meditation teacher what it was all about. She told me that meditation was simply a conscious effort to create awareness of the present moment. She gave me examples of meditation techniques like looking at a picture, feeling the wind on my skin or focusing my attention on my breath. I had to laugh when she told me that last one. After I told her I had been practising breath training three times a day for three years, she laughed with me.

There are many ways to create awareness of the present moment. The breath is the most simple and universal approach to meditation. It is at the core of almost all meditation techniques. Your goal is not to change the shape or flow of your breath with meditation. Rather, you just need to observe the breath. Watch the air flow in and out of your body.

In the beginning, your attention drifts away from the breath. You may find yourself daydreaming, thinking of problems, or thinking thoughts of anything else. That is completely normal. You do not want to try stopping these thoughts. Redirecting them is the best option. When you catch yourself thinking about other things, congratulate yourself. You are now aware that you were not aware of the present moment. With this new awareness, return your attention to your breath. Watch it flow in and out of the body. Observe the nuances of it. Enjoy your breath. Once your time is up or you've become overwhelmingly frustrated by the process, stop and come back to it again after a break or the next day.

Technique

1. Practise meditation after a breathing technique or on its own
2. Make sure you are in a comfortable environment. You may want a pillow for your head and a blanket to make it a cosy experience
3. Technically, meditation can be practised sitting up but I prefer lying down as it reduces pains and distractions in the body. Lie down on your back, rest your legs out on the floor and relax
4. Focus your attention on the tip of your nose. Observe your breath being pulled into your body and then watch it flow back out effortlessly. You can keep your attention here or you can move through different aspects of the breath, noticing the belly and chest move with the breath wave. Pay attention to the temperature of the air. Become aware of other sensations in your body as you breathe
5. Stay relaxed; keep your attention on your breath. If it wanders, that is fine. Congratulate yourself for noticing your breath wandering and then return your focus to the tip of the nose again
6. Continue this process until you feel like you are finished, your timer is up or you become frustrated with the exercise. Ideally, you want to leave the exercise feeling good if you can

> **PRO COACHING TIP**
>
> - Set a timer for your session. That way you don't need to be worrying about getting lost in time or missing appointments during the day. If you need to stop before the timer is up, that is ok too. There is no 'winning' here; just practise.

ULTIMATE VISUALISATION PROCESS

Visualisation is known to help you create the life you want for yourself.

Improving your health, getting the job you want, buying the house of your dreams, or performing at your peak in sport when it counts, are things many of us want in life. We often set goals around them to help us achieve them. These goals are achieved more easily when you use visualisation techniques regularly. The point of a visualisation technique is twofold:

1. It helps you to achieve your goals by having you feel good about them right now
2. It helps you see your goal with great clarity

When you feel good about your goal and you can see the minute details of it, a part of your brain, called the reticular activation system, is alerted to seek the things you want throughout your daily life. With this full alignment, you'll find yourself achieving them as if they were inevitable. The process of visualisation involves taking time out of your day to specifically think about your goals and imagine achieving them as if they were already achieved.

In my ultimate visualisation process, I change how you feel first so that you feel great before you visualise your goal. Using breathwork and images from your past. you can profoundly change your state. This preparation creates a more powerful experience for your mind, helping you clarify your goal and envision it more clearly.

The Technique

1. Perform the technique in a safe and comfortable environment. Lie down on your back and make yourself as comfortable as possible. Your bed is an ideal place to perform the technique
2. Set a clear intention before you begin. Choose the goal you want to envision
3. Use Wim Hof Style breathing during the full session
4. After two rounds of Wim Hof breathing think of a memory that makes you feel really, really good (examples: wedding day, a beach you love to visit, a loved one, etc.)
5. Be specific with the memory – vividly imagine the memory

6. Feel the memory as if you're living it now
7. Focus on the feeling for a little while. Make the feeling very strong. If you need to tap into more memories to create a stronger good feeling then do so
8. Once you feel great, then switch your attention to your goal
9. Continue the breathing technique and picture your goal as if you are watching it take place right now in your mind
10. Once more, be specific and see your goal clearly. Tap into the feeling of living your goal right now
11. When you're finished envisioning your goal, finish the last round of your breathing technique, let go of the goal in your mind and sink into relaxation
12. Relax and allow the mind to wander for the rest of the session

SUPPLEMENTARY TECHNIQUES

In my research I have reviewed over one hundred and thirty techniques and distilled them into this 'phase' and 'block' training framework. The idea of the blocks of training is to focus your effort on improving certain aspects of your breathing system. Not all the techniques I have researched are included in this framework and there are probably countless other techniques out there that I don't even know about yet. However, from a breathing perspective, what I have found through the years is that newer techniques simply fit into one of these three categories: mechanics, resilience, and rhythm.

This means that there are techniques out there that may work better for you but I haven't included them in the programme. If you find other techniques and want to know how they fit into an overall plan, simply substitute them for similar ones in this framework, then use them accordingly.

EXAMPLE 1: Balloon breathing is a set of techniques I came across through my personal training work. In this technique you use a balloon as a feedback mechanism to feel how you breathe in different postures. I've seen them used by DNS, Paul Gagne, Art of Breath and excellent colleagues of mine like Scott Tate, Alex Nurse and Joel White. This is a fine supplement to training breathing mechanics. I find it much more applicable when I'm coaching movement and core stabilisation functions of breathing, as opposed to the foundations of breathing described here. There'll be more of those techniques in the follow-up book to this one.

EXAMPLE 2: The 4-7-8 breathing technique from Dr. Andrew Weil isn't included in this programme. It's a rhythmical technique and there is no progression to it to build CO_2 tolerance. It's a slow, 19-second breath or almost 3 BPM rhythm, so it is an advancement of the 4:6 or box breathing technique, with a base of four seconds.

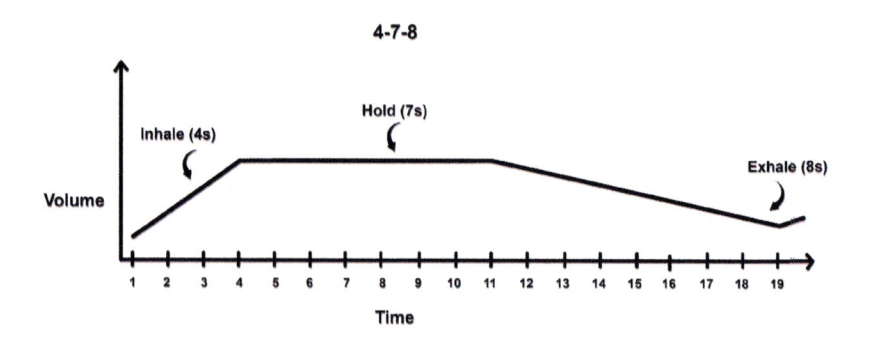

4-7-8

Inhale (4s), Hold (7s), Exhale (8s) — Volume vs Time

EXAMPLE 3: Using the free diving apnoea tables is an alternative way to train CO_2 tolerance. These are a supplement for the breath-holding technique in Phase 2.

EXAMPLE 4: I came across saw breathing in the *Knowles Breathing Method*. This is a 'cleansing breath' and fits into the rhythm category of breathing techniques. Here, the exhale sounds like you're sawing a piece of wood. You exhale sharply, inhale slightly, exhale sharply, inhale slightly, and repeat until your exhale is finished. You inhale and start again. It's great for dumping CO_2 and for the energiser techniques of the rhythm section.

Saw Breathing 1

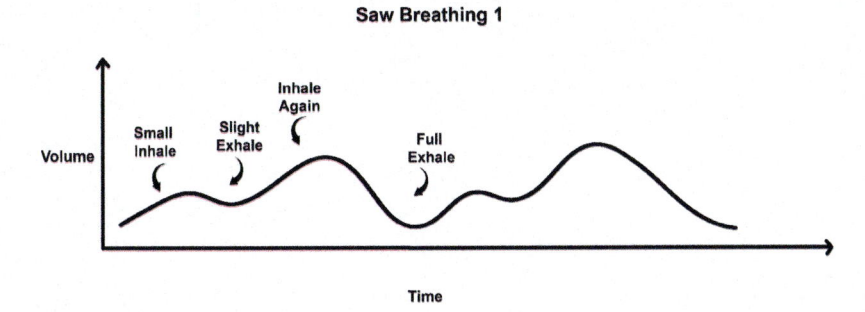

(Graph: Volume vs Time, showing Small Inhale, Slight Exhale, Inhale Again, Full Exhale)

EXAMPLE 5: Shamanic breathing is a staccato-type breath I first learnt from Dan Brulé. You can perform the staccato on the inhale, exhale, or both. On the inhale it sounds like the breath is going up a flight of stairs – small inhale, slight hold, small inhale, slight hold, small inhale.

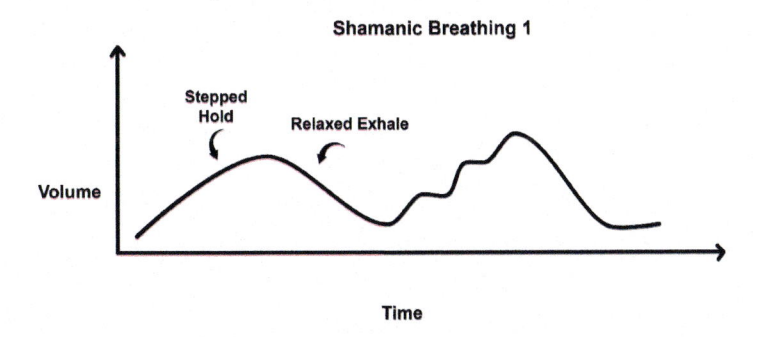

Shamanic Breathing 1

(Graph: Volume vs Time, showing Stepped Hold, Relaxed Exhale)

On the exhale you travel down the stairs. When done on the inhale it helps to increase the capacity of the lungs, on the exhale it dumps CO_2. Overall, it fits in with the energising – rhythm techniques like the Wim Hof or connected breathing.

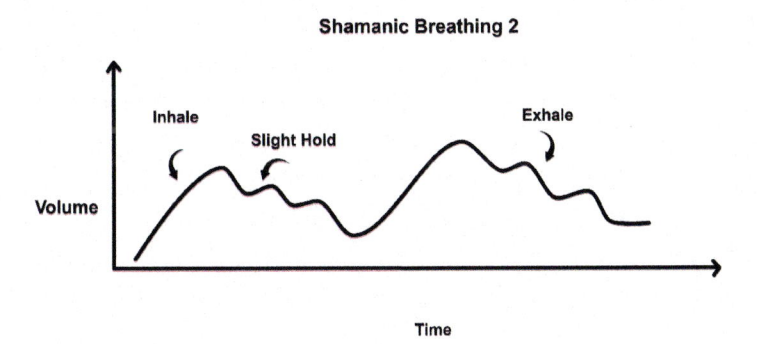

Shamanic Breathing 2

(Graph: Volume vs Time, showing Inhale, Slight Hold, Exhale)

THE MAGIC OF BREATHWORK

17

The breath knows how to go deeper than the mind

WIM HOF

Breathwork is a generic term floating around the internet to encompass all things breathing. Breathwork and breath training are not the same, necessarily. Dan Brulé described breathwork as a 'formula for personal transformation'. In his book, *Just Breathe,* he defined it as 'the use of breath awareness and conscious breathing for healing and growth, personal awakening and transformation in spirit, mind and body'. Brulé identified three basic skills to breathwork: awareness, relaxation, and breathing. By this definition, breathwork can be seen as a one-off breathing experience (a session, workshop, or retreat). Its purpose is to transform the whole person through breathing, awareness and relaxation. A successful session requires the person's experience to be integrated with the rest of their life; the person needs to make sense of what just happened in order to benefit fully from it. Breathwork is not the same as breath training, in my opinion. It is more about connecting deeply with yourself, other people, and nature than about restoring the physical breathing system. In that sense, I use breathwork sessions to connect people with the deeper aspects of themselves and bring themselves into alignment in spirit, mind, body, community, and nature. Breathwork alone may not restore the breathing system fully. It is more of a catalyst for connecting with the spirit and bringing the body and mind into alignment. To return your breathing to its natural centre, you need to make sense of the session (integrate it) and combine it with the rest of the breath training.

Phase 3 in the training programme contains the foundation of all breathwork techniques – Wim Hof breathing. The method is broken into two techniques: connected breathing and breath-holding. These two parts are the primary techniques in all breathwork methods. Think of them like the primary colours in a colour palette. Exploring variations of these techniques creates a whole spectrum of colours which you can use to create your art and enjoy your session. Breathwork is not just about the breathing technique itself, it's also about everything that goes into the session. It is said you can never stand in the same river twice. Well, it's the same for a breathwork session. You will never have the exact same breathwork session twice because the conditions to create that point in time never appear identically. The seven factors that influence a session are:

1. The chosen technique(s)
2. The session length
3. Your state of mind
4. The facilitator's intentions (if they have one)
5. The environment – the room or space itself together with other sensory stimuli
6. The other people in the room
7. The music – track choice and acoustics

To begin, I recommend you keep things simple. A nice warm room and a comfortable space like your own bed, combined with a single speaker playing a pre-chosen track list at a moderate-high volume. If you're looking to create a very powerful experience you simply combine more – and more powerful – stimuli. However, I recommend you go to an experienced and qualified breathing facilitator for a few sessions before playing with these more potent stimuli, as the experience can be overwhelming for some people. To get you started with your own breathwork, I've included a few tips on creating a more potent and stimulating breathing session.

SENSORY STIMULATION

All of this breath work in Phase 3 is performed with eyes closed to enable you to travel into your mind and spirit more easily. Providing other stimuli can either enhance the experience or detract from it and so it is important to control the other elements first and then strategically introduce more elements into your sessions. The stimuli I've found that carry the most potency include:

- Performing a session with other people
- Altering the rhythm and volume of the music
- Introducing live music into your sessions
- Introducing light stimuli throughout the session
- Performing the techniques in a heated space

MUSIC

All rhythms or beats entrain the body and mind into synchronicity. Some of the most primordial beats are the beats of a drum, clapping hands, stamping feet, chanting, singing and the rhythm of our breath. Once we feel that rhythm, we become part of it and we join as one with ourselves, our community, and the beat. This is the power of music in breathwork. Music and breathwork go hand in hand. Together with breathing, the music helps us entrain to states of consciousness which help us discover more about ourselves. There are three types of music that work particularly well with breathwork:

1. Heavy beats
2. Journeying beats
3. Calming tunes

Typically, the music is arranged in order one, two, three. This order entrains the breath from our noisy, busy world into the quietness of the mind most efficiently. If you want to explore your own mind, none of the music you choose should have lyrics you comprehend in them – they should not influence you. If you'd rather perform contemplation or a visualisation, you can choose songs with lyrics, but be very careful that all of the lyrics complement the purpose of the session.

SETTING AN INTENTION

Breathwork sessions in Phase 3 can be performed with intentions or without. An intention is a purpose and a focus for what you are seeking in your session. Relaxation, love and peace are some words people use to help them drop into a more relaxed state. Deeper intentions may be focusing on what you want to do with your life or who you are in your essence. If you know what it is you want, then by all means set an intention before the session. The intention should be very specific to what you want to know.

While we speak about intentions, it is important to know two things. The first is that your mind talks in images, not words. Words help to find the image you're after but it's the image that evokes feeling in you. This is why dreams can seem so bizarre. Images you see, people you meet in your mind or circumstances you encounter are your mind's way of giving you information. The only caveat is that the meaning is very rarely literal; rather, it is figurative. And so you need to ask yourself questions like: What does that image mean to me? What does that person represent in my life?

The second thing to know with intentions is that you may receive part of an answer. The rest of the answer comes in your dreams and in your waking life over the coming days and weeks. Awareness of synchronicities, feelings and things out of the ordinary in the lead-up to your session, during your session and afterwards all become part of the process of unravelling your intention. The best way to understand these phenomena is to journal and create art daily for four to six weeks.

Sometimes it is best not to set an intention. Just let it happen. Allow your breath to give you what you need without trying to control everything. As long as you integrate the process, your body will guide you in understanding your life as it presents here and how.

BREATH MASTERY

In Phase 3, there is no right or wrong way to breathe. As Wim Hof says, 'Just breathe'. This form of breathwork is more like art than following a structured format. All of the methods I use in this phase can bring you to a similar space in your mind. Holotropic breathwork uses just the circular breathing; Wim Hof likes to add in breath-holding, and Dan Brulé mixes in yawning and staccato breathing patterns. The connected circular breathing is the foundation to get you started, and once you're going, you can use your breath almost any way you like to create your own art and dive into different aspects of your mind. Once you get a handle on the Phase 3 techniques I've listed, feel free to explore other similar methods or create your own forms.

No matter which technique you choose, you will find that there comes a point in time when the breath takes over. Allow this to happen, go with the flow of the breath, and move your body if it desires to move. Have fun with it all.

COMMUNITY

With art and journaling, community is another highly under-rated yet vital aspect of breathwork. It is so important that you have people you can open up to about your experience and share it with them so that you can gain insights into your experience and begin to understand it for integration into your life. The role of the community is not to offer its insights or to give you advice; it is simply to be there for you. This support helps you to have a safe session and to make sense of what is happening for you. The shared experience of breathing together with other people creates a very tight bond for everyone. It truly is magical to behold.

BREATHING FACILITATORS

The breathing facilitator is the person who leads your session. For people new to this form of training, it is important to find a qualified and experienced guide for your first few sessions. Breathwork, as I've said, can unravel emotions and unlock parts of your memory you never knew existed. Having someone there to guide you through this experience is very important for your mental and physical health, so you can make sense of your experience and integrate it back into your life.

There are so many great breathing facilitators out there nowadays from various different methods. No one guide or method is the best; it is simply a question of who is the best for you. You need to do your research first. Find out if they have what you need by means of support and guidance in their sessions. Then, go with your gut feeling about the person. Your intuition is always right.

COMPLIMENTARY BREATHING AND LIFESTYLE HABITS 18

As a human, you were created to be able to walk barefoot, run for miles, swim seas, lakes and rivers, jump from heights, sleep soundly, perform demanding labour/exercise regularly, overheat in the summer, get cold in the winter, nourish yourself with good food, and go hungry now and then. As a spiritual being, you yearn to talk to others, listen to music, gather in groups, celebrate life, mourn death, create with your talents, and live a life with purpose. If you lived in harmony with your biological system, your communities, and Mother Nature, there would be no need for breath training. By default, your lifestyle would cultivate your natural centre. From this perspective, there are only three needs for breath training:

1. You live a life removed from your innate biology which results in a perceived centre and adapted breathing patterns
2. You suffered a trauma in the past which you haven't processed fully
3. You want to use your breath for performance in some field of life

Ingraining lifestyle components – in alignment with your natural biology – is an absolute requirement to restoring your breath fully. Nowadays, breath training may have become the most critical piece of the jigsaw; but that is only because we have strayed so far from our natural lifestyle. Breath training is insufficient on its own to restore your natural centre. To restore your breath, be healthy and feel fully alive, you need to include other elements of our natural lifestyle which we have stripped from ourselves, unknowingly, in modern times. Some lifestyle habits are compulsory for everybody to include in their lives, like nose breathing at rest, exercising hard, sleeping soundly, and exposing yourself to varying temperatures. It is beyond the scope of this book to delve deeply into the details of lifestyle, but just know that it is highly recommended to try as many as you can over time. The ones that are most useful to you will show up in your life.

DAILY BREATHING HABITS

It is vital to the health of your body that you breathe through your nose at rest and during low-level activities – always. The role of mouth breathing is to alleviate stress, express emotion, communicate, or use a mouth breathing technique for a specific purpose. Your body loves nose breathing for so many reasons. The biggest and best reason why it loves nose breathing so much is because:

NOSE BREATHING IS THE NATURAL WAY TO BREATHE AT REST

Here are just some of the benefits you'll feel when you nose breathe all day and all night:

- ✓ Nose breathing has more filters for air than Instagram has for pictures
- ✓ Nose breathing generates nitric oxide to relieve blood pressure
- ✓ Nose breathing de-stresses you quicker than meditation
- ✓ Nose breathing is a monitor for endurance capacity in sport better than any fitness wearable, HRV or heart rate monitor

PART 3   THE INNATE-STRENGTH BREATH TRAINING PROGRAMME

Essentially, the nose's job is to prepare the air for the body to use easily. It warms and filters the air, dilating the smooth muscles of the arteries and airways to allow more air to be transported to the cells of the body.

Nose breathing is 50% harder to do initially but it increases oxygen in your cells by up to 20%!

Switching from mouth to nose breathing can be a pretty hard cycle to break. Some people give up after a day or two because they find nose breathing tougher to do than mouth breathing. People feel like they're struggling to get air into their system and, in a way, that is what's happening. But that's what is supposed to happen; it's just a matter of getting a feel for breathing less air until your body adapts to its new breathing pattern.

Think of it the same as wanting to lose weight

To lose weight, you need to reduce your calories and eat mindfully (i.e. chew your food). It's the same with optimising your respiratory system – you need to breathe less and prepare the air better for your body. You need to nose breathe.

When you initially switch to nasal breathing and begin to incorporate some breath training exercises, you will notice that you will yawn, sigh, and cough more. This is a good sign. It means that you have created the need to breathe, that you have a higher than usual CO_2 level in your system, and your body is looking to return itself to normal.

But beware: normal for your body is not necessarily healthy!

So suppress the urge to take a big breath or even breathe through the mouth in an effort to reset your CO_2 tolerance level and return your body to a healthy state. Once your respiratory system is healthy, yawning, sighing, and all those wonderful relaxation reflexes become important to do once more.

These benefits sound great, but have you ever tried to nose breathe all day? It takes some time to train. In conjunction with your breath training exercises, you should also cultivate an awareness of nose breathing during the day, exercising with nose-only breathing and nose breathing at night too.

NOSE BREATHING DURING THE DAY

Becoming aware of your breath during the day is one of the most potent tools you can have in your wellbeing toolbox. Everyone from yogi masters to Olympic coaches recommends breath awareness. The simple next step to this process is to switch to nose breathing once you are aware you are mouth breathing.

Switching to nose breathing at every opportunity will double down on the physical and mental benefits of becoming aware of your breath. Just remember to go easy on yourself. Some people tend to be hard on themselves when they catch themselves mouth breathing initially. Don't fall into this trap. Make a game of it, and stay light about it. Every time you catch yourself mouth breathing, give yourself a pat on the back – say well done for catching it, and now return to nasal breathing again.

NOSE BREATHING AT NIGHT

Ingraining the nasal breathing pattern at night is critical for your health and overall success in this programme. Night-time nose breathing is associated with a decrease in sleep-disordered breathing, sleep apnoea, and it helps you to have a deep, restful night's sleep. The benefits of a deep rest are beyond the scope of this book, but let's just say without it, you will not be healthy.

Correcting breathing at night is one of the first habits I address when coaching sleep habits to people. In order to entrain a nose breathing pattern at night, you need three main factors in place.

The first is that your day-time lifestyle is set up well – you rise, breathe well throughout the day, get outdoors into nature, exercise daily, and eat well. All the good stuff you know to do for health in general. The second and more specific habit you need to address is your sleep posture. The final habit you may need to instil is helping the mouth to remain closed with tape.

BED-TIME POSTURE

Ensure you have a firm pillow that fits your body. If your pillow is too small or soft, your head posture will lead to mouth breathing. If in doubt, use two pillows.

Secondly, sleeping on your back tends to lead to mouth breathing at night due to gravity. Encourage better sleep posture by placing another pillow or foam roller behind your back and lying on your side.

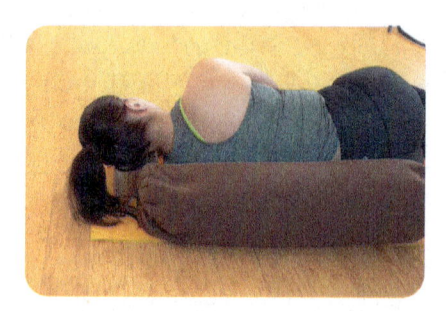

If you do have to sleep on your back, place a pillow under your knees to improve your posture and support your breathing.

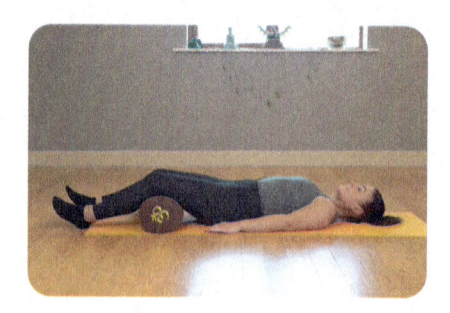

TAPING YOUR MOUTH AT NIGHT

It's the more controversial option for sure, but its safety and effectiveness are superb. It's been used since the 1970s in breathing methods, orthodontics, sleep clinics and myofunctional therapy clinics for enhanced breathing mechanics and better sleep. If you're a mouth breather at night, you'll notice the difference in your mood and energy with just one night of mouth taping. Here's a basic process for mouth taping at night:

- Buy some 3 m Micropore paper tape from your local pharmacy
- Tear off a 4' to 6' strip
- Fold over a tab on one end
- Stick the tape horizontally across your lips
- When you wake in the morning, pull the tab, and the tape will come straight off

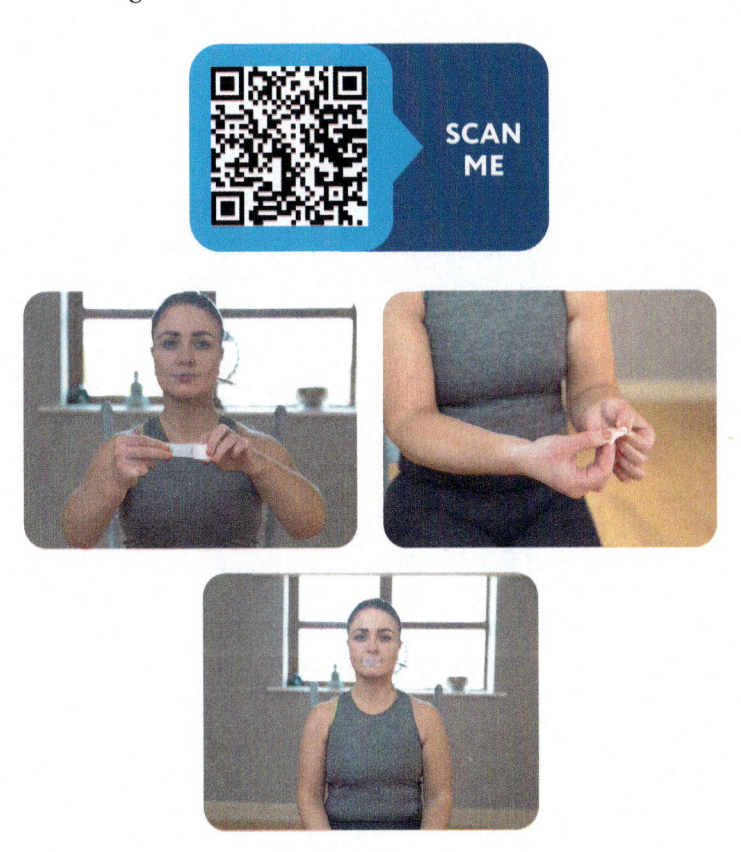

If you're anxious at all, start by taping up during the day to get you comfortable with the idea. You can also buy the 1.25 cm thickness tape and stick it vertically across your lips. This still keeps the mouth closed, but allows some wiggle room to mouth breathe if you really feel the need.

> *Please only tape yourself! Never tape up children, the infirm, people under the influence of alcohol or drugs or people who don't want to tape up*

An alternative to paper tape came on the market in 2020. One of my teachers, Patrick McKeown, produced an excellent product called 'Myotape'. The tape is placed around the mouth on a stretch. The stretched material closes your lips together when you relax, but if you feel the need to consciously open your mouth, you can. It's a fantastic product to use with children and adults alike.

Finally, please be aware that mouth taping is not the ultimate goal of breathing at night; rather, it is a means to an end. You tape your mouth to improve your sleep as you train your breathing during the day. You should no longer require the tape once you have ingrained your natural centre. At this point, feel free to remove it. You will only need to return to mouth taping if your life becomes hectic and your breathing adapts once more. Then you may tape temporarily as you improve your lifestyle again. Typically, this process takes three to six months.

EXPRESSING THE BREATH

Vocal communication is another vital function of breathing. Most people know this but not many realise the importance of it. Whispering, humming, talking, singing, shouting and roaring are expressions of the breath. Breathing is the foundation of communication. As air is exhaled out of the body, it passes through the vocal cords in the throat. The air is spun and vibrated through the cords to produce vibrations and sound. The nasal passages, tongue, and the shape of the mouth provide tone and texture to the breath to finish off the sound being expressed. Most people, even singers, think of sound coming from the voice box alone, and forgetting the impact of quality breathing patterns on sound. Developing the foundations of a quality breath, then, is extremely important in the production of quality sound and communicating effectively. Equally important to your breath and health is the expression of your emotions. Joy, love, happiness, anger, resentment, fear, guilt, rage and sadness are emotions that you need to let go of and possibly communicate to others. Having quality breathing patterns and performing breathwork helps to free you of the personal, familial, social, and societal norms, which result in emotions being locked inside us and the breath becoming adapted.

BREATHING WHEN TALKING

Inhale through the nose and speak through the mouth. When inhaling, breathe into the lower ribs and flare them out to the side. Slow down the breath, speak fewer words per breath, pause after each sentence, and enjoy the conversation. Learning to animate your breath through voice training is an excellent complement to breath training and will really enhance your breathing practise's benefits.

COUGHING AND SNEEZING

Both coughing and sneezing are innate autonomic reactions of your body to an irritant. Dust particles, respiratory infections, and food particles can all cause one of these reactions to occur. Both reactions are a strong eccentric contraction of the diaphragm, designed to expel the particle or move the infection immediately. If your body continues to signal the reaction, you can end up in a fit of coughing or sneezing, impacting your long-term CO_2 tolerance and overall breathing pattern. The key to stopping an attack naturally and clearing the particles from your respiratory system is to cough and sneeze through your nose!

Yes, I said that right; cough and sneeze through your nose. By doing this, you'll not only clear your lung of irritating particles, but you'll clear your whole upper respiratory system too. Remember, all of that disgusting foreign pollution will be bound up in some lovely mucus, so make sure to have a tissue handy to catch it all.

Rest assured, coughing and sneezing through your nose will reduce and even eliminate all extended reactions, clear your system, and maintain healthy breathing habits.

CLEARING A RESPIRATORY INFECTION

Movement of your lungs is really important for clearing primary viral infections and preventing bacterial infections. However, you can't exactly run or lift weights when you have an infection because your immune system is too compromised. You can add heat, rest, quality nutrition, supplementation, and some light breathing exercises to your repertoire. Over the years, I have found hot baths combined with traditional essential oil therapy to be the most effective treatment for a respiratory infection. It forms the foundation of my recovery protocol.

The hot bath part is easy. Simply draw a bath twice daily and soak for up to 20 minutes. Add Epsom salts, candlelight and some music to really enhance the experience, and calm the body and mind. This part of the protocol aims to place the body in a resting and recovering state to enable your immune system to do its best work fast.

Essential oil therapy is an old-school practice I used to do as a kid before drugs and inhalers were common. I was inspired to restart this practice quite recently and found it extremely helpful in shifting infections and speeding up my recovery. I have added some very useful breathing tips to the old-school practice to enhance the whole experience.

For the essential oil therapy, I'll take a bowl of steaming water and add a few drops of eucalyptus and menthol essential oils to the steaming water. Next, I dip my head over the bowl and cover both my head and the bowl with a towel. Then I sit and breathe in the fragrant steam. Smelling the steaming essential oils is a great way to open up the lungs and move an infection. In the early minutes of the treatment, your body will react vigorously and cough profusely. Stick with it though. Eventually, you'll cough up the parts of the infection in phlegm. This clears out your lungs of the infection and enhances gas diffusion into and out of the body. The result is that you breathe and feel much better. Once the coughing has subsided, I'll always finish the treatment with reduced breathing patterns, like the breath-calming technique from Workout 4. I usually do this treatment for 10-20 minutes, three times a day until the infection is cleared, and I feel able to start some walking breath-hold training.

EXPRESSING EMOTION

Positive and negative emotions need to be expressed regularly. I understand that it might not always be acceptable to tell others what you're feeling at a given time, but you must express those emotions at some stage during the day nonetheless. Breathwork, sport, ice baths, loved ones, close friends, and nature are brilliant practices, supports and environments to help you express emotion healthily. These are widely accepted places in society for you to safely express your emotions in a healthy manner. Your breathing will return to its natural centre as you express those emotions. A more complete list of society-accepted places to balance emotions is listed on the next page:

PART 3 THE INNATE-STRENGTH BREATH TRAINING PROGRAMME

	BALANCING EMOTIONS	
	Negative Emotions	**Positive Emotions**
Emotion	Fear Guilt Shame Rage Anger Resentment Frustration	Love Joy Happiness Appreciation
Lifestyle solutions to balance the emotions	Judo BJJ Combat & aggressive sports (e.g. Rugby) Ice baths and cold water swimming Talking with loved ones and friends Connecting with animals talk therapy Journalling	Nature walks Being creative in your work Talking to people Being of service to people Connecting with animals Making people laugh Supporting others

BREATHING DURING EXERCISE

Many people ask me how they should breathe during exercise. Is it through the nose, the mouth or does it matter? Let me answer quickly and then explain myself. If you are interested in getting the most out of your body, whether for a power sport, an endurance sport or anything in between, then, yes, learning to breathe effectively in your exercise matters. Through the last five years of research and coaching, I have realised that there are many more nuances to performance breathing than nasal breathing alone. If you want to learn more deeply about breathing in training and sports performance, then you're going to have to wait for my next book, I'm afraid.

For the time being, it is important to understand that, regardless of the nature of your exercise, nasal breathing is the foundation of all breathing patterns. You must learn to ingrain a foundation level of nasal breathing into your system if you want to make the most of your breathing system to benefit your exercise.

Allow your breathing to be your guide to stop exercising. This will help you build up your own internal compass for the energy systems you use while training and your fatigue factor. Better than any fitness-wearable technology, your breath guides you to your training capacity when you get used to breathing through your nose whilst exercising.

When you need to open your mouth for any reason during exercise, stop exercising. Recover your breath and go again when you're ready. After that, there are many multiple layers to breathing when discussing sports and physical performance.

For athletes in power sports, like weightlifting or strongman events, be mindful, stick with your normal breathing patterns during your training and competition. Your diaphragm and breathing system provide the basis of strength for your entire lift. If you alter your breathing patterns during your lift, you will increase the risk of an injury until you have properly developed the skill.

When you are warming up for exercise, it is a great idea to layer up your clothing (especially in cold climates) and perform four to six repetitions of a strong breath hold at the beginning of the warmup. This will prepare your cardio and respiratory systems excellently for the work that is to follow, and it reduces the need for a second wind, and improving endurance too.

HEAT EXPOSURE TRAINING

Next to breathing, heat regulation is one of the most under-rated modes of training in physical preparation today. Maintaining core and peripheral temperature are fundamental processes in your body. When you train temperature regulation specifically, you will reap many rewards in your breath training and in your health, these include:

- ✓ More efficient breathing system
- ✓ Better CO_2 tolerance
- ✓ Promotion of a more relaxed body and mind
- ✓ Sleep more soundly
- ✓ Improved immune function
- ✓ Stronger cardiovascular system
- ✓ More supple joints and injury prevention
- ✓ Reduce pain
- ✓ Feel better
- ✓ Reduced warm-up time for sport
- ✓ Better endurance levels

Temperature training is also known as exposure training. This is because you are exposing your body to a different temperature than it is used to, be it a hot stimulus or a cold one. The net result of exposure training is an adaption process from your body. In other words, it gets used to the contrasting environments and responds accordingly. Much like all forms of training, exposure training has many purposes and layers. When you include this training mode in your programme, you will reap all of the benefits I listed above. I suggest you train heat exposure concurrently with Phases 1 and 2 of the breath training programme.

HOW TO TRAIN GRADUAL HEAT EXPOSURE

Showers

- Start with taking two hot showers daily. Start with at least a two-minute shower and then build it from there to as long as you like. Make the showers as hot as possible. Finish with a cool shower for 30 seconds if you are feeling mentally up to the challenge! Trust me, it's worth it, you'll feel amazing getting out. Just remember – nose breathing only and calm your breathing as quickly as possible!

- After a week of twice daily hot showers, start taking Contrast Showers, where you alternate hot and cold temperatures. Try three minutes hot and thirty seconds cold, then repeat two to four times. Maintain contrast showers throughout the programme or advance to cold showers if you dare!

Baths and Saunas

- Rather than two-a-day showers, you can make the stimulus more potent by including a hot bath or sauna.
- If you're taking a hot bath, include one to three cups of Epsom salts to further enhance the benefits of the exposure training.
- *Stay in the bath/sauna as long as you can nose breathe only*! If you need to mouth breathe, then your body is under too much heat stress and you need to get out. That may mean you only last a minute or two initially and that's ok. Try and set the temperature so you can stay in for at least ten minutes.

Two Hot showers per day

or

One hot shower and one hot Epsom salt bath/sauna per day

COLD EXPOSURE TRAINING

The exact opposite of heat training is cold exposure training [CET]. Heat training is more foundational than cold training, and it gives your body a helping hand to relax after many years of being stuck in a stressed state. CET, on the other hand, shocks your system into a relaxed state. CET is a stressor but when it's used wisely, it can be extremely therapeutic and even enjoyable. In science, they call it a hormetic effect; in strength training they call it the principles of overload and adaption, but for us, it simply means we gain a myriad of direct and indirect benefits to our breathing system and health when done well.

- ✓ More efficient breathing system
- ✓ Promote a more relaxed body and mind
- ✓ Sleep more soundly
- ✓ Lowers inflammation throughout the body
- ✓ Stronger cardiovascular system
- ✓ Improved immune function
- ✓ More resilience to stress
- ✓ Enhanced recovery from exercise and sports training
- ✓ Feel better

To do cold training well and for it to benefit you, we need to establish some breathing and immune system criteria first.

- Never perform supra-ventilation techniques (Phase 3) before you get in or while in water of any kind
- I recommend people to begin CET when their BOLT score rises above 25 seconds (before that, it should all be heat training)
- CET is best trained with Phase 3 techniques
- A person with Raynaud's Syndrome and cardiovascular disease should be careful using CET. They should start gently and progress slowly. CET is a shock to your system, and you don't want it to shock you too much, after all!
- CET is trained gradually. Do not 'man up' or jump straight into freezing water without any prior experiences
- The training focuses on controlling your breathing as you expose yourself to the cold. Your body may automatically take a few extra big breaths to cope with the cold but your goal is to reduce your breathing as soon as possible, and calm it under the stress of the cold
- Any water temperature below 15 degrees Celsius is considered CET, and you will gain benefits from it

There are four types of CET modalities, each with a different stimulus to the body. There are air baths, cold showers, ice baths and Mother Nature (the sea, a lake, a river or full immersion in moving water).

HOW TO TRAIN COLD EXPOSURE TRAINING

Air bathing

Simply get outside, take your shoes and socks off and walk on the grass/sand barefoot. Over time, reduce the number of layers you are wearing. Begin to expose yourself to the cold elements and feel the cold.

Air bathing can then be progressed as far as you like by increasing your time in the cold and decreasing your layers. I've climbed a mountain in minus ten degrees Celsius temperatures topless and wearing a pair of shorts. Anything is possible, but be smart; I was fully supervised and trained to perform the event.

Cold Showers

Begin by taking contrast showers and then progress to a cold shower. Contrast showers are like interval training for hot and cold. Spend up to three minutes under a hot shower then turn it cold for 30 seconds. Week-on-week, you can progressively turn it colder for longer. Once you've reached a two-minute cold contrast shower, you should give the straight-up cold shower a try.

There are two ways to immerse yourself into a straight-up cold shower. The first (and easiest) is the cold shower Hokey-Cokey. Gradually place your right foot into the shower, then remove it. Do the same with the left foot, then move onto your arms, your body and eventually your head. When taking a cold shower, you want to fully soak all of your body and head. The second way to take a cold shower is just to get straight under. It's certainly more potent initially to take a cold shower this way but you get the discomfort over and done with.

Ice Baths

Easier, more convenient, and safer than Mother Nature, ice baths provide the ultimate stimulus for CET. They've been used by athletes and in therapy for centuries and they're finding a revival of popularity of late, thanks to the Wim Hof method. To take an ice bath, you simply fill a tub with cold water and top it up with ice. The water temperature should fall below 15 degrees to avail of the benefits from CET. Typically, the temperature of an ice bath will fall as low as six degrees Celsius. Tap water temperatures vary depending on the time of year and where you are located in the cold and so the amount of ice required will also vary. I've used anywhere from 10 kg of ice in a bath to 100 kg. In Ireland and the UK you can conveniently buy ice pretty cheaply from one of the big supermarkets. Some people who really get into ice bathing end up converting a deep freezer in their home to save on cost and the environment. There are many websites that show you how to set these up easily.

Mother Nature Cold Exposure

The final way to CET is by using the greatest resource of them all – Mother Nature. Jumping into the seas, lakes and waterfalls provided by Mother Nature has been used as a therapy to humans for eons. There are written accounts dating back hundreds of years in Japan and France of people jumping into cold bodies of water to benefit the body, mind, and spirit. Japanese Shinto practitioners, Judoka and the German Naturopathy method, and the Kneipp method, are three famous examples of these accounts. Bathing in bodies of cold water is a different challenge to bathing in an ice bath. The water moves, it changes depth, and there are other safety aspects to consider. These changes in environment can challenge both your concentration levels and your ability to stay warm. Moving water feels up to thirty times colder than a still body of water due to convection. It's why a cold and wet winter's day in Ireland (at possibly 5 degrees Celsius) feels much colder than a dry cold day in the arctic (at -5 degrees Celsius).

VARIABLES IN MOTHER NATURE'S COLD EXPOSURE TRAINING		
Location	Temperature	Speed
Sea	Various temperatures	Varying speeds
River	Various temperatures	Varying speeds
Mountain River	Cold temperature	Fast
Lake	Cold temperature	Still
Waterfall	Cold temperature	Very fast
Ice Waterfall	Very cold	Varying speeds

No matter which stimulus you choose, always remember to be safe. The aim of CET is not to stay in the harshest conditions for as long as you can but to use the CET to benefit your body. Your breath is the first key to unlocking CET's benefits for you.

Allow your body to breathe after the initial exposure. This may mean some mouth breathing for a handful of breaths, then calming your breath as quickly as possible, staying relaxed. You may find humming to be a useful breathing technique when exposing yourself to the more extreme ranges of CET. Once your breath is relaxed and calm, it's time to do the same with your body. Squeeze and release the muscles of your body, drop your shoulders, and bring as much relaxation into the experience as possible. The more relaxed you are during CET and the more you enjoy it, the more benefits you will gain from the experience. The third and final key to CET is to get out while you still feel good. This is hugely important.

The danger of CET is that you stay in the cold for too long. For a training effect, you only need to be exposed to cold water for thirty seconds to two minutes. Typically, you will get a shock when you first get in and then your body calms down after about sixty seconds. Between minutes one to two is the most fruitful time to gain the benefits of CET. Cold shock can set in after three minutes of exposure, and hypothermia after twenty minutes, depending on the water temperature and your training.

The most recent science on the benefits of CET were published in late 2021 by a Danish researcher named Susanna Soeberg in *Cell*, a highly prestigious peer-reviewed journal. During her research, Soeberg found the golden amount of time required per week for CET to benefit you. It didn't matter if you performed the CET all in one go or in multiple exposures but, according to her, eleven minutes per week is the ideal frequency of CET required for positive mental and physical health benefits. In an Instagram interview with Dr. Andrew Huberman in December 2021, she elaborated on her research. She told the viewers that the water itself does not have to be particularly cold; anything under fifteen degrees Celsius is enough to reap the rewards.

Wim Hof is the modern-day guru of ice training. He has set over 26 Guinness World Records in the cold; everything from an almost two-hour ice bath to climbing to the death zone of Everest in a pair of shorts and boots. I am one of his students in breathing, mindset and cold exposure therapy. As Wim has often acknowledged, nature is a powerful force, we need to respect her. Feeling good is your guide to staying on the safe side.

- From a BOLT of 15 seconds – focus on heat training and air bathing only
- From a BOLT of 25 seconds progressively train CET – daily contrast showers, daily cold showers, a weekly ice bath, or CET in mother nature

NUTRITION AND BREATHING

Energy is produced in the presence of both oxygen and nutrients. The oxygen we get from our breathing, and the nutrients are extracted from the food we eat. When you improve your food, you relieve your breathing system of some pressure and generate energy more efficiently. Everything works together, as one unit in the body. It is very difficult to optimise your breathing system without improving all other systems of the body, especially the digestive system.

Now I know there are many diverse and opposing views of nutrition out there, and it usually falls between vegan, meat-eating, or something in between. How you eat and your reasons for doing so are none of my business. I long ago learnt that no matter what science or counter-argument is presented to someone about their nutrition habits, it is very difficult for them to change their minds, usually because one's eating pattern has been developed for a cultural or moral reason. I'm ok with all of that. I understand that food plays a very important role in both human society and the Earth's ecology. With almost a trillion of us on the planet, if we all ate the same way, the planet would not be able to cope very well for very long. The important thing for me to impart to you about nutrition is that it serves three roles for humans:

1. Support the health of your body and your lifestyle
2. Enjoyment on social occasions with your community
3. Emotional release from stress

Your food should provide you with the nutrients your body requires for it to work well and for you to live your lifestyle. If you are suffering with low energy, mood swings, or any disease of the body, you are most likely eating food that is out of alignment with the health of your body. This also has significant impacts on your breathing system because it is your breathing system that has 70% of the responsibility to eliminate the toxins and the ash left over from metabolism.

Scenario 1: Eating for Social Reasons

Think of it like this; it's Christmas Day and you've just finished a feast for all the ages. Four hours, five courses, and several helpings of everything on the table later and you plonk yourself on your couch. Sit there and listen. Listen to your breath. Is it calm, gentle and relaxed, or are you heaving and gasping for air? The untold pressure of eating so much food has knock-on effects into your breathing system from this one big meal. Your body finds it difficult to cope with all the calories you ate, the diversity of food in one sitting and the foods you ate which it doesn't like. The same logic is applied when you eat too much food, or foods your body doesn't like over the course of your life. It has direct knock-on effects into the health of your breathing system. Your breathing system can then become dysfunctional, and a host of diseases can develop as a result. A clear-cut example of this is when we eat so much we become obese. Obesity is linked with mouth breathing at night. The disturbances of our breathing at night leads to increased snoring, sleep-disordered breathing, and obstructive sleep apnoea (OSA). If obesity and OSA were not bad enough, we are now more likely to develop type 2 diabetes and cardiovascular disease. It's pretty grim, right? And the two links in the chain which we have control over are our nutrition and our breathing.

Scenario 2: Emotional Eating

You are sitting down on a Thursday night after a tough day at work. Being the leader of an important project, your boss has been down your throat about failure to make a deadline. To make matters worse, your team just aren't gelling together, there's in-house fighting, and everyone is out for themselves. The commute home was the same disaster as always, two hours to make a journey you'd do in twenty-five minutes at the weekend. All day you've been sustaining yourself on coffee and sandwiches on the go from the deli because you've been that busy. Now that you're home, you've forgotten to do the shopping for the week. You open the cupboards and there's nothing in them. You go to the freezer and luckily you find a frozen pizza there. Even though you know eating the pizza will have repercussions tomorrow, tomorrow can wait. You deserve it; it's been a tough day. You gobble up the pizza and proceed to the couch to flake out for the evening. As you sit there with a belly swelling up from the pizza, you feel happy and content. Like an itch that's been scratched, you finally feel ok.

The above two scenarios can play out in numerous ways. Take a look at your own life and see how it works. Either way, it is so easy for us in this modern world to overconsume food and to eat foods that our bodies will suffer from. We can be vegan, meat-eating or anything in between; that's just the nature of human beings. I have found the key to nutrition is first to look after your emotional stressors (breathing, physical activity and finding purpose in life), then build your resilience through mini-challenges and finally realign why you eat the foods you are eating. You can do all of this within the context of your culture, your social occasions, and your moral choices.

Most important things to address for nutrition:

1. Know why you are eating – health, emotions, social
2. Address general stress first through breathing and lifestyle
3. Find another, more beneficial, way to release emotions – Phase 3 breathing techniques, walking, sport, art, music, boxing, singing, etc.
4. Put in the good foods for health first
5. Support your food choices within your cultural and moral context
6. Prepare your food in advance – plan, shop, and prepare for the unexpected
7. Enjoy your food, enjoy your social occasions

From this point, diving deeper into nutrition becomes contentious and requires much more depth of explanation. This is not a place I want to go with this book and so I am not going to recommend particular nutrition strategies or foods to eat. Just know that any return to more natural foods and high-quality foods is good for your body. Quality water, quality vegetables, fruit, nuts, seeds, herbs, spices and high-quality meat, fish, and poultry are what the human body is designed to process for energy. Eat mostly these foods and you'll find a noticeable difference in your breathing and health.

Finally, know that if you've been eating foods that your body doesn't like for a long time, you may need to rehabilitate your digestive system, just as you have done with your breathing system. This may entail anything from fasting to specific protocols to supplements. Health is a continual journey over a lifetime for modern people. Feeling great may be the goal, but maintaining it for as long as you live, takes as long as you live. This is not a sprint, it's a marathon. Take your time, do each phase well, and enjoy the journey.

SLEEP AND BREATHING

Last, but definitely not least of the lifestyle components to health and better breathing, is sleep. Poor quality sleep is one of the biggest red lights for an unhealthy body. Snoring, mouth breathing at night, sleep-disordered breathing, insomnia, and sleep apnoea are huge risk factors for co-morbidity diseases like cardiovascular disease, diabetes, ADHD, and cancer to name a few. For many, in recent times, sleep has become the number one lifestyle habit to fix. For me, it's way down the list. It's down the list not because it's not very important – it is extremely important – but because it is more important to address what happens to you during the day first, which then impacts your sleep. The latest sleep science is finding the same results.

The most important things to address for sleep are:

1. Prepare your bedroom like a bat cave – pitch-black
2. Night-time breathing pattern – nose breathing only and mouth tape if necessary
3. Rise at a similar time every day, including weekends
4. Get daylight into your eyes first thing in the morning and at sunset too
5. Exercise vigorously early in the day
6. Reduce coffee to morning times only and possibly eliminate it
7. Regulate your eating times – breakfast, lunch, dinner
8. Prepare for sleep 1-3 hours in advance by dimming lights, turning off TV, phones, laptops, and Wi-Fi

BREATHING FOR LIFE PERFORMANCE

19

Once you have trained your breathing system for health and returned your system back to its natural centre, we can then apply breathing techniques to help you perform better in life. The idea behind breathing for life performance is to give you breathing tools to upregulate your system in preparation for periods of intense psychological stress and to downregulate your system once those periods have passed. They are techniques to give you a boost of energy and focus when required, or help to chill you out. Think of downregulate as the process of taking your system down from a high, without a crash. Examples could include calming yourself after an emotional conflict with someone, relaxing after a day's work before you get home, or even chilling out after a big meal. Upregulation, on the other hand, is like having a coffee to kick-start your day, or needing to get in the zone for a high-powered meeting. Throughout our modern lives, each of us comes across these situations.

Downregulation techniques calm your system through nasal-only breathing, reduced breathing, lengthening your breath and increasing carbon dioxide in the blood. The brain responds to these techniques by activating the parasympathetic branch of the nervous system and calming us down. Upregulation techniques perform the exact opposite way on the body and brain. These techniques decrease carbon dioxide in the blood, change the blood pH, and signal the brain to initiate a stress response. The stress response secretes adrenaline and prepares blood sugar to be used as energy. Just as a cup of coffee does, it gives us the feeling of energising the body, and it focuses our mind to perform a task. The techniques you've already practiced in your training program can also be used beyond training in breathing for life performance. They can also be classified as upregulation or downregulation techniques, as shown below.

When choosing the right technique for you, you should ask yourself the following questions:

Do I need to relax and stay calm?

or

Do I need to energise and focus?

Once you answer these questions, select a technique from each category: relax and calm or energise and focus. Any of the techniques will deliver the effect you desire. Some are more potent than others but one approach is not better than another. Your job is to experiment with the different techniques and find out which ones work best for you in a given situation. I've added additional techniques here for more variety and individualisation of your breath practice. You could also stack the techniques one on top of the next to create a more powerful breathing session and have much more fun with your training.

BREATHING FOR LIFE PERFORMANCE

CLASSIFICATION OF THE INNATE-STRENGTH BREATH TRAINING PROGRAMME TECHNIQUES

Relax, and think calmly and clearly	Energise and focus
Downregulate	Upregulate
Intentional Yawn	
Breath of Freedom	
Diaphragm Release Technique	
Breath Hold 1	Progressive Wim Hof Breathing
Breath Hold 2	Wim Hof Breathing
4:6 Breathing	
Humming Breath	
Breathing Bands	
Breath Calming	

CLASSIFICATION OF BREATHING FOR LIFE PERFORMANCE TECHNIQUES

Relax, and think calmly and clearly	Energise and focus
Downregulate	Upregulate
Use nose only for most techniques	
Tornado Breath*	
4, 5 ,6 ,7 Basic Tempo	*Use mouth only for all techniques*
1111 (Box Breathing)	142
1121	Coffee Breath
Warrior Breath	Breath Pumping
Yoga Alternate Nostril Breathing	
Saw Breathing*	

*uses both nose and mouth

ADVANCED BREATHING TECHNIQUES TO RELAX AND CALM

All of the techniques for relaxing and calming extend the length of each breath. A longer breath can deliver several ways to calm the body, depending on how you practice it. Generally, a longer breath:

- ✓ Reduces the number of breaths you take per minute
- ✓ Activates the parasympathetic branch and dampens the sympathetic branch of your nervous system

If you think of your breath as a box with an inhale, a hold across the top, an exhale, and a hold across the bottom, then you can manipulate the length of your breath by lengthening any side of it. This is the basic premise to all calming techniques and it's the first way I lengthen the breath here.

TORNADO BREATH

I first learned of the tornado breath from Dan Brulé. He didn't have a name for it at the time, so I began calling it a tornado because that's how it looked. Dan worked with the Russian Ministry of Psychiatry for over ten years researching this breath pattern. In an interview with me, he told me that during this research, they found that nobody who could perform the tornado breath was clinically depressed, and nobody who was clinically depressed could perform this breath. The benefits of the tornado breath are:

- ✓ Lengthens the inhale
- ✓ Uses the full lung capacity
- ✓ Teaches relaxation of the exhale, mouth, jaws, throat and tongue
- ✓ Good for positive mental health and relaxation

The tornado breath is an all-mouth breath with two parts to it – the inhale and the exhale. To begin, shape your mouth into a very small hole, like you've wrapped your lips around a straw. The pressure from the small hole will force you to use more of your diaphragm than you'd traditionally use with mouth breathing. In fact, it will work more like a nasal inhale (only better) because the hole is so small. Suck the air in through the mouth. As your lungs begin to fill, slowly open your lips wider and wider. At the top of your inhale, your mouth will be fully open and your lungs filled with air. In this sense, the breath is funnelled in through your lips in the same shape as a tornado.

Once you've reached the top of your inhale, let go of the exhale. Relax the mouth and jaws completely and allow the breath to fall out of your body. Then begin your next breath.

Total Time: 2 – 10 minutes

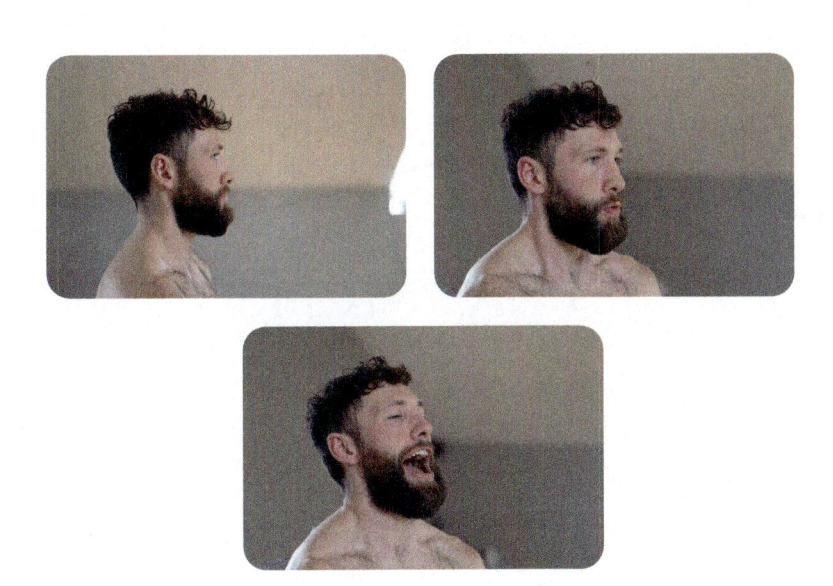

PART 3 THE INNATE-STRENGTH BREATH TRAINING PROGRAMME

4, 5, 6, 7 BASIC TEMPOS

These breathing techniques are all practised with nose breathing. Feel free to breathe into Zones 1 and 2 – belly and chest. Each of the tempos builds on the last to lengthen the breath and reduce the number of breaths you take in a one minute. As with all of these advanced techniques, the basic tempos can be practised anywhere, for from two minutes up to an hour, depending on how drastic an effect you seek. Obviously, the effect is more potent the longer you practice the technique.

Total Time for all Tempos: 2 – 10 minutes

Method: 4040 TEMPO   *7.5 breaths per minute*

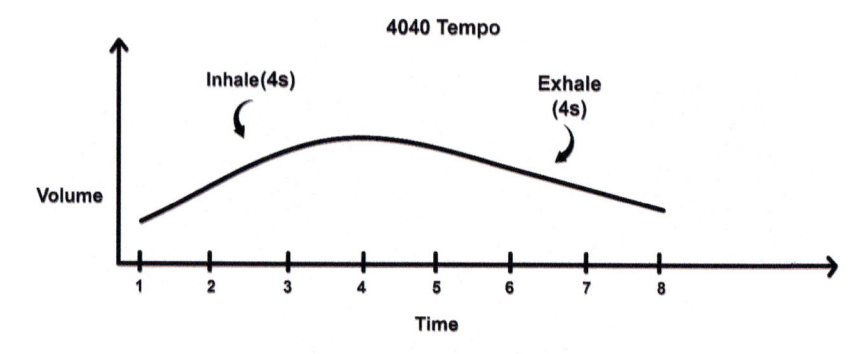

4040 Tempo

Inhale(4s)   Exhale (4s)

Volume

Time

1. Inhale for 4 seconds
2. No pause at the top
3. Exhale for 4 seconds
4. No pause at the bottom

   a. Keep a pendulum or continuous breath – no pauses

Method: 5050 TEMPO *6 breaths per minute*

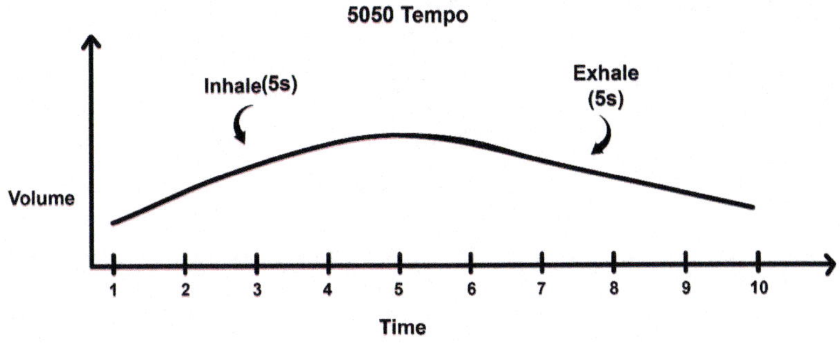
5050 Tempo
Inhale(5s)
Exhale
(5s)
Volume
1
2
3
4
5
6
7
8
9
10
Time

1. Inhale for 5 seconds
2. No pause at the top
3. Exhale for 5 seconds
4. No pause at the bottom

    a. Keep a pendulum or continuous breath – no pauses

Method: 6060 TEMPO *5 breaths per minute*

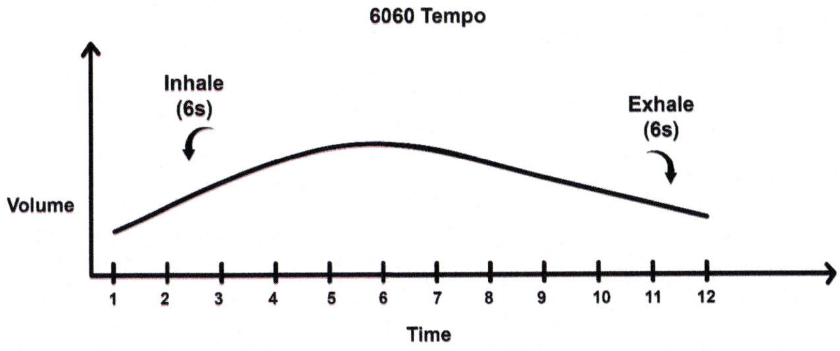
6060 Tempo
Inhale
(6s)
Exhale
(6s)
Volume
1
2
3
4
5
6
7
8
9
10
11
12
Time

1. Inhale for 6 seconds
2. No pause at the top
3. Exhale for 6 seconds
4. No pause at the bottom

    a. Keep a pendulum or continuous breath – no pauses

Method: 7070 TEMPO *4.2 breaths per minute*

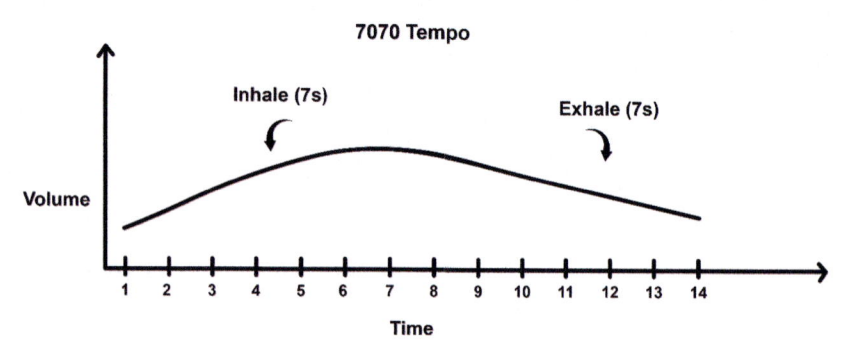

7070 Tempo

Inhale (7s) — Exhale (7s)

Volume / Time

1. Inhale for 7 seconds
2. No pause at the top
3. Exhale for 7 seconds
4. No pause at the bottom

   a. Keep a pendulum or continuous breath – no pauses.

1111 TEMPO TECHNIQUE (BOX BREATHING)

Imagine being a soldier in the heat of a raging battle, and you're rescuing an innocent hostage from a terrorist. Your heart is pumping, your hands are sweaty, and gunfire surrounds you. Imagine that you've just forced your way through the gunfire to come face-to-face with your enemy. It's down to you to take the shot to kill the enemy or risk losing the hostage. A calm trigger finger and a clear mind are obviously critical to the success of your objective.

This is a situation many Special Forces soldiers find themselves in. Mark Divine is one of them, and as a US Navy Seal, he was taught box breathing to help him remain calm and make a critical decision to save lives. You mightn't be an elite soldier and may never need to rescue a hostage but you too can practice box breathing and link your breath, body and mind to remain calm during stressful situations, like in a board room meeting or an argument.

BREATHING FOR LIFE PERFORMANCE

Box Breathing

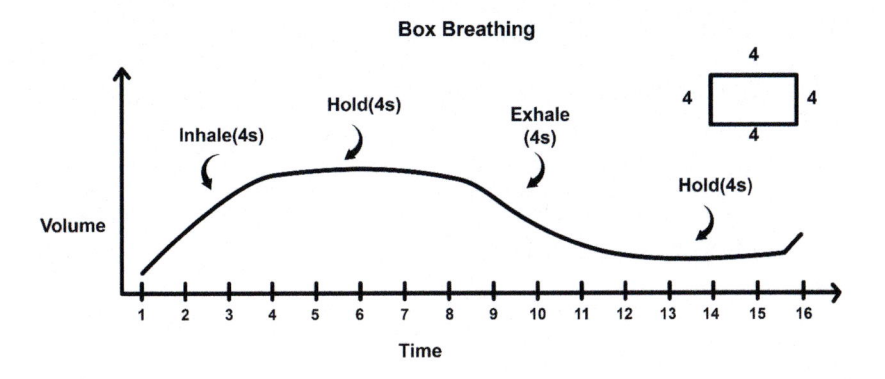

Graph showing Volume vs Time: Inhale(4s), Hold(4s), Exhale(4s), Hold(4s), with a box diagram labeled 4 on each side.

Technique

1. This technique can be performed in daily life, sitting, standing or moving
2. Use nose-only breathing for this technique
3. Make your breath into the shape of a box by inhaling, holding, exhaling and holding for an even amount of time
4. Begin with a base number of four seconds which means you inhale for four seconds, hold your breath at the top of the inhale for four seconds, exhale for four seconds, then hold at the bottom for four seconds
5. Repeat three to six times
6. If you're comfortable, then progress to a base five
7. You can continually advance this technique to challenge your CO_2 tolerance levels and your ability to handle physical and mental stress. I've worked my way up to a base of fifteen seconds, but I find a base of seven to ten seconds to be best for this technique

Total Time: 2 – 10 minutes

PART 3   THE INNATE-STRENGTH BREATH TRAINING PROGRAMME

1121 TEMPO TECHNIQUE

1121 is a progression on box breathing. I like to begin using it when my box breath is over seven seconds. It challenges you slightly differently to the box breath by lengthening your exhale twice as long as any other part of the breath. This provides a different stimulus to the box breath but a similar overall effect.

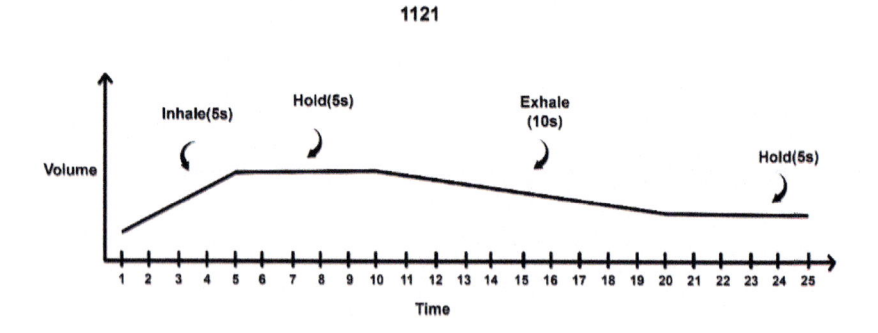

Technique

1. This technique can be performed in daily life, sitting, standing, or moving
2. Use nose-only breathing for this technique
3. Begin with a base number of five seconds. This means you inhale for five seconds, hold your breath at the top of the inhale for five seconds, exhale for ten seconds, then hold at the bottom for five seconds
4. Repeat three to six times
5. If you're comfortable then progress to a base six. The maximum useful base I've found is seven seconds. After that, I feel the amount of time you spend on the technique outweighs the perceived benefits you may get from it

Total Time: 2 – 10 minutes

WARRIOR BREATH TECHNIQUE

So far you have extended your breath by humming, slowing your exhale and using a variety of breath holds. This time you'll partially constrict your throat muscles to lengthen your breath. Like with the box and 1121 techniques, practicing the warrior breath helps you to control your breath under physical and mental pressure. The difference now is that you don't hold your breath after the inhale or exhale; rather, a partial muscle constriction is practised on the inhale, exhale, or both. Think of warrior breath like placing your finger over a part of a running garden hose. Normally, the water flows out of the hose easily, but when you place your finger over it, the finger forces the water out of a smaller gap in the hose. In the warrior breath, when you partially close your throat, you produce a similar pressure on your breath. By doing this, we end up extending our exhale. The trick now is to practice extending your exhale as long as you can and remain calm at the same time.

Technique 1 – exhale only

1. Begin with a small inhale
2. No pause at the top
3. Exhale with a partially closed or constricted throat

    a. This will sound like Darth Vader
    b. Another way to think of this technique is when you fog a mirror with your breath. Now close your mouth and do the same. Just do it slowly

4. Repeat this exercise and gradually increase the size of your inhale

Total Time: 2 – 10 minutes

Technique 2 – inhale and exhale

1. Inhale with a constricted throat
2. No pause at the top
3. Exhale with a constricted throat
4. Repeat

Total Time: 2 – 10 minutes

YOGA ALTERNATE NOSTRIL BREATHING

According to ancient yoga traditions, the alternate nostril breathing technique balances out the parasympathetic and sympathetic branches of the nervous system. This wisdom is starting to be confirmed by research in more recent times too. Anecdotally, people seem to love this technique to boost energy and clear the mind.

Technique

1. You can perform this technique in any posture
2. Use the nose only for breathing
3. To begin, block your right nostril with the thumb of your right hand. This will force the air in through the left nostril when you breathe
4. Inhale fully through the left nostril
5. At the top of the breath, let go of your right nostril, and immediately block your left nostril with one of your fingers on the same hand
6. Exhale out of the right nostril
7. Inhale through the same right nostril
8. At the top of the inhale, switch over again
9. Exhale through the left
10. Repeat eight to ten times

Total Time: 2 – 10 minutes

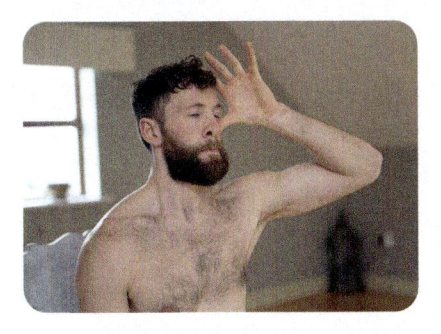

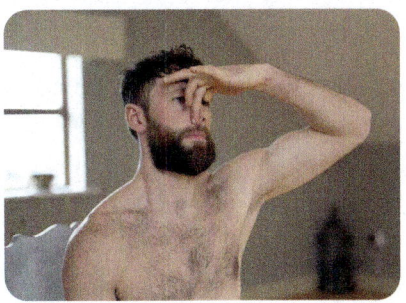

SAW BREATHING TECHNIQUE

The saw breath is another technique designed to lengthen your exhale, fill your lungs, calm your body and clear your mind. The full technique can be broken into two different breathing techniques: Part 1 focuses on the inhale, and Part 2 on the exhale. Like with almost all breathing techniques, the saw breath has been around a long time. Recently, part one of the technique was rebranded and received notoriety online as being the fastest way to calm your body. They now call this aspect of the technique the physiological sigh.

Part 1 tricks your body into using more of your lungs than you'd normally access. This trick enhances blood flow, ventilation, and movement in the smaller or outer parts of your lungs, thereby improving your ability to use your lungs. It calms the mind at the same time. The trick to this part of the technique is to break your full inhale into several steps. That means your inhale now looks like a staircase and sounds like somebody sawing a piece of wood.

Part 1 (focus on the inhale)

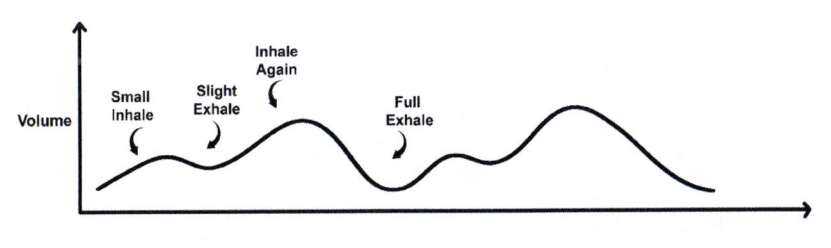

Technique

1. Breathe with a nasal inhale. You can use a nasal or mouth exhale
2. Instead of breathing fully in, break your inhale into two parts. Inhale halfway, stop, inhale again
3. I prefer breaking the inhale into three or four parts to fill the lungs completely and maximise the inhale
4. Just let go of the exhale
5. Repeat for a minimum of two minutes to calm your body

Total Time: 2 – 10 minutes

Part 2 of the saw breath focuses on the exhale. Similar to part one, it tricks your body into lengthening your exhale more than it would normally do. The extra-long exhale improves diaphragm contraction and the use of your full lungs. Just like with Part 1, the trick is breaking up your exhale by pausing it. Again, it looks like a staircase and sounds like somebody sawing a piece of wood.

Part 2 (focus on the exhale)

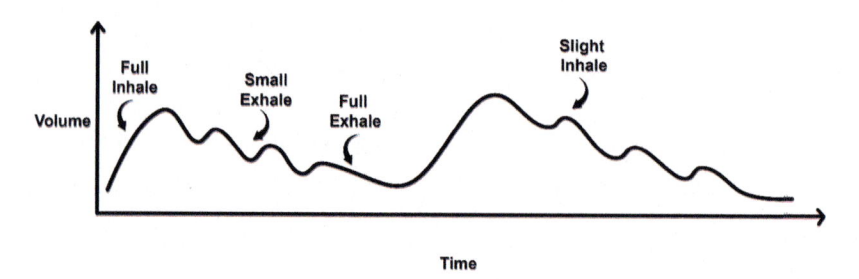

Technique

1. As with part one, breathe with a nasal inhale. You can use a nasal or mouth exhale
2. Inhale fully
3. Instead of exhaling fully in one go, break your exhale into two or more parts. When you stop your breath in the middle of an exhale, you'll notice that it is more comfortable to take a sip of air in.

That's ok; the sip of air with the pause gives the exhale the sound of a sawing a piece of wood
4. I prefer breaking the exhale into three or four parts only
5. Finish the exhale by emptying your lungs completely of air
6. Allow the inhale to rebound naturally
7. Repeat for a minimum of two minutes to calm your body

Total Time: 2 – 10 minutes

Finally, you can combine the whole technique to produce one powerful saw breathing technique. Practising this technique for a minimum of two minutes is a great way to improve your diaphragm, enhance your usable lung capacity, relax the body, and calm your mind.

ADVANCED BREATHING TECHNIQUES TO FOCUS AND ENERGISE

The purpose of the techniques in this section is to upregulate your nervous system quickly so that you can be alert to working during the day. That might mean physical work, as in the gym or during sport, or mental work, like being switched-on during a meeting. All of the techniques decrease CO_2, alert the brain and generate adrenaline. The difference is in their power to do that job. Progressive Wim Hof breathing and the Wim Hof breathing exercises can be added to this category of techniques. These would be the most powerful of all the upregulation techniques. I begin here with 142 Tempo Breathing, move onto a Coffee Breath, and finish with Breath Pumping.

142 TEMPO BREATHING TECHNIQUE

The 142 Tempo Breathing Technique is the only strong breath hold technique I've included in this category. It is more of an upregulation technique than a downregulation because the main breath hold is performed after the inhale. A breath hold at the top will generate a lot of pressure in your ribcage and is very stressful for your body compared to an exhaled-breath-hold.

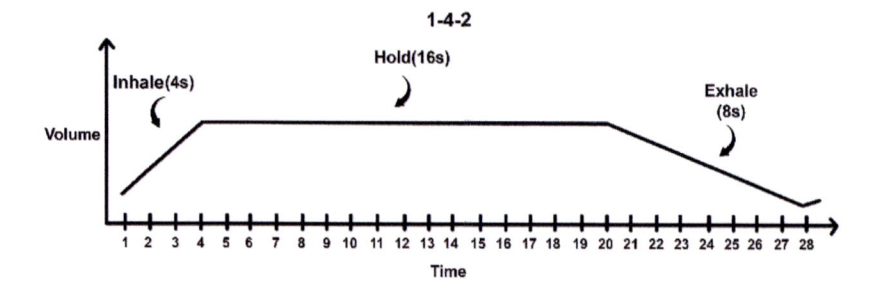

1-4-2

Inhale(4s) — Hold(16s) — Exhale (8s)

(Volume vs Time graph, time axis 1–28)

Technique

1. This technique is usually performed with nose-only breathing but you could use your mouth if you wish
2. Start with base number 4 seconds
3. Inhale (4s) – hold top (16s) – exhale (8s) – no hold bottom (0s)
4. Repeat three to six breath cycles
5. If comfortable, then progress your base

Total Time: 2 – 10 minutes

COFFEE BREATH

Named for its benefits, the coffee breath does exactly what it says on the tin – it feels like you just had a cup of coffee. It perks you up, energises you, and helps you to focus for the day. Unlike its namesake, the coffee breath doesn't leave you in a slump hours later. This technique simply makes you feel great; just be cognisant you don't over-use it as an energy-crutch for too long. For example, this breath will help energise you if you had a rough night's sleep, but no amount of breathing will help you replace continuous lost sleep.

Coffee Breath

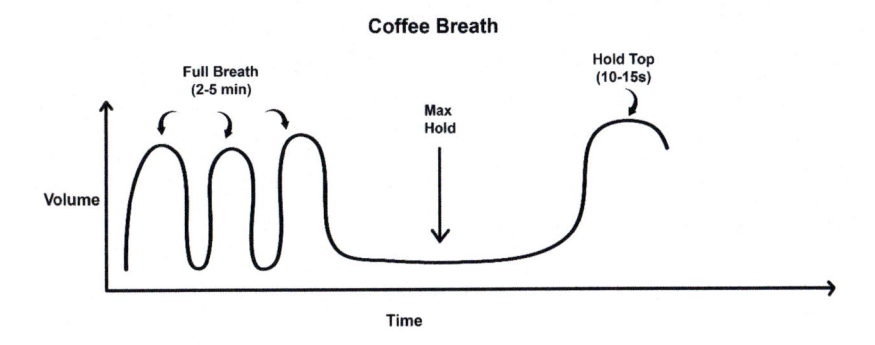

[Diagram showing volume vs. time with Full Breath (2-5 min), Max Hold, and Hold Top (10-15s)]

Technique

1. Performed best when seated or lying on your back
2. Inhale through your nose and exhale through mouth
3. Breathe full continuous breaths for two to five minutes
4. After the breathing time is up, balance the breath with a breath hold after the exhale
5. Hold your breath for as long as you're comfortable
6. Finish the technique by inhaling and holding your breath at the top for ten seconds

Total Time: 2 – 10 minutes

BREATH PUMPING

Breath pumping is a more intense version of the coffee breath, and it falls into the breathwork category of techniques. As with all big and fast breathwork techniques, do not perform breath pumping if you are pregnant or have epilepsy. Don't perform it in water, or when operating heavy machinery, and be conscious of the emotional component of the technique.

The focus of this technique is to exhale strongly out of your body. The strong exhale gets rid of CO_2 and strengthens the diaphragm too. A loss of CO_2 signals the brain to generate adrenaline. The adrenaline then gives you a feeling of increased energy and enhanced focus. Generally, you'll feel better and pain sensitivity is decreased with techniques like breath pumping. Intensifying the speed of your breath and lengthening your breathing time increases the amount of CO_2 you expend and all the positive feelings that come with that. I suggest you start slow and find a pace you can sustain for ten to twenty minutes. You can increase the intensity of the technique by exhaling to a faster rhythm.

Breath Pumping

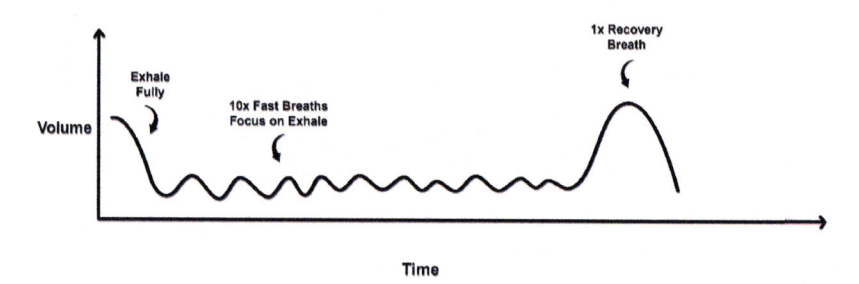

Technique

1. Start with nasal-only breathing
2. Exhale fully
3. Pump the breath with an active exhale and passive inhale
4. Breaths should be rhythmical
5. Start slowly and keep control
6. Begin with 10 breaths followed by one full recovery breath (full inhale and exhale)
7. Repeat six times
8. Speed up gradually to technical failure (you can't keep your breathing rhythm)
9. Inhale fully at the end and slowly exhale all the way to the bottom
10. Once you become competent with ten breaths, you can increase your breaths to as many as you like. Whenever you lose your rhythm, perform a recovery breath
11. Advance to mouth breathing when you become competent with the nose breathing

Total time: 10 – 20 minutes

EPILOGUE

There is nothing prettier in the whole wide world than a girl in love with every breath she takes

ATTICUS

Take a breath.

Without a doubt, when you practise breath training consistently as per the programme, you will breathe free. It may take you only a few sessions to reap the rewards, or it may take several months. Typically, training takes 12-16 weeks to optimise your breath. Stick with it, and you will meet with surprising benefits and insights into your breath, body, and mind.

If you find yourself getting stuck, hitting a plateau, or becoming frustrated with the process, know that this is natural. Persist.

When you do eventually come to know your breath, it'll be time to let go of it. You won't need to tape yourself up at night forever and you won't need to do breathing exercises daily. Awareness of your breath in the moment will be sufficient. Remember, your breath will always be with you as you do every other activity in life, so go and enjoy your life.

Like a wave in the ocean, your breath increases in size and volume with greater levels of excitement, activity, and pleasure. It also falls like a wave when you want to slow down in life, recover, regenerate, and relax.

EPILOGUE

Like a well-trained dog, your breath will become your best friend for the remainder of your life. It'll guard you against long-term stress and being overwhelmed. It'll protect you through the traumatic times of life, and it'll be a superpower to focus and energise your efforts on the greatest life you want to live.

When you train it and learn to breathe free, your breathing becomes all this and more.

The science behind the breath is ever-evolving, just as we are. While it doesn't fundamentally change how I coach people, it helps me understand people better and why someone's breathing may be adapted. Just recently, I connected the science of dopamine and breathing in my studies. Dopamine is commonly known as the 'molecule of more' in the brain. It controls our motivation, reward, craving, pleasure, pain and addiction pathways in the brain. The science is too young yet to make definitive statements about dopamine and breathing, but let's say for now that the roles of breathing and energy are connected at a higher level to general motivation, reward, pain, and pleasure. The more we live our life to the full, the more dopamine is generated in our brain to motivate us to keep going. After we get a dopamine hit, energy in the form of adrenaline, noradrenaline, and even blood sugar is subsequently released downstream to give us the ability to perform life at full throttle. Adrenaline, as it turns out, is even created from dopamine. This is all good news in general, but just as our breath adapts to a perceived centre with a high-octane lifestyle, so does our dopamine system.

Did you ever notice that one cup of coffee used to be enough to feel great, but now it takes four? A pizza used to taste amazing, but because you eat it too often, you now crave more? Sex, drugs, video games, movies, a high-paced career, and overtraining; all produce a similar short-term spike in dopamine and a chronic decline in long-term circulating levels. The good news is that quality lifestyle practices, like breathing free, taking cold dips, and exercising regularly raise dopamine levels just as effectively as other substances without the less desirable long-term outcomes. However, there are two key differences:

1. The rise in dopamine is slower with quality lifestyle practices
2. You repeat lifestyle practices daily, so you're continually raising your baseline dopamine levels

The result of improving your breath and lifestyle is that the overall baseline levels of circulating dopamine improve rather than reduce – you feel better, become more motivated by life, find more joy in the simple pleasures of life and you enjoy peak experiences for what they are – a fleeting moment of pure joy in time. Afterwards, you return to the contentment of life.

Just like with the breath, your baseline level of dopamine needs to be restored to get more love out of the life you live. This insight is the connection between the subtle benefits of breathing free and enhanced lifestyles with the science of dopamine. Over the years, I've noticed that as clients restore their breathing to its natural centre, they become more motivated by doing things that are meaningful to them for no other reward than the pleasure of doing it. They don't need a trophy, social applause or any accolades. They simply do and enjoy. They take great pleasure in the simple things life has to offer, like driving a van with no radio blaring, noticing the energy of a city or the smile of a child, or playing sport without inhibition. This is the feedback I get the whole time; it's not something I can advertise on Instagram too successfully but these are the benefits that make a real difference to people. These simple everyday moments become more joyful for my clients, and in turn, they become more grateful as a natural by-product of breathing free.

Additionally, the exciting things in life become even more exciting for people who breathe free. The goals they hit and the achievements they earn become peak experiences of life. These experiences are cherished in the moment and released just as quickly.

When you breathe free, these strong baselines and unbridled joy become your new way of life. It feels amazing at first, and then it just becomes the norm for you. This is the way of dopamine, the way of our neurobiology, and the way of breathing free. It's science. It's nature. It's life.

EPILOGUE

For now, you need to have faith, hope, and commitment. You need to believe that you, too, can breathe free and be strong. All the answers are inside of you. Commit to breath training and live your greatest life.

Initially, this book was supposed to fully explain all that I know about breathing. But alas, it was too much for one book. My next book will focus on breathing for sports performance. This is a subject dear to my heart. If you remember, my breathing story has always been intertwined with sport. From my desire to play football for Dublin, to becoming a trainer, running a marathon with my mouth taped, becoming a black belt in judo and coaching countless clients to their goals and achievements in sport. Since 2017, I have discovered many things about the integration of breathing and training that are still cutting-edge. Safe to say, breathing for health is the foundation of any sports breathing programme. It accounts for approximately 90% of the benefits to breathing for sports performance. A further book on 'sport performance breathing' enhances your training and performance by about another 10% on top of the knowledge contained here.

Living a great life is the second area I will write about in the future. We are living at the leading edge of life. We are the most intelligent species on the planet. We are evolving faster than ever because we are connected more than ever through technology. However, we have forgotten our biological and spiritual needs. Regardless of how advanced a civilisation we become, we still need to meet those needs to thrive in life. Breathing free, exercising often, eating well, living in harmony with nature, having meaning in our life, being kind and sharing with others are just some of those needs that must be met. I am in a unique position in my career where I see people who are broken apart because they have forgotten those needs in the demands of achieving more. The awareness on a societal level is coming, though. It's a fascinating time to be alive, and I look forward to sharing my experience with the world.

Breathe free.

Inhale and exhale.

APPENDIX

Here are twenty-one of the life-changing learnings and experiences from some of my clients over the years. I have written them here in the hope that they will help you in the course of your own training.

Breath training has been one of the most uplifting and, at the same time, infuriating experiences of my life.

Breath training has helped me understand my body on such a deep level, to listen to it, and give it what it needs.

Through breath training, I started to realise the main issue for me personally was my body was in a stressed state. Anyone looking at me would never think I am stressed, I come across as the most calm and relaxed person you could meet but when you take time to really connect with your breath, it can tell you so much more about yourself, even on a daily basis.

I have been using heart rate variability to track how my body is recovering for years but now I feel I can use the BOLT score, which has been superior, in my opinion.

The breath training helped me tackle anxious feelings once I made it a priority each day, especially as I started to approach the latter stages of my menstrual cycle. It has also helped decrease night sweats, increase energy, and reduce pain and bloating.

Some of the benefits I experienced include: finally improving and understanding my nasal congestion, learning how to listen to my body, and completely changing my philosophy on the body and mind.

I found myself getting a much better quality of sleep every night. My recovery from hard strength training sessions was better, which is due to the better sleep and respiratory function. I also had much more energy to play with my daughter and even decreased my reliance on my asthma medication.

The breath training was also helping to release pent-up stress and emotions. I found emotions bubbling to the surface when I least expected it. After letting them go, I felt calmer and able to focus on the day's task.

I really noticed breathing is huge for digestion and for losing weight. My body will prioritise stress over digestion so if you are also wondering why you might be struggling to lose weight even though you may be eating less ... maybe look at your stress levels?

I am a numbers guy and wanted to track the data. Leo and I decided to track both breath-related and strength-related metrics. I went from being able to hold my breath and walk only fifteen paces to walking one hundred paces after about four and half months of training.

When Leo explained to me on Day One 'With the breath, less is more', I didn't expect it would take me eight months to finally 'get it'.

My unrelenting competitive brain wouldn't allow me to back off despite my body's clear indications I needed to relax. This was rooted in an unwillingness to accept stepping backwards as I detested the feeling of perceiving myself as a failure.

My training was performed on my own. Nobody cheering, no teammates, just me and my breath. Immense feelings of aloneness came over me at times on the road where I would practise my steps every day. My busyness of life never allowed me to face this emotion so squarely before. There was nowhere I could hide.

The breath training took me out of my head and got me back in my body allowing me to start feeling emotions properly again for the first time in decades – this alone may have been the most crucial change supporting me to save my marriage.

I started this journey as a man unwittingly full of fear. I completed this programme with a sense that nothing is impossible. Explained in practical terms: On Day One, I achieved forty-two steps breath hold maximum. During this technique I thought I was going to black out and hit my head off the road. Yes, I literally feared this in the last three steps Day One! Today, I did one hundred and fifty steps and had my breath calm within the first two breaths. Two hundred steps is my personal best when playfully testing my limits. During the breath calming exercise I started with a breath count six times higher than normal. These days, my breath is almost imperceptible during my ten-minutes of breath calming. There are no limits.

I reconnected with the overwhelming joy it is to be able to have my wife lying naked on top of me in bed and actually being able to take a whole effortless breath as a powerful man once again.

The first benefit that I noticed from these breath exercises was that I had more energy throughout the day and that I was starting to sleep more soundly. Whenever I was feeling tired, I would go for a walk and do a few breath holds and immediately feel that I had more energy to continue about my day. I also started to feel more in control at work and better able to regulate myself and my moods. I felt that, as a result, I was better able to work through problems again, and I had a much clearer head to deal with problems. I also noticed that I was a lot calmer during the day and was better able to deal with difficult issues that arose at work and at home.

APPENDIX

I could not believe the impact breathing had on stress and anxiety straight away.

Friends and colleagues also started to notice these positive changes that I was experiencing.

Most enjoyment was only in hindsight, as most of the learning involves high doses of learned humility!

We think doing nothing and just breathing is a waste of time when, more often than not, it's actually the most beneficial thing you could do for yourself. The breath has helped me to cope so much better, even just from a mood perspective.

'I can see so far, not because I am so tall but because I stand on the shoulders of giants'

I express my heart of loving appreciation to my breath coach Leo for his life's dedication to embodying his mastery of breathwork – extending this to his teachers of the principle-based approach used in my program, Patrick McKeown, Wim Hof and Dr. Buteyko. I cannot repay you for the gift of getting my life. Thank you.

INNATE-STRENGTH CLIENTS

Thank you for reading this book, taking responsibility for your health and performance, training your breath and breathing free. Now it's your turn to spread the good news about breathing.

Leo Daniel Ryan. 9/1/2023

GLOSSARY OF TERMS

Adapted Breathing: Breathing patterns resulting from trauma or a variety of stressors over time. These patterns help you deal with stress in the short-term but promote dis-ease, pain and illness in the long term. For example, mouth breathing.

Apnoea (Breath-Holding): A subconscious breathing pattern or a conscious technique where you hold your breath. It is usually held after an inhale or exhale but can be held at various points throughout the breath wave.

Baselines: The level of energy and health you start out with at the beginning of a day/challenge. It is also the state you should return to after the event.

Breathe-Ability: A combination of a naturally centred breathing pattern and deliberate breathing.

Breath Awareness: Your conscious recognition of your own breathing.

Breathe Free: The awareness and process of developing your breathe-ability.

Breathing Continuum: A model describing the interconnectedness of all breathing techniques on the human body, mind and spirit.

Breathing Mechanics: muscular recruitment for the purpose of breathing.

Breathing Rhythms: Breathing techniques that alter the size and speed of the breath, without using breath holds. (i.e. 5050 or 6060)

GLOSSARY OF TERMS

Breathing System: The interconnectedness of every system in the human body from the perspective of breathing.

Breathing Zones: A practical division of the thorax to describe how you see the breath move. There are three breathing zones: abdominal region, mid-chest, and upper-chest.

Breath Training: The structured and progressive approach to training your breathing system for health and/or performance in life.

Breathwork: A breathing session designed to change your state. It is typically used to help you feel good and/ or help with trauma therapy. From the state change you can also use breathwork to solve problems creatively.

Carbon Dioxide: Originally thought of as a waste gas, it is now redefined as so much more. It is responsible for helping oxygen diffuse into the cell, and it has effects on fear, panic anxiety, concentration, focus and fatigue.

Cleansing Reactions: Short-term immune responses arising from any mode of training. These are common reactions for people new to breath training or practising potent techniques they aren't accustomed to.

CO_2 Sensitivity: A reading in the body and brain of CO_2 levels. A high sensitivity to CO_2 means you react fast to CO_2 and breathe more often. Typically, this results in an increased likelihood of fear, panic, anxiety, asthma, allergies, low endurance and a host of other adaptations in the body. A low sensitivity means you are slower to respond to rising levels of CO_2.

CO_2 Tolerance: The brain's maximum ability to handle CO_2. Typically, the higher the tolerance the better the result for you. A high tolerance leads to calmness, focus, concentration, quality energy levels, and endurance.

Chest Breathing: Typically using Zone 3 as the dominant breathing muscles. Also known as clavicular or upper chest breathing.

GLOSSARY OF TERMS

Deliberate Breathing: Your ability to use your breath competently through life. Typically, it is used to express emotions, generate strength, play sport, and concentrate intently.

Deep Breathing: Breathing with your diaphragm as the prime mover (best practised with nasal breathing).

Dis-ease: A state of physical health where the body is stressed. In this state, you typically show signs and symptoms of adaptation to the stress in the form of pain, illness, mood swings, fluctuating energy, and possible disease.

Downregulation: The parasympathetic system is activated. The body and mind slows down to recover, repair and restore themselves.

Dysfunctional Breathing: A term used in general scientific research to describe breathing patterns that have adapted to life with perceived negative consequences. It's not a term I like to use because it suggests something is wrong with your breath. There's nothing wrong with it, it's just shaped itself to the demands of your life, and now it is no longer serving you positively.

Fast Breathing: Breathing more breaths per minute than needed.

Full Breathing: Filling your whole breathing system with air. The belly moves and the rib cage expands to maximum capacity with a full breath. Also known as big breathing.

Heightened Breathing Pattern: A form of adapted breathing patterns related to chronic activation of the sympathetic nervous system and a reduced ability to relax (fight/flight response). For example, hyperventilation.

Human Performance Pyramid: A hierarchical model describing the power of lifestyle on the human body, mind and spirit.

Hormesis: The science of researching the positive effects of stress on the human body.

Hyperventilation: Breathing more than your metabolic needs. Typically, it is a medically-termed breathing pattern with negative consequences to your health. Also known as over-breathing.

GLOSSARY OF TERMS

Hypoventilation: A chronic breathing pattern that reduces your ability to breathe deliberately.

Inflammation: An immune system response to stress. It keeps you alive in the short term, and it can lead to secondary disease if continually secreted in the long term.

Let Go: Your ability to release the exhale. It is also used analogously to describe the release of tension, emotions, stress, and trauma from the body.

Light Breathing: Reducing the amount of air you inhale whilst maintaining relaxation.

Lowered Breathing Pattern: A form of adapted breathing pattern related to chronic activation of the parasympathetic nervous system and a reduced ability to become aroused (freeze response). For example, inflexible rib cage.

Mouth Breathing: Inhaling and/or exhaling with the mouth. Also a synonym for an inability to focus, or poor cognitive comprehension of a situation.

Nasal Breathing: Inhaling and exhaling with the nose only.

Natural Centre: A state of being throughout the day from which you can then energise yourself effectively or drop into deep states of rest with ease.

Naturally Centred Breathing Pattern: Nasal-only breathing combined with a low, slow, and deep breathing pattern as a subconscious breathing pattern.

Natural vs normal: Natural is the most efficient and effective way you move and think. Normal is the way you are used to moving. Natural may not feel normal if your normal is adapted.

Nitric Oxide: For our purposes, it is a gas produced in the nose and the body. Its role is to filter air, and dilate airways and blood vessels.

Oxygen: The main nutrient required for creating energy in the body. It travels from the environment through the nose/mouth to your lungs. From there, oxygen is extracted by the body and transported by the blood. The important part of the process is to get oxygen from the blood to the cell, where it is used to create energy in the form of ATP.

Slow Breathing: Reducing the number of breaths you take per minute.

Supraventilation: A short-term hyperventilating breathing pattern practised intentionally to arouse your nervous system and energise you. It can be practised as faster breathing, full breathing or a combination of both.

The Edge of the Cliff: The state of being where you are about to tip from a positively stressful state (i.e. a challenge) into a fearful and negative state (i.e. a panic attack).

Training Block: A small period of training, typically one to six weeks long.

Training Effect: The hormetic effect of training the body. It is positive/negative response to a training programme. For example, when you practise a breath-holding programme, you develop your ability to hold your breath. You'll also remain calmer, think clearer, and feel better from the programme. These are all training effects.

Training Phase: A longer period of training made up of several smaller blocks.

Unified respiratory system: The nose, trachea, bronchi, alveoli, and lungs are one system joined from the start to the end.

Upregulation: The sympathetic nervous system is activated. Energy is produced in the body, and the body prepares for fight/flight.

BIBLIOGRAPHY

RECOMMENDED EXPERTS, READING AND VIEWING

My knowledge is distilled from various books, research papers, courses, fellow professionals and experiences. I think writing out every resource I've used in this book would take up more paper space than the book itself! For this reason, I've only listed the resources that I think are of significance to you, the reader, and will contribute to your knowledge of breathing, health, coaching and life in general.

EXPERTS TO SEEK OUT

Patrick McKeown – respiratory physiology and practice of 'lowering' breathing techniques

Wim Hof – Cold training, mindset training and finding you

Dan Brulé – Breathwork

Brian MacKenzie & Rob Wilson – Human performance, stress tolerance, breathwork and temperature exposure. www.shiftadapt.com

Robin Rothenberg – Yoga therapy

Shereen Yusuf – Breathing for women's health

Jill Miller – Self-myofascial release www.YogaTuneUp.com

Dr. Eric Serrano – All things health and performance related

Patrick Wright – Life coaching

John Connors – All things strength and conditioning. www.isipersonaltraining.com

Eoin Lacey – Functional medicine made understandable. www.eoinlaceyeducation.com

Dr. Andrew Huberman – Science protocols applied to life. The Huberman Lab Podcast

Victoria Felkar – Women's health, Canada.

Joy Ryan – Women's health, Ireland.

TEXTBOOKS

Principles of Anatomy & Physiology. Gerard J. Tortora & Sandra. R. Grabowski (2003). 10th Ed. John Wiley & Sons Inc

West's Respiratory Physiology. The Essentials. John B. West & Andrew M. Luks. (2016) 10th ed. Wolters Kluwer

Textbook of Natural Medicine. Joseph Pizzorno Jnr & Michael Murray (2020). 5th Ed. Vol 1. Churchill Livingstone.

Textbook of Natural Medicine. Joseph Pizzorno Jnr & Michael Murray (2020). 5th Ed. Vol 2. Churchill Livingstone.

Anatomy Trains: Myofascial Meridians for Manual Therapists and Movement Professionals. Thomas Myers (2020). 4th Ed. Elsevier.

Exercise Physiology. Nutrition, Energy, and Human Performance. William D. McArdle, Frank I. Katch & Victor L. Katch (2015). 8th Ed. Wolters Kluwer

BREATHING BOOKS

Shut Your Mouth and Save Your Life – Primary Source Edition. George Caitlin (1882). Trubner & Co, London.

The Hindu-Yogi Science of Breath. Ramacharaka (1903).

Behavioural & Psychological Approaches to Breathing Disorders. Beverly Timmons & Ronald Ley (1994). Plenum Press

Recognizing and Treating Breathing Disorders. A Multidisciplinary Approach. Leon Chaitow, Dinah Bradley & Christopher Gilbert (2014) 2nd Ed. Elsevier

Asthma-Free Naturally. Patrick McKeown (2003). AsthmaCare

Anxiety Free: Stop Worrying and Quieten Your Mind. Patrick McKeown (2010). Asthmacare

Jaws: The Story of a Hidden Epidemic. Sandra Khan & Paul R. Ehrlich (2018). Stanford University Press

GASP!: Airway Health – The Hidden Path to Wellness (2016). Michael Gelb & Howard Hindin. Create Space Independent Publishing Platform

Buteyko Meets Dr. Mew. Patrick McKeown (2010). Asthmacare

The Oxygen Advantage. Patrick McKeown (2015). Piatkus

The Breathing Cure: Exercises to Develop New Breathing Habits for a Healthier, Happier and Longer Life. Patrick McKeown (2021). OxyAtBooks

Wim Hof Method: Activate Your Potential, Transcend Your Limits. Wim Hof (2020). Rider

The Healing Power of Breath. Richard Brown & Patricia Gerbarg (2012). Shambhala Publications.

Just Breathe. Mastering Breathwork for Success in Life, Love, Business and Beyond. Dan Brulé (2017). Atria Books

Breathe Deep, Laugh Loudly: The Joy of Transformational Breathing. Judy Kravitz (1999). Ini Free Press

Holotropic Breathing. A New Approach to Self-Exploration and Therapy. Stanislav Grof & Christina Grof (2010). State University of New York Press

Big Fat Myths. Ruben Meerman (2016). Random House Australia

Beyond Stuttering: The McGuire Programme – for Getting Good at the Sport of Speaking. Dave McGuire (2019). 3rd Ed. The McGuire Programme California LLC.

Breath. The New Science of a Lost Art. James Nestor (2020). Penguin Random House UK

Breathe. The simple, Revolutionary 14- Day Program to Improve Your Mental and Physical Health. Belisa Vranich (2016). St. Martins

Freediving Manual. Learn How to Freedive 100 Feet on a Single Breath. Mike McGuire (2014). First Printing

PERSONAL DEVELOPMENT BOOKS

The Midnight Library. Matt Haig (2021). Canongate Books

Going Right: A Logical Justification for Pursuing Your Dreams. Logan Gelbrich (2019). Gelbrich Development LLC

Ikigai: The Japanese Secret to a Long and Happy Life. Héctor García & Francesc Miralles (2017). Hutchinson

Man's Search for Meaning. Viktor E. Frankl (2004). Rider

The Celestine Prophecy. James Redfield (1994). Bantam

The Tenth Insight. James Redfield (1997). Bantam

The Alchemist. Paulo Coelho (1995). Harper Collins

Ask and it is Given – Learning to Manifest Your Desires. Esther & Jerry Hicks (2004). Hay House

BIBLIOGRAPHY

The Comfort Crisis: Embrace Discomfort to Reclaim Your Wild, Happy, Healthy Self. Michael Easter (2021). Rodale

Roppo No Kuzushi Lesson. Jigoro Kano. Bu-sen Judo. http://www.busenmilano.org/judo-educazione/

BOOKS ON STRESS AND TRAUMA

Why Zebra's Don't Get Ulcers. Robert Sapolsky (2004). St. Martins Press

The Burnout Gamble: Achieve More by Beating Burnout and Building Resilience. Hamza Khan (2017). Hamza Khan

The Body Keeps The Score: Brain, Mind and Body in the Healing of Trauma. Bessel Van Der Kolk M.D. (2015). Penguin

The Polyvagal Theory: Neurophysiological Foundations of Emotion, Attachment, Communication and Self-Regulation. Stephen Porges (2018). W. W. Norton & Company

YOUTUBE VIDEOS

Matthew McConaghey – This is Why You're Not Happy. This is One of The Most Eye Opening Speeches. https://youtu.be/L9Cgaa8U4eY

The Power of Believing You Can Improve Carol Dweck TED Talk. https://youtu.be/_X0mgOOSpLU

The Hidden Meanings of Yin Yang. John Bellaimey. https://youtu.be/ezmR9Attpyc

The Power of Words. https://youtu.be/Hzgzim5m7oU

https://youtu.be/a5HjYUBLhxo

Abraham Hicks – Negative Emotions Exist for Two Reasons Only. https://youtu.be/D57wsNTFIlg

BIBLIOGRAPHY

Being Brilliant Every Single Day. Dr. Alan Watkins. TedXPortsmouth. Part 1. https://youtu.be/q06YIWCR2Js

Being Brilliant Every Single Day. Dr. Alan Watkins. TedXPortsmouth. Part 2 https://youtu.be/Q_fFattg8N0

The Superhuman World of Wim Hof: The Iceman. https://youtu.be/VaMjhwFE1Zw

Less Breath: Better Health? Mouth Breathing vs Nose Breathing. https://youtu.be/wgwxn9mRpAY

The Challenges of Mouth Breathing. Paul Chek Part 1 https://youtu.be/k6vVJw3qg94

The Challenges of Mouth Breathing. Paul Chek Part 2 https://youtu.be/mm2KAPqCfAc

The Challenges of Mouth Breathing. Paul Chek Part 3 https://youtu.be/E4w-0fVtj18

The Challenges of Mouth Breathing. Paul Chek Part 4 https://youtu.be/PWr1D-dBHpU

The Neuroscience Behind Breathwork with Patricia Garberg and Dan Brulé. https://youtu.be/8Ol5otIhBQU

Documentary on the Buteyko Method, QED, BBC1, 1998. https://youtu.be/ADf6Ol1KmmY

Dr. Buteyko Interview 1998 Talking About His Breathing Method. www.TheBreathingMan.com https://youtu.be/zpu8uVdFWz4

Respiration Gas Exchange. https://youtu.be/qDrV33rZlyA

Control of Respiration. https://youtu.be/9j6BpanhpKY

Mechanism of Breathing. https://youtu.be/GD-HPx_ZG8I

PODCASTS

The High Performance Podcast. E83 – Mel Robbins: Can you Really High 5 your Way to Happiness?

Redbull, How to Be Superhuman Podcast. Series 2 Episode #1. The Man Who Travelled Up Everest Twice without Oxygen: Killian Jornet.

The Huberman Lab Podcast. Episode 35. Dr. Robert Sapolsky: Science of Stress, Testosterone & Free Will.

The Huberman Lab Podcast. Episode 54. Dr. Jack Feldman: Breathing for Mental & Physical Health & Performance.

JRE MMA Show #114 with Rickson Gracie

The Gen. Pop. Podcast #13. Breath Training, The Overlooked Essential with Leo Ryan.

WeMove Podcast #2. Overcoming Asthma and Breathing for Performance with Leo Ryan.

SIGNIFICANT RESEARCH PAPERS

Basheer, B., Hegde, K.S., Bhat, S.S., Umar, D., Baroudi, K. (2014). *'Influence of Mouth Breathing on the Dentofacial Growth of Children: A Celphalometric Study'.* Journal of International Oral Health. Vol. 5. Issue. 6. Pp: 50-55

Bernardi, L. *'Slow Breathing. So Simple – So Complex'.* Presentation

Bernardi, L., Gordin, D., Bordino, M., Rosengård-Bärlund, M., Sandelin, A., Forsblom, C., and Groop, P-H. (2017). *'Oxygen-induced Impairment in Arterial Function is Corrected by Slow Breathing in Patients with Type 1 Diabetes'.* Scientific Reports. DOI: 10.1038/s41598-017-04947-4

Bohr, C., Hasselbalch, K. And Krogh, A., (1904). *Concerning a Biological Important Relationship – The Influence of Carbon Dioxide Content of Blood on its Oxygen Binding.* Skand. Arch. Physiology. 16 401-412. Translated by Marquardt, U., (1997). CHEM 342 Introduction to Biochemistry.

Bordoni, B., and Zanier, E. (2013). *'Anatomic Connections of the Diaphragm: Influence of Respiration on the Body System'*. Adv. Resp. Med. 85.PP:290-291 DOI: 10.2147/JMDH.S45443

Bordoni, B., and Morelli, F. (2016). *'Failed Back Surgery Syndrome: Review and New Hypothesis'*. Journal of Pain Research. Vol. 9. Pp: 17-22. DOI: 10/2147/JPR.596754

Bordoni, B. (2017). *'Network of Breathing. Multifunctional Role of the Diaphragm: A Review'*. Adv. Resp. Med. 85.PP:290-291 DOI: 10.5603/ARM.20170047

Bordoni, B., Morabito, B. (2018). *'Symptomatology Correlations between the Diaphragm and Irritable Bowel Syndrome'*. Cureus. Vol. 10. Issue. 7. DOI: 10.7759/cureus.3036

Bordoni, B., Simonelli, M., and Morabito, B. (2019). 'The Fascial Breath'. Cureus. Vol. 11. Issue 7. DOI: 10.7759/cureus.5208

Bordoni, B., Morabito, B., and Simonelli, M. (2020). *'Ageing of the Diaphragm Muscle'*. Cureus. Vol. 12. Issue 1. DOI: 10.7759/cureus.6645

Bowler, S.D., Green, A., Mitchell, C.A. (1998) *'Buteyko Breathing Techniques in Asthma: A Blinded Randomised Controlled Trial'*. MJA. Vol. 169. Pp: 575-578

Brocherie, F., Girard, O., Fais, R., and Millet, G.P. (2017) *'Effect of Repeated Sprint Training in Hypoxia on Sea-Level Performance: A Meta-Analysis'*. Sports Med. Vol. 47. Pp: 1651-1660. DOI: 10.1007/s40279-017-0685-3

Burgess, J., Ekanayake, B., Lowe, A., Dunt, D., Thien, F., and Dharmage, S.C. (2011). *'Systemic Review of the Effectiveness of Breath Retraining in Asthma Management'*. Expert Review. Respiratory Medicine Vol 5. Issue 6. Pp: 789-807

Courtney, R. (2008). *'Strengths, Weaknesses and Possibilities of the Buteyko Breathing Method'*. Association for Applied Psychophysiology and Biofeedback. Vol. 36. Issue 2. Pp: 59-63

Cowie, R.L., Conley, D.P., Underwood, M.F., Reader, P.G. (2007). *'A randomised Control Trial of the Buteyko Technique as an Adjunct to Conventional Management of Asthma'.* Respiratory Medicine. DOI: 10.1016/j.rmed.2007.12.012

Dallam, G.M., McClaran, S.R., and Foust, C.P. (2018). *'Effects of Nasal versus Oral Breathing on VO2Max and Physiological Economy in Recreational Runners Following an Extended Period Spent using Nasally Restricted Breathing'.* International Journal of Kinesiology and Sport Science. DOI: 10.7575/aiac.ijkss.v.6n.2p.22

Drigas, A., and Mitsea, E. (2022). *'Conscious Breathing: a Powerful Tool for Physical & Neuropsychological Regulation. The Role of the Mobile Apps.'* Technium Social Sciences Journal. Vol 28. P135-158

Draheim, C., Hicks, K. L., & Engle, R. W. (2016). *Combining Reaction Time and Accuracy The Relationship Between Working Memory Capacity and Task Switching as a Case Example.* Perspectives on Psychological Science, *11*(1), 133-155. doi: 10.1177/1745691615596990

Feinstein, J., Gould, D., and Khalsa, S.S. (2022) *'Amygdala-driven Apnea and the chemoreceptive Origin of Anxiety'.* Review. Biological Psychology. https://doi.org/10.1016/j.biopsycho.2022.108305

Foroughi, C. K., Werner, N. E., Nelson, E. T., & Boehm-Davis, D. A. (2014). Do interruptions affect quality of work?. *Human Factors: The Journal of the Human Factors and Ergonomics Society, 56*(7), 1262-1271. doi: 10.1177/0018720814531786

Girard, O., Brocherie, F., and Millet, G.P. (2017) *'Effects of Altitude/Hypoxia on Single- and Multi-Sprint Performance: A Comprehensive Review'.* Springer International Publishing. Switzerland. DOI: 10.1007/s40279-017-0733-z

Grassmann, M., Vlemincx, E., Von Lupoldt, A., Mittelstädt, J.M., and Van Den Bergh, O. (2016). *'Respiratory Changes in Response to Cognitive Load: A Systemic Review'.* Neural Plasticity. DOI: 10.1155/2016/8146809

Heck, D.H., McAfee, S.S., Babajani-Ferremi, A., Rezaie, R., Freeman, W.J., Wheless, J.W., Papincolaou, A.C., Ruszinkó, M., Sokolov, Y., and Kozma, R. (2017). *'Breathing as a Fundamental Rhythm of Brain*

Function'. Front. Neural Circuits 10:115. DOI: https://doi.org/10.3389/fncir.2016.00115

Holloway, E., and West, R.J. (2007). '*Integrated Breathing and Relaxation Training (The Papworth Method) for adults with Asthma in Primarycare: A Randomised Control Study*'. Thorax. Vol. 62. Pp: 1039-1042. DOI: 10.1136/thx.2006.076430

Illi, S.K., Held, U., Frank, I., Spengler, C.M. (2012). '*Effect of Respiratory Muscle Training on Exercise Performance in Healthy Individuals*'. Sport Med. Vol. 42. Pp: 707-724.

Janssens, L., Brumagne, S., McConnell, A.K., Hermans, G., Troosters, T., Gayan-Ramirez, G. (2013). '*Greater Diaphragm Fatigability in Individuals with Recurrent Low Back Pain*'. J. Resp. Phys & Neurob. Vol. 188 DOI: 10.1016/j.resp.2013.05.028

Khana-Zweig, R., Geva-Sagiv, M., Weissbrod, A., Secundo, L., Soroker, N., Sobel, N. (2016). 'Measuring and Analysing the Human Nasal Cycle'. Plos One. DOI: https://doi.org/10.1371/journal.pone.0162918

Kox, M., Hopmna, M., Pickkers, P. Et al. (2012). '*The Influence of Concentration / Meditation on Autonomic Nervous System Activity and the Innate Immune Response: A Case Study.*' Psychosomatic Medicine. Vol. 74. Iss 5. P489-494. DOI: 10.1097/PSY.0b013e3182583c6d

Kox, M., Van Eijk, L.T., Zwagg, J., and Pickkers, P. (2014). '*Voluntary Activation of the Sympathetic Nervous System and Attenuation of the Innate Immune Response in Humans.*' PNAS. Vol. 111. No. 20. DOI: https://doi.org/10.1073/pnas.1322174111

Kulur, A.B., Haleagrahara, N., Adhikary, P., Jeganathan, P.S. (2013). '*Effect of Diaphragmatic Breathing on Heart Rate Variability in Ischemic Heart Disease with Diabetes*'. Araq. Bras. Cardiol. Vol. 92 (6). DOI: 10.1590/S0066-782x2009000600008

Litchfield, P., (2006). *Good Breathing. Bad Breathing. Breathing is behaviour, a unique behaviour that regulates body chemistry, pH.* Self-Published

LoMauro, A., and Aliverti, A. (2018). *Sex Differences in Respiratory Function*. Breathe. Vol. 14. Pp: 131-140.

Lum, L.C., (1975). *Hyperventilation: The Tip and the Iceberg*. Journal of Psychosomatic Research. Vol 19 pp 375-383

McHugh, P., Aitcheson, F., Duncan, B., and Houghton, F. (2003). '*Buteyko Breathing Technique for Asthma: An Effective Intervention*'. The New Zealand Medical Journal. Vol. 116. No. 1187

Melnychuk, M., et al. (2018). '*Coupling of Respiration and Attention via the Locus Coeruleus: Effects of Meditation and Pranayama.*' Society for Psychophysiology Research

Monti, A., Porciello, G., Tieri, G., and Aglioti, S.M. (2020). '*The 'Embreathment' Illusion Highlights the Role of Breathing in Corporeal Awareness*'. Journal of Neurophysiology DOI: https://doi.org/10.1152/jn.00617.2019

Morais-Almeida, M., Wandalsen, G. F., Solé, D. (2019). '*Growth and Mouth Breathers – Review Article*'. Journal Paediatria. Vol. 95. Issue. 1. Pp: s66-s71. DOI: https://doi.org/10.1016/j.jped.2018.11.005

Peper E., and Gibney, K.H. (2003). '*Taking Control: Strategies to Reduce Hot Flushes and Premenstrual Mood Swings*'. Biofeedback. Vol. 31. Issue. 3. Pp: 20-24

Ramirez, J.M., (2014). '*The Integrative Role of the Sigh in Psychology, Physiology, Pathology and Neurobiology*'. NIH. National Library of Medicine. DOI: 10.1016/B978-0-444-63274-6.00006-0

Ricoy, J., Rodríguez-Nuñez, N., Álvarez-Dobaño, J.M., Toubes, M.E., Riveiro, V., and Valdés, L. (2019). *Diaphragmatic Dysfunction. Review*. Pulmonology. Vol. 25. Issue. 4. Pp: 223-235. DOI: https://doi.org/10.1016/j.pulmoe.2018.10.008

Rocha, T., Souza, H., Cunha Brandão, D., Rattes, C., Ribeiro, L., Lima Campos, S., Aliverti, A., Dornelas de Andrade, A. (2015). '*The Manual Diaphragm Release Technique Improves Diaphragmatic Mobility, Inspiratory Capacity and Exercise Capacity in People with Chronic*

Obstructive Pulmonary Disease: A Randomised Control Trial'. JPhys 187. DOI: 10.1016/jphys.2015.08.009

Sano, M., (2019). *Global Burden of Cardiovascular Diseases and Risk Factors, 1990–2019*. Journal of the American College of Cardiology. 9 December 2020. doi: 10.1016/j.jacc.2020.11.010.

Sikter, A., Faludi, G., and Rihmer, Z. (2009) *'The Role of Carbon Dioxide (and intracellular pH) in the Pathomechanism of Several Mental Disorders. Are the diseases of Civiilzation Caused by Learnt Behaviour, Not the Stress Itself?'.* Theoretical Article. Neuropsychopharmalogica Hungary. pp161-173. DOI: 10.1016/B978-0-444-63274-6.00006-0

Sikter, A., Rihmer, Z., and De Guevara, R. (2017) *'New Aspects in the Pathomechanism of Diseases of Civilization, Particularly Psychosomatic Disorders. Part 1. Theoretical Background of a Hypothesis.* Review Article. Neuropsychopharmalogica Hungary. Pp95-105. PMID: 28918418

Sikter, A., and Sonne C. (2021) *'A New Hypothesis on Vascular Calcification: The Exhausting Buffer Syndrome (EBS)'*. Neuropsychopharmalogica Hungary. 23 (1). Pp215-220.

Sikter, A. (2022) *'Chronic Psychic Stress Can Cause Metabolic Syndrome through Mild Hypocapnia'*. Review Article. Neuropsychopharmalogica Hungary. 24(3) Pp126-133.

Van Middendorp, H., Kox, M., Pickkers, P., Evers, A.W.M (2014). *'The Role of Outcome Expectancies for a Training Program Consisting of Meditation, Breathing Exercises, and Cold Exposure on the Response to Endotoxin Administration: A Proof-Principle Study.'* Proc Natl Acad Sci USA. DOI:10.1073/pnas.1322174111

GENERAL RESEARCH STATS AND FACTS FROM THE WEB

Basic Medical Key (2017). Chapter 15. Respiratory Disease. Found at: https://basicmedicalkey.com/respiratory-disease-4/

BIBLIOGRAPHY

Brady, J., (201). 'Mental Health Issues Cost State €8.2 Bn Each Year, Says Harris'. The Irish Times. Found at: https://www.irishtimes.com/news/health/mental-health-issues-cost-state-8-2bn-each-year-says-harris-1.4001595#:~:text=Minister%20tells%20conference%20stress%2C%20anxiety%20and%20depression%20have%20impact%20on%20Irish%20economy&text=Mental%20health%20issues%20cost%20the,services%20industry%20conference%20on%20Thursday.

Center for Disease Control and Prevention (2015). Fact Sheet. Found at: https://data.cdc.gov/NCHS/NCHS-Top-Five-Leading-Causes-of-Death-United-State/mc4y-cbbv

Devane, C.L., Chiao, E., Franklin, M., Kruep, E.J., (2005). *'Anxiety Disorders in the 21st Century: Status, Challenges, Opportunities, and Comorbidities with Depression'*. AJMC. Vol. 11. Issue 12. Found at: https://www.ajmc.com/view/oct05-2158ps344-s353

Khaodhiar, L., McCowen, K.C., Blackburn, G.L. (1999). *'Obesity and its Comorbid Conditions'*. Review. DOI: 10.1016/s1098-3597(99)90002-9

Levine, H. (2020). 'How Stress Can Hurt Your Chances of Having a Baby'. Grow by WebMD. https://www.webmd.com/baby/features/infertility-stress#1

Mental Health Reform (2018). The Mental Health Reform Pre-Budget Submission 2019. Found at: https://www.mentalhealthreform.ie/wp-content/uploads/2018/08/Mental-Health-Reform-Pre-Budget-2019-Submission.pdf

National Institute of Mental Health. Anxiety Disorder Statistics. Found at: https://www.nimh.nih.gov/health/statistics/any-anxiety-disorder#:~:text=Prevalence%20of%20Any%20Anxiety%20Disorder%20Among%20Adults,-Based%20on%20diagnostic&text=An%20estimated%2019.1%25%20of%20U.S.,than%20for%20males%20(14.3%25).

Raferty M.N., Sarma K., Murphy, A.W., De La Harpe, D., Normand, C., & McGuire, B. (2010). *'Chronic Pain in the Republic of Ireland*

– *Community Prevalence, Psychosocial Profile and Predictors of Pain-related Disability: Results from Prevalence, Impact and Cost of Chronic Pain (PRIME) study, Part 1'.* PAIN Volume: 152. DOI: 10.1016/j.pain.2011.01.019

The Authors (2020). 'Mental Health Matters'. The Lancet Editorial. Vol 8. DOI: https://doi.org/10.1016/S2214-109X(20)30432-0

World Health Organisation (2020). Top 10 Causes of Death Factsheet. Found at: https://www.who.int/news-room/fact-sheets/detail/the-top-10-causes-of-death#:~:text=The%20world's%20biggest%20killer%20is,8.9%20million%20deaths%20in%202019.

World Health Organisation (2021). Obesity Factsheet. Found at: https://www.who.int/health-topics/obesity#tab=tab_1

ACKNOWLEDGEMENTS

I recently heard it said that survival takes one skillset and thriving a completely different one. This saying has rung true in my life. Medication and medical care helped me to survive asthma. Love, community, faith, hope, training, and lifestyle choices have helped me to thrive and strive for my greatest life. Thank you to all who have helped me on my journey.

To:

The doctors and the creators of the drugs for keeping me alive, thank you.

My mam and dad for being my parents, for having hope when I had none and for supporting me on my journey, thank you.

My wife Joy for encouraging me to be my best self, for loving me and always standing with me. Thank you Joy, for encouraging me to write this book and continually motivating me over five years and many government lockdowns as I managed to piece it together slowly but surely. Thank you to the girls, Beatrice, Genevieve and Juliette. I know I drive you mad with my idiosyncrasies. Hopefully, one day, you will understand that I do these things out of love – I love you all very much and I am grateful you chose us as parents.

My parents-in-law John and Teresa, for always supporting Joy and I since the day we met. Your kindness, compassion, and support know no bounds. We thank you deeply for everything you do for us and the girls. And to Sr. Collette, for all of your love, and support to us.

ACKNOWLEDGEMENTS

Patrick McKeown, for having the courage to go to Russia in the 1990s and learn from Dr. Buteyko, when hardly anybody in the Western world knew of him. Thank you for your journey to health. Thank you also for starting a business in breathing when nobody else was doing it. Thank you for teaching me personally. Thank you for your vision, your heart, your kindness, your passion, and your dedication to spreading the news about breathing better and having the Oxygen Advantage.

Wim Hof for being a beacon of love and a pillar of happiness, health, and strength in the world. Thank you for teaching me personally and sharing your method with me through your academy. Through your community I have found many friends, I have come to know myself so much better, and I have helped many people find more of themselves too. Thank you for these gifts.

Brian MacKenzie and Rob Wilson for being curious about the breath. Through our conversations back in 2017 we discovered that breathing was about more than methods, rather it was the principles that are important. Thank you for sharing your knowledge and experience of breathing with the world.

The breathing communities I've been lucky to be part of: my fellow Oxygen Advantage Master Instructors, Wim Hof Method Instructors, Buteyko Instructors and all of the wonderful breathing teachers I have met over the years. Thank you for influencing me and shaping my experience of the breath.

My mentors and colleagues in the fitness industry for giving me my breaks, teaching, guiding and sharing with me along the way, thank you. A special thanks to Noeleen Gregory for her guidance throughout my whole career. Thank you Derry Temple for hiring me in my first full-time position as personal trainer, you changed my life. John Connors and Eoin Lacey, for your passion in health and fitness, your knowledge and your influence on my career. Darren Katz, for your faith in this Irish guy, and friendship with me over the years. Brendan Prior, for being the most awesome gym owner in Ireland and allowing me to coach my clients under your roof. Dr. Eric Serrano, for your

ACKNOWLEDGEMENTS

friendship and mentoring over the years. And finally, thank you to all my wonderful colleagues and friends in the fitness industry over the years. You all mean the world to me and I thank you for making me a better coach and person. Thank you all.

My fabulous clients, I wouldn't have developed myself as a coach without you. Thank you for your trust in me. A special thank you to everyone who was generous enough to give a testimony to the power of the breath. It is your success stories that will drive the health of the world forward.

This book would not have been possible without the help of so many people. Chris from writerservices.co.uk. You paired me with my editor and guided me in the self-publishing route, thank you so much. Many thanks to my editor for giving me the structure and language I needed to express my thoughts.

To Cathy Wyer for reading, editing, rereading and re-editing many manuscript versions over the years. This book would not be a reality without your help.

The images you see in the book were created with the help of Marcus Quinn. Thank you for designing and delivering them. They look awesome and really bring the book alive for the reader. Thank you for everything.

The photos were taken by Rob Fay. Thanks, Rob, for all of your help with the photos featured here and in the rest of my business. Thank you to Yoga Boann for the beautiful studio and extra help with the photo shoot. Thank you to the models, Stefan McDonnell and Martha Moussally. I really appreciate the time and energy you gave to the shoot.

To Steve Taber of ItsEeze, my awesome go-to web guy. You designed the Innate-Strength website and helped me build the Innate-Strength brand's foundations. I couldn't have done it without you, so thank you. To the team at Innate-Strength – Marcus and Jason – I am so excited to have you on board recently, and I look forward to working with you and watching you grow as breathing coaches.

ACKNOWLEDGEMENTS

A special thank you to everybody that contributed financially to getting this book into your hands. The final push to have it designed and printed was financed by the generous contributors below. Thank you for your donations from the bottom of my heart.

Níall Kane	Tomasz W.
Lynn Shannon	Chantal and Jonathan
Christopher Todd	Anonymous
Claire Conway	Leo & Deirdre Martin
James McCormack	Emma Hickey
Yvonne and Tristan McMichael	Noel Q
Cathal Keaney	Rob
Trevor Byrne	Andreas Gustafsson
Anita & Gary Power	Anonymous
Ursula Hake	Marianne Eaton
Angela Eaton	Walter Martin
Mr. Jasper Chow	Mrs. Kathleen Smith
Dave H.	Cathy Wyer
Tom	Liam O'Mahony
Rachel	Steve Taber
Ian McNeill	Ed
James Cashen	Leo and Paula Ryan
Katie Millett	Robert K.
Geraldine Davies	Teresa and John McMahon
Tracy Lennon	Andy Cuthbert
Anonymous	Sr. Collette Keane

Thank you also for any contributions received after the printing of the book. Finally, to you the reader, thank you for investing in this book. I hope you see your investment return one hundred-fold in health and joy.

Leo Daniel Ryan, Ireland.

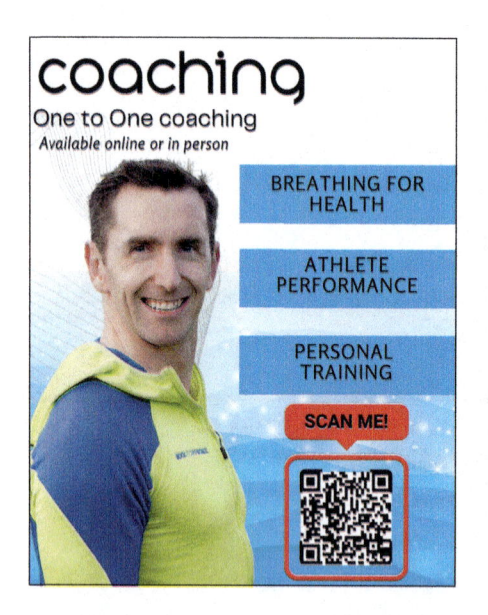

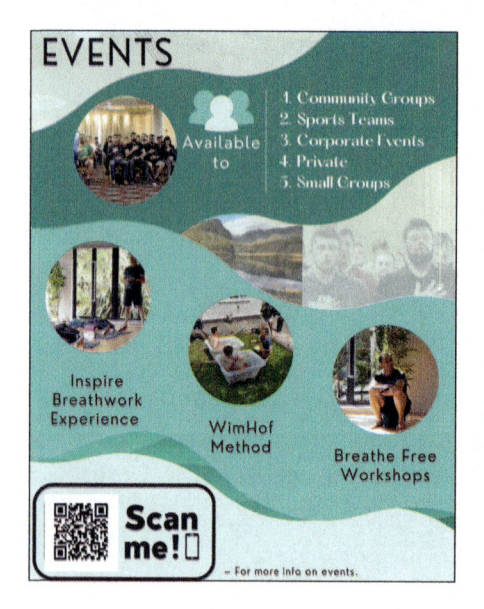

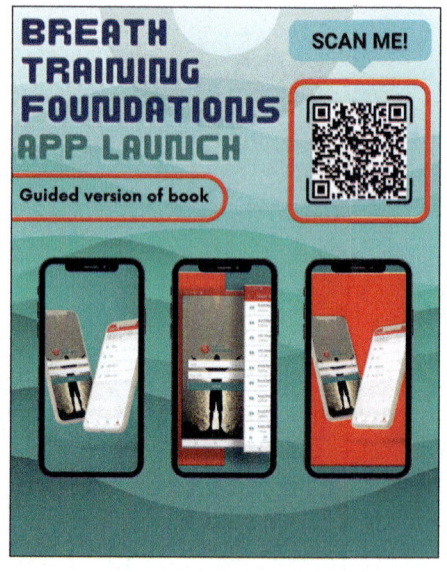

coaching
One to One coaching
Available online or in person

- BREATHING FOR HEALTH
- ATHLETE PERFORMANCE
- PERSONAL TRAINING

SCAN ME!

THE OXYGEN ADVANTAGE AFFILIATE FOR 5% OFF
SCAN ME

EVENTS
Available to:
1. Community Groups
2. Sports Teams
3. Corporate Events
4. Private
5. Small Groups

- Inspire Breathwork Experience
- WimHof Method
- Breathe Free Workshops

Scan me!
– For more info on events.

BREATH TRAINING FOUNDATIONS APP LAUNCH
Guided version of book

SCAN ME!

ABOUT THE AUTHOR

Leo Daniel Ryan is a Breath and Performance Coach. He is the founder of Innate-Strength.com. Leo has studied athletic training, health and breathing since healing himself of asthma in 2004. After graduating with an MSc from University College Dublin, he continued to educate himself prolifically throughout his professional career in Ireland and internationally. He has attained multiple diplomas and certificates from elite personal training, physical therapy and breathing schools including Diploma Buteyko Method, Wim Hof Instructor, Oxygen Advantage Master Instructor, Fascial Stretch Therapist, Strength and Conditioning Specialist, and Pilates teacher.

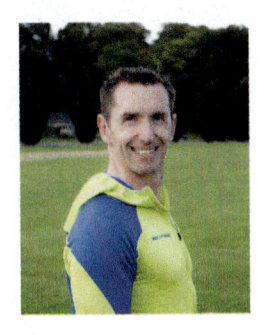

Leo's love for health and physical performance has seen him research more than 100 breathing techniques, mentor with coaches to Olympians and World Champions, and undertake several internships with the world-renowned Dr Eric Serrano.

Up to 2019, Leo spent much of his time coaching one-to-one in a personal training environment and testing his training methodology on himself. He played senior club GAA football in Dublin with St. Sylvester's. He is a 2nd Dan black belt in judo, ran marathons without any specific training, gained more than 52 lbs of muscle, and even climbed a mountain with nothing on but a pair of shorts and boots. His clients have healed cardiovascular disease, asthma, and anxiety.

ABOUT THE AUTHOR

They've reduced symptoms of depression, panic, colitis, and rheumatoid arthritis. Some have gained weight purposely, and others have intentionally lost weight. The best thing is, that they've also gone on to return to their passions in life, or achieve feats of their dreams. Some notable achievements include becoming intercounty GAA stars, being professional athletes, climbing Mt. Everest, swimming the English Channel, becoming an Olympian, and achieving a Guinness World Record.

Above all, Leo is a family man. He is married to Joy and they have three fantastic children – Beatrice, Genevieve and Juliette. There is nothing more Leo loves than sharing his passion and knowledge of breathing, health and life with his family, friends, clients, and now, the world.

Printed in Great Britain
by Amazon